Autoinflammatory Disorders

Editors

WILLIAM ABRAMOVITS
MARCIAL OQUENDO

DERMATOLOGIC CLINICS

www.derm.theclinics.com

Consulting Editor
BRUCE H. THIERS

July 2013 • Volume 31 • Number 3

ELSEVIER

1600 John F. Kennedy Boulevard • Suite 1800 • Philadelphia, Pennsylvania, 19103-2899

http://www.theclinics.com

DERMATOLOGIC CLINICS Volume 31, Number 3
July 2013 ISSN 0733-8635, ISBN-13: 978-1-4557-7588-0

Editor: Stephanie Donley
Developmental Editor: Teia Stone

Dermatologic Clinics (ISSN 0733-8635) is published quarterly by Elsevier Inc., 360 Park Avenue South, New York, NY 10010-1710. Months of publication are January, April, July, and October. Business and editorial offices: 1600 John F. Kennedy Blvd., Suite 1800, Philadelphia, PA 19103-2899. Customer service office: 11830 Westline Drive, St. Louis, MO 63146. Periodicals postage paid at New York, NY, and additional mailing offices. Subscription prices are USD 346.00 per year for US individuals, USD 532.00 per year for US institutions, USD 404.00 per year for Canadian individuals, USD 636.00 per year for Canadian institutions, USD 473.00 per year for international individuals, USD 636.00 per year for international institutions, USD 159.00 per year for US students/residents, and USD 230.00 per year for Canadian and international students/residents. International air speed delivery is included in all *Clinics* subscription prices. All prices are subject to change without notice. **POSTMASTER:** Send address changes to *Dermatologic Clinics*, Elsevier Health Sciences Division, Subscription Customer Service, 3251 Riverport Lane, Maryland Heights, MO 63043. **Customer Service: 1-800-654-2452 (U.S. and Canada); 314-447-8871 (outside U.S. and Canada). Fax: 314-447-8029. E-mail: journalscustomerservice-usa@elsevier.com (for print support); journalsonlinesupport-usa@elsevier.com (for online support).**

Reprints. For copies of 100 or more, of articles in this publication, please contact the Commercial Reprints Department, Elsevier Inc., 360 Park Avenue South, New York, New York 10010-1710. Tel.: (212) 633-3813; Fax: (212) 462-1935; Email: reprints@elsevier.com.

The *Dermatologic Clinics* is covered in *MEDLINE/PubMed (Index Medicus)*, *Current Contents/Clinical Medicine*, *Excerpta Medica, Chemical Abstracts,* and *ISI/BIOMED*.

Printed and bound by CPI Group (UK) Ltd, Croydon, CR0 4YY

Transferred to digital print 2012

Contributors

CONSULTING EDITOR

BRUCE H. THIERS, MD
Professor and Chairman, Department of
Dermatology and Dermatologic Surgery,
Medical University of South Carolina,
Charleston, South Carolina

EDITORS

WILLIAM ABRAMOVITS, MD, FAAD
Assistant Clinical Professor (Dermatol),
Department of Medicine, Baylor University
Medical Center and Texas A&M Medical
School; Departments of Dermatology and
Family Practice, University of Texas
Southwestern Medical School; Dermatology
Treatment and Research Center, Dallas, Texas

MARCIAL OQUENDO, MD
Dermatology Treatment and Research Center,
Dallas, Texas

AUTHORS

WILLIAM ABRAMOVITS, MD, FAAD
Assistant Clinical Professor (Dermatol),
Department of Medicine, Baylor University
Medical Center and Texas A&M Medical
School; Departments of Dermatology and
Family Practice, University of Texas
Southwestern Medical School; Dermatology
Treatment and Research Center, Dallas, Texas

JOAQUIN J. RIVAS BEJARANO, MD
Senior Clinical Science Manager, Global
Medical Affairs, Immunology, AbbVie, Chicago,
Illinois; Adjunct Faculty, Biology Department,
LoneStar College, Houston, Texas

DANIEL BUTLER, BS
Clinical Research Investigator, University of
Arizona School of Medicine, Tucson, Arizona

MICHAEL C. CHEN, PhD
Galderma Laboratories, LP, Fort Worth,
Texas

EDWARD W. COWEN, MD, MHSc
Head, Dermatology Consultation Service,
Dermatology Branch, Center for Cancer
Research, National Cancer Institute, National
Institutes of Health, Bethesda, Maryland

JOHN J. CUSH, MD
Director of Clinical Rheumatology, Baylor
Research Institute, Rheumatology Research,
Dallas, Texas

FATMA DEDEOGLU, MD
Assistant Professor, Program in
Rheumatology, Division of Immunology,
Boston Children's Hospital, Boston,
Massachusetts

JONATHAN S. HAUSMANN, MD
Fellow in Rheumatology, Program in
Rheumatology, Division of Immunology,
Boston Children's Hospital, Boston,
Massachusetts

KIERON S. LESLIE, DTM&H, FRCP
Department of Dermatology, University of California San Francisco, San Francisco, California

THOMAS MANDRUP-POULSEN, MD, DMSc
Professor, Department of Biomedical Sciences, Faculty of Health and Medical Sciences, University of Copenhagen, Copenhagen, Denmark; Adjunct Professor, Department of Molecular Medicine and Surgery, Karolinska Institutet, Stockholm, Sweden

MATTHEW H. MECKFESSEL, PhD
Galderma Laboratories, LP, Fort Worth, Texas

HALEY B. NAIK, MD
Clinical Research Fellow, Dermatology Branch, Center for Cancer Research, National Cancer Institute, National Institutes of Health, Bethesda, Maryland

MARCIAL OQUENDO, MD
Dermatology Treatment and Research Center, Dallas, Texas

KANADE SHINKAI, MD, PhD
Assistant Professor of Clinical Dermatology, Department of Dermatology, University of California San Francisco School of Medicine, San Francisco, California

GARY STERBA, MD, FACP, FACR
Miami Medical Consult, Coral Gables, Florida

YONIT STERBA, MD
Pediatric Rheumatology Fellow, Children's Hospital at Montefiore, Bronx, New York

SHIVANI V. TRIPATHI, MD
Department of Dermatology, University of California San Francisco, San Francisco, California

WENDELL C. VALDECANTOS, MD
Associate Medical Director, Immunology, Global Medical Affairs, AbbVie, North Chicago, Illinois

Contents

> Autoinflammatory syndromes and diseases are a group of disorders of innate immunity. This group has grown rapidly in recent years as a result of research advancements in molecular biology and genetics. These diseases often present with skin manifestations and the dermatologist may not recognize the constellation of symptoms and medical history as a systemic inflammatory disease. Dermatologists would benefit from a deeper understanding of these diseases and the new treatments available for them.

> Autoinflammatory diseases, including CAPS, TRAPS, HIDS, FMF, Blau, and CANDLE, have unique dermatologic presentations that can be a clue to diagnosis. Although these conditions are rare, the morbidity and mortality can be severe, and well-informed physicians can place these conditions in their differential diagnosis when familiar with the dermatologic manifestations. This review article presents a brief overview of each condition, clues to diagnosis that focus of dermatologic manifestations and clinical images, basic laboratory tests and follow-up, a brief review of treatments, and concludes with an overview for these autoinflammatory conditions and their differential diagnoses.

> This article provides a new categorization of inflammatory pustular dermatoses in the context of recent genetic and biological insights. Monogenic diseases with pustular phenotypes are discussed, including deficiency of interleukin 1 receptor antagonist, deficiency of the interleukin 36 receptor antagonist, CARD14-associated pustular psoriasis, and pyogenic arthritis, pyoderma gangrenosum, and acne. How these new genetic advancements may inform how previously described pustular diseases are viewed, including pustular psoriasis and its clinical variants, with a focus on historical classification by clinical phenotype, is also discussed.

> Pyoderma gangrenosum (PG) is a neutrophilic dermatosis characterized by ulcerating skin lesions with rapid onset and recalcitrant treatment course. PG treatment targets an array of inflammatory pathways with variable success. One of the hallmark

features of PG is its association with a broad spectrum of systemic disorders. The authors hypothesize that there are common inflammatory pathways linking these systemic disorders to neutrophilic dermatoses. Rare autoinflammatory diseases offer insights into the understanding of inflammatory skin conditions. This article explores observations of the natural history of PG that illuminate aspects of PG pathogenesis, highlighting the role of autoinflammatory mediators.

Interleukin-1 (IL-1) is a potent inflammatory cytokine that plays a central role in the innate immune response. IL-1 mediates the acute phase of inflammation by inducing local and systemic responses, such as pain sensitivity, fever, vasodilation, and hypotension. It also promotes the expression of adhesion molecules on endothelial cells, which allows the infiltration of inflammatory and immunocompetent cells into the tissues. The release of IL-1 from the epidermis after activation is a primary event that promotes inflammatory skin conditions through the induction of various cytokines, proinflammatory mediators, and adhesion molecules.

This article presents a summary of the evidence for a link between autoinflammatory diseases and psoriasis. The main concepts regarding the disease state of psoriasis are discussed and these lead to a change in the perspective on the clinical and pathophysiologic nature of psoriasis as a chronic, recurrent disease with important genetically defined features, and an associated or concomitant systemic inflammatory state that involves a multifactorial cellular and molecular network, transforming the old perception of psoriasis as a localized autoimmune skin disease, to one of psoriasis as a systemic inflammatory disease with autoinflammatory features and severe associated comorbid conditions.

Autoinflammatory disorders are disorders of the innate immune system that are distinct from autoimmune disorders. Dysregulation of the innate immune system, specifically an increase in interleukin-1 beta (IL-1β), gives rise to a spectrum of symptoms marked by inflammation and pain. Identification of causative gene mutations led to the discovery of the inflammasome. Many autoinflammatory disorders also have a strong pain component. The contribution of IL-1β to pain and neural involvement is underappreciated. This article provides an overview of the current autoinflammatory disorders and highlights the contribution IL-1β makes to pain in these disorders.

Autoinflammatory syndromes comprise a diagnostically challenging group of systemic inflammatory disorders uniquely related by (1) dysregulation of innate immunity, (2) inflammasome activation, (3) dramatic clinical features (high fevers, neutrophilic rashes, and bone or synovial involvement), (4) impressive acute phase responses, and (5) effective treatment with cytokine inhibitors. This review details some of the more common autoinflammatory disorders, their distinguishing features and dermatologic manifestations, and how an accurate diagnosis can be established in patients presenting with periodic or intermittent febrile disorders.

DERMATOLOGIC CLINICS

Dedication

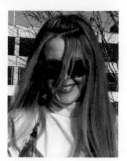

Kimberly Dawn Vincent, MD

This issue of Dermatologic Clinics is dedicated to Kimberly Dawn Vincent, MD. Dawn is the inspirational colleague who has kept me on my academic and personal toes since I met her 3 years ago. I can tell she practices excellent dermatology and is an angel to her patients and all the lives she touches.

William Abramovits, MD
Department of Medicine
Baylor University Medical Center
and Texas A&M Medical School at Dallas
3500 Gaston Avenue
Dallas, TX 75246, USA

The Departments of Dermatology and
Family Practice
University of Texas Southwestern Medical School
5323 Harry Hines Boulevard
Dallas, TX 75235, USA

Dermatology Treatment and Research Center
5310 Harvest Hill Road
Dallas, TX 75230, USA

E-mail address:
drA@dermcenter.us

Dermatol Clin 31 (2013) ix
http://dx.doi.org/10.1016/j.det.2013.05.003
0733-8635/13/$ – see front matter © 2013 Published by Elsevier Inc.

Preface
Autoinflammatory Diseases and Syndromes in Dermatology

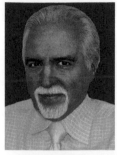 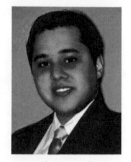

William Abramovits, MD   Marcial Oquendo, MD
Editors

Medical Dermatologists, assuming that they are all like me, and I am like them, take diagnostic and therapeutic challenges as fun and exciting. A series of coincidental events led me to discover that long-time patients of mine, and some personal friends, with puzzling clinical findings not matching a syndrome or disease I could recognize (nor could other specialists) fit into a newly identified category of entities named autoinflammatory. It felt so good for me to be able to call them and tell them that I found not only an explanation for their symptoms and a diagnosis but also a treatment!, something called anti-IL-1, for example.

As luck would have it, one after another, within a short period of time, with the contribution of referring colleagues who found out about my interest in autoinflammatory disorders involving the skin, I started to develop a cadre of patients with these, and a keen eye for their diagnosis.

But, with increasing knowledge comes increasing awareness of one's ignorance, and with that for me came increased concern and desire to understand things. This was further stimulated by the realization that pain and rashes of particular morphologies could be alleviated by specific medication, be it colchicine, well-selected disease modifiers, or biologics against the trigger of their inflammation, ones that intervene at almost gene level.

Obviously, I am not the only one itching to identify patients with these syndromes, as in the process of classifying them, first for my own benefit and then for this issue, I recognized that, case after case, with all kind of variants, were being reported about in every issue of every journal familiar to me

as a dermatologist. The seemingly impossible task of creating a practical review for a dermatology journal became a possibility when the consulting editor of this series suggested that I invite some experts to contribute to my effort and make it a reality.

With the invaluable help of my coeditor, Marcial Oquendo, MD, I believe that I have managed to bring together a group of brilliant and expert minds to competently present to the usual dermatology readership of this series, and to those attracted by the subject of autoinflammation, a useful source of information on this field, not yet a decade old, where they can begin to comprehend, diagnose, and treat patients with syndromes and diseases caused by autoinflammation.

William Abramovits, MD
Department of Medicine
Baylor University Medical Center and
Texas A&M Medical School at Dallas
3500 Gaston Avenue
Dallas, TX 75246, USA

The Departments of Dermatology and
Family Practice
University of Texas Southwestern Medical School
5323 Harry Hines Boulevard
Dallas, TX 75235, USA

Dermatology Treatment and Research Center
5310 Harvest Hill Road
Dallas, TX 75230, USA

E-mail address:
drA@dermcenter.us

Dermatol Clin 31 (2013) xi
http://dx.doi.org/10.1016/j.det.2013.05.002

Introduction to Autoinflammatory Syndromes and Diseases

William Abramovits, MD[a,b,c,d],*, Marcial Oquendo, MD[d]

KEYWORDS

- Autoinflammation • Inflammasome • Interleukins • Recurrent fever • Familial Mediterranean fever

KEY POINTS

- Autoinflammatory syndromes and diseases are an expanding, usually poorly understood, and difficult to treat group of conditions.
- They underlining pathophysiology revolves around the overactivation or underregulation of the inflammatory process resulting in multisystemic tissue damage.
- New insights into the molecular mechanisms of inflammation and genetic profiling have led to the development and use of anticytokine therapies with a level a success not previously achieved.

Autoinflammatory syndromes and diseases are a group of disorders of innate immunity that are often inherited, sometimes acquired, characterized by febrile episodes, recurrent, of variable duration, seemingly unprovoked, and with multidistrict inflammation of variable severity.[1,2] Unlike the classic autoimmune diseases in which the immunopathogenesis occurs primarily in lymphoid organs, that of the autoinflammatory disorders develops and occurs in the affected tissues, implying that tissue-specific factors in the target organs contribute to disease expression. A direct association between defective immune responses to bacterial components and these diseases has not been clearly established.[3] Excessive or protracted signaling, or both, by cell surface or intracellular innate immune receptors is central to their pathogenesis.

Most classic autoinflammatory syndromes are generally dependent on germline or de novo gene mutations that cause or facilitate the assembly of a protein complex called inflammasome, capable of detecting cellular danger signals generated by infectious agents or metabolic stressors. Consequent production of proinflammatory cytokines, principally interleukin (IL)-1β, leads to the creation of autoamplifying feedback loops that explain their chronicity.[4] These diseases and syndromes were initially cataloged as periodic fever syndromes.[5–7]

Clinical classification of autoinflammatory diseases and syndromes is presented in **Table 1**. A classification based on molecular insights garnered over the past decade was recently proposed; it is intended to supplant the classification shown in **Table 1**, which is opaque to the genetic, immunologic, and therapeutic interrelationships that have become evident of late. Intrinsic inflammasomopathies represent molecular lesions in the constituent proteins of the inflammasome; extrinsic inflammasomopathies denote disorders of various upstream or downstream regulatory elements (**Table 2**).[8]

Authors have no conflict of interest to disclose.

[a] Department of Medicine, Baylor University Medical Center and Texas A&M Medical School, 3500 Gaston Avenue, Dallas, TX 75246, USA; [b] Department of Dermatology, University of Texas Southwestern Medical School, 5323 Harry Hines Boulevard, Dallas, TX 75235, USA; [c] Department of Family Practice, University of Texas Southwestern Medical School, 5323 Harry Hines Boulevard, Dallas, TX 75235, USA; [d] Dermatology Treatment & Research Center, 5310 Harvest Hill Road Dallas, TX 75230, USA
* Corresponding author. Dermatology Treatment & Research Center, 5310 Harvest Hill Road, Dallas, TX 75230.
E-mail address: drA@dermcenter.us

Table 1
Clinical classification of the autoinflammatory syndromes and diseases

Hereditary recurrent fevers	Familial Mediterranean fever (FMF)
	Mevalonate kinase deficiency syndrome (MKDS)
	Tumor necrosis factor receptor-associated periodic syndrome (TRAPS)
	Cryopyrin-associated periodic syndromes (CAPS)
	   Familial cold-associated syndrome (FCAS)
	   Muckle-Wells syndrome (MWS)
	   Neonatal-onset multisystem inflammatory disease (NOMID)/chronic infantile neurologic cutaneous articular syndrome (CINCA)

Idiopathic febrile syndromes	Systemic-onset juvenile idiopathic arthritis (SJIA) Periodic fever, aphthous stomatitis, pharyngitis and adenitis or periodic fever, aphthous pharyngitis and cervical adenopathy syndrome (PFAPA) Pyoderma gangrenosum, acne, and suppurative hidradenitis syndrome (PASH) Behçet disease Nakajo-Nishimura syndrome Chronic atypical neutrophilic dermatosis with lipodystrophy and elevated temperature (CANDLE) syndrome
Pyogenic disorders	Pyogenic arthritis, pyoderma gangrenosum (PG), and acne syndrome (PAPA) Chronic recurrent multifocal osteomyelitis (CRMO) syndrome Majeed syndrome Deficiency of IL-1 receptor antagonist (DIRA) Deficiency of IL-36 receptor antagonist (DITRA) CARD14-mediated pustular psoriasis (CAMPS)
Immune-mediated granulomatous diseases	Blau syndrome Crohn disease
Autoinflammatory diseases of the bones	Cherubism
Complement disorders	Atypical hemolytic uremic syndrome (aHUS) Age-related macular degeneration (AMD)
Hemophagocytic and vasculitic syndromes	Familial hemophagocytic lymphohistiocytosis (FHLH) Secondary hemophagocytic lymphohistiocytosis
Miscellaneous	Atopic dermatitis Psoriasis Vitiligo Alopecia Rosacea Atherosclerosis Multiple sclerosis Diabetes

Data from Masters SL, Simon A, Aksentijevich I, et al. Horror autoinflammaticus: the molecular pathophysiology of auto-inflammatory disease. Annu Rev Immunol 2009;27:621–68.

CLINICAL CLASSIFICATION OF THE AUTOINFLAMMATORY SYNDROMES AND DISEASES
IL-1β Activation Disorders and Other Inflammasomopathies

IL-1β secretion has emerged as a central mechanism in the pathogenesis of many inflammatory diseases. Genetically defined syndromes such as cryopyrin-associated periodic syndromes (CAPS) and Familial Mediterranean fever (FMF), as well as diseases associated with NLRP3 activation by danger signals such as gout, pseudogout, Alzheimer disease, or diabetes mellitus, are included in this group. Drugs directed against IL-1 activity contribute to the identification and treatment of a

Table 2
Molecular/immunologic classification of the autoinflammatory diseases

IL-1β activation disorders and other inflammasomopathies	Intrinsic: FCAS, MWS, NOMID/CINCA Extrinsic: FMF, PAPA, CRMO, Majeed syndrome, HIDS, recurrent hydatidiform mole, DIRA, DITRA, MKDS Complex/acquired: gout, pseudogout, fibrosing disorders, type 2 diabetes mellitus, Schnitzler syndrome, multiple sclerosis, Nakajo-Nimura syndrome, CANDLE syndrome, joint contractures, muscular atrophy, microcytic anemia, and panniculitis-associated lipodystrophy syndrome (JMP), alopecia areata
Nuclear factor kappa-β (NF-Kb) activation disorders	Crohn disease CAMPS Blau syndrome Guadeloupe periodic fever (FCAS2)
Protein folding disorders of the innate immune system	TRAPS Spondyloarthropathies
Complement disorders	aHUS AMD PFAPA
Cytokine signaling disorders	Cherubism
Macrophage activation disorders	Still disease, IJS Chediak-Higashi syndrome Griscelli syndrome X-linked lymphoproliferative syndrome Hermansky-Pudlak syndrome FHLH Secondary HLH Atherosclerosis
Miscellaneous	Atopic dermatitis Psoriasis Gout Diabetes Vitiligo Rosacea (cathelicidins) Behçet disease

Data from Masters SL, Simon A, Aksentijevich I, et al. Horror autoinflammaticus: the molecular pathophysiology of autoinflammatory disease. Annu Rev Immunol 2009;27:621–68.

broad spectrum of disorders beyond those characterized as autoinflammatory.[9]

NF-kappaB Activation Syndromes

Inappropriate activity of NF-kappaB is linked to autoimmune and autoinflammatory diseases. Multiple mechanisms ensure proper termination of NF-kappaB activation. Recent genetic studies have shown a clear association between several mutations in the gene responsible for downregulation of NF-kappaB and immunopathologies such as Crohn disease (CD), rheumatoid arthritis (RA), systemic lupus erythematosus (SLE), psoriasis, and type 1 diabetes mellitus.[10]

Protein Misfolding Syndromes

Misfolding of proteins can lead to structures that may be nonfunctional, have suboptimal functioning, or be degraded by cellular machinery, or structures in which exposed epitopes lead to dysfunctional interactions with other proteins. Several serious diseases seem to involve misfolding of particular proteins (in parentheses) including cystic fibrosis (cystic fibrosis transmembrane conductance regulator [CFTR]), Marfan syndrome (fibrilin), Fabry disease (α-galactosidase) and Gaucher disease (glucocerebrosidase). Others caused by insoluble protein deposition on or inside cells include Alzheimer disease (amyloid β and tau), type 2 diabetes mellitus (amylin), Parkinson disease (α-synuclein) and prion diseases. Certain cancers are associated with misfolded proteins (eg, tumor suppressor protein gene p53).[8,11,12]

Complement Regulatory Diseases

The complement cascade is an important mediator of the inflammatory response to infection; this pathway is tightly regulated by membrane-bound and soluble factors to prevent uncontrolled activation that can lead to damage to host tissues. Absence or mutation of the transcriptional regulation of the soluble complement regulatory genes, C1 inhibitor, complement factor I, complement factor H, and C4 binding protein, are associated with specific diseases; their contribution is often poorly understood.[13]

Disturbances in Cytokine Signaling

Cytokine signaling via a restricted number of genetic pathways positively or negatively regulates cell types involved in initiation, propagation, and resolution of inflammation. Because components of such pathways are closely associated with inflammatory diseases, cytokine-targeted therapies are increasingly used to suppress inflammation.[14]

Macrophage Activation Syndromes

Exaggerated immune response can develop as a primary condition or secondary to infections, some drugs, and various diseases, resulting in liver dysfunction, encephalopathy, pancytopenia, and disseminated intravascular coagulation (DIC).[15] The development of macrophage activation syndrome (MAS) has been reported in patients with inflammatory bowel disease (IBD), after liver transplantation, and is triggered by medications, particularly sulfasalazine and antitumor necrosis factor (TNF) biologics.[15]

MOLECULAR AND BIOLOGICAL COMPONENTS OF AUTOINFLAMMATORY SYNDROMES AND DISEASES

- IL-1: IL-1, a cytokine first cloned in the 1980s, rapidly emerged as a key player in the regulation of inflammatory processes. It is a powerful inducer of fever and inflammation, angiogenesis, tissue remodeling, and other features of the acute phase response.[16,17] Highly conserved throughout evolution, IL-1 comprises 11 proteins (IL-1F1 to IL-1F11) encoded by 11 distinct genes.[18] More than any other cytokine family, IL-1 is closely linked to the innate immune response as shown by the discovery that the cytoplasmatic domain of

IL-1 receptor type I (IL1R1) is highly homologous to the cytoplasmatic domains of all toll-like receptors (TLRs). Thus, fundamental inflammatory responses such as induction of cyclooxygenase type 2, overexpression of adhesion molecules, and nitric oxide synthesis are indistinguishable, whether triggered by IL-1 or TLR ligands; both nonspecifically affect antigen recognition and lymphocyte function. Although both families evolved to assist in host defense against infection, unlike the TLR family, the IL-1 family includes members that suppress inflammation.[19] IL-1 acts on T-lymphocyte regulation and includes IL-1α and IL-1β, encoded by 2 separate genes.[1,16] IL-1α or IL-1β rapidly increases the messenger RNA expression of hundreds of genes in multiple different cell types. IL-1 activities occur at 3 levels: (1) synthesis and release, (2) membrane receptors, and (3) intracellular signal transduction. Ligand binding to the receptor responds with a complex sequence of combinational phosphorylation and ubiquitination events resulting in activation of NF-kappaB signaling, Janus kinase (JNK), and p38 mitogen-activated protein kinase pathways, which cooperatively induce the expression of canonical IL-1 target genes (such as IL-6, IL-8, MCP-1, cyclooxygenase [COX]-2, IkappaB-α, IL-1α, IL-1β, MKP-1) by transcriptional and posttranscriptional mechanisms. Most intracellular components that participate in the response to IL-1 also mediate responses to IL-18, IL-33, and TLRs. Positive and negative feedback mechanisms are in place to amplify or terminate cellular responses to IL-1.[18]

- ○ IL-1α: IL-1α is a cytokine with many metabolic, physiologic, and immunologic effects. Although produced by several cell types, it is characteristic of epithelial cells. Its synthesis in bulk by healthy keratinocytes is part of the immunologic function of the epidermis to maintain the cutaneous barrier and prevent entrance of pathogens.[20] IL-1α interacts with several other cytokines; the most clinically relevant is its synergism with TNF.[21,22]
- ○ IL-1β: IL-1β, a cytokine produced as a pro-protein, is proteolytically activated by caspase-1 in macrophages. An important mediator of the inflammatory response, it is present in proliferation, differentiation, and apoptosis processes.[23]
- ○ IL-1 receptor antagonist: IL-1 receptor antagonist (IL-1Ra) is a naturally occurring

inhibitor of IL-1 and an important negative regulator of the inflammatory response. A genetic deficiency of IL-1Ra was recently shown to be the cause of a severe inflammatory syndrome in humans.[24] IL-10 activates the signal transducer and activator of transcription 3 (STAT-3) and modulates IL-1Ra transcription in lipopolysaccharide (LPS)-treated phagocytes by making IL-1Ra promoter accessible to readily available nuclear NF-kappaB.[24]

  o IL-1 receptor type II: IL-1 receptor type II (IL-1 RII) is a naturally occurring inhibitor of IL-1. It binds to IL-1α and β and acts as a distractor, inhibiting the activity of such ligands. It is thought that IL-4 works as an antiinflammatory agent by activating IL-1RII, thus antagonizing IL-1 activity.[16,25]

• IL-17: IL-17, a cytokine produced by a subset of CD4+ T-helper cells called Th-17 that mount a protective immune response to several microbial pathogens, is implicated in a wide range of autoimmune, allergic, and autoinflammatory diseases such as eczema, RA, psoriasis, multiple sclerosis, IBD, and the enthesitis of psoriasis.[26,27] Missense mutations of the gene encoding for NLRP3 are connected to excessive production of IL-1β, likely caused by a diminished inflammasome activation threshold resulting in neutrophilic infiltration and an IL-17 dominant response from augmented Th-17 cell differentiation.[28] A major source of IL-17 is a T lymphocyte that constitutively expresses the IL-23 receptor, like splenic lymphoid tissue inducer-like (LTi-like) cells, which might contribute to the dynamic organization of secondary lymphoid organ structure and host defense.[29]

• TLR: TLRs are a class of membrane receptors that sense extracellular microbes and trigger antipathogen signaling cascades.[30] Positive feedback loops triggering immune activation can occur when TLR signaling pathways stimulate host cells in an unchecked manner. On occasions, endogenous molecules such as heat-shock protein trigger specific immune responses that create a TLR-dependent autoamplification loop; this can lead to persistent immune activation.[31,32]

• Regulatory B cells: Regulatory B cells (B-reg) are lymphocytes that produce antiinflammatory cytokines, like IL-10, and suppress Th1 and Th2 inflammatory responses. In some multiorgan inflammatory disorders with infiltration, where autoantibodies are not detected, B-regs seem to play a critical early role in T-cell priming or expansion.[33,34]

• Regulatory T cells: Regulatory T cells (T-reg) are lymphocytes that play a crucial role maintaining control of other leukocytes. Depletion may result in autoimmune disorders such as thyroiditis, gastritis, diabetes mellitus, and colitis, at the same time improving the response to antitumor vaccines.[32] T-regs maintain peripheral tolerance in healthy individuals and suppress immune responses during infections to prevent tissue damage. To allow for effective infection elimination, T-regs themselves need to be regulated; the presence of pathogens is communicated to T-regs via TLRs, T-regs respond to ligands for TLR-2, 4, 5. Different TLRs have different effects on T-reg function, resulting in more or less suppression or abrogation.[32]

• Cytotoxic T-lymphocyte antigen 4: Cytotoxic T-lymphocyte antigen 4 (CTLA4, CD152), a costimulatory molecule expressed on activated T cells, plays a key inhibitory role during T-lymphocyte activation. The gene encoding for CTLA4 has been suggested as a candidate to confer susceptibility to autoinflammatory diseases and is associated with Behçet disease.[35]

• Antimicrobial peptides: Cutaneous production of antimicrobial peptides (AMPs) is a primary system for protection against skin infections; their expression further increases in response to microbial invasion. Defensins are a type of AMP first characterized for their antimicrobial properties and include the cathelicidins.[36]

  o Cathelicidin: Cathelicidin is a unique AMP that protects the skin through direct antimicrobial activity and initiation of cellular responses resulting in cytokine release, angiogenesis, reepithelialization, and inflammation. Underexpression is a factor in Alzheimer disease; in rosacea, it is abnormally processed to forms that induce inflammation; in psoriasis, it converts self-DNA into a potent stimulus in an autoinflammatory cascade. Vitamin D_3 is a major factor in the regulation of cathelicidin.[36,37]

• Caspase-1: Caspase-1 is a protein member of the cysteine-aspartic acid protease (caspase) family. Sequential activation of caspases plays a central role in the execution phase of cell apoptosis. Activated by inflammasomes, caspase-1 processes the secretion and maturation of IL-1β and IL-18.[6,38]

• Danger receptors: Danger receptors are sensors of microbial invasion, cell stresses, and physiologic perturbations that can elicit inflammatory responses.[39]

- ○ Nucleotide-binding oligomerization domain: Nucleotide-binding oligomerization domain (NOD) is a danger receptor that recognizes intracellular patterns capable of activating transcription of inflammatory cytokines.[40]
- ○ Nucleotide-binding oligomerization domain-2: Nucleotide-binding oligomerization domain-2 (NOD-2) is a cytosolic innate receptor able to sense peptidoglycan from gram-positive and gram-negative bacteria, triggering receptor interacting protein-2 (RIP2)-mediated and NF-kappaB-mediated proinflammatory and antibacterial responses. Mutations in the gene encoding NOD-2 in humans have been associated with CD and Blau syndrome.[40,41]
- ○ NOD-like receptor: NOD-like receptors (NLR) are intracellular microbial sensors; some sense nonmicrobial danger signals and assemble into inflammasomes, linking the sensing of microbial products and metabolic stresses to proteolytic activation of IL-1β and IL-18.[30]
- Putative nucleotide-binding (nucleoside triphosphatase) domain: The putative nucleotide-binding (nucleoside triphosphatase) domain (NACHT) is found with other domains in a variety of proteins involved in the regulation of inflammation and/or apoptosis.[42] The acronym stands for: neuronal apoptosis inhibitor protein, major histocompatibility complex (MHC) class 2 transcription activator, incompatibility locus protein from *Podospora anserina*, and telomerase-associated protein.
- Nucleotide-binding domain, leucine-rich repeat containing family: Nucleotide-binding domain, leucine-rich repeat containing family (NLR) include intracellular proteins, generally formed by a leucine-rich repeat (LRR) near the C-terminal and a NATCH. Several function in the innate immune system as sensors of pathogen components and participate in immune-mediated cellular responses via the caspase-1 inflammasome.[40] The NLR network provided pivotal genetic and molecular insights into diseases previously regarded as autoimmune. NLR-related disorders include CAPS, CD, gout, and pseudogout, principally associated with increases in TNF or IL-1.[3] The protein linked to their N-terminal differentiates NLRs. The largest group possesses a pyrin domain (PYD), known as NLRP (previously NALP). More than 14 subtypes of have been described.
  - ○ Inflammasomes: Inflammasomes are large multimeric protein complexes linking the sensing of microbial products and metabolic stresses (intracellular danger) to production of some proinflammatory cytokines. As a cytosolic sensor, it is the signaling platform required for the activation of IL-1β by proteolysis of prointerleukin (proIL)-β to the active form. The activation and mechanism of action varies depending on the components forming the complex. The first inflammasome described was named NLRP1.[43,44]
  - ○ Inflammasome NLRP3: Initially identified in a group of rare autoinflammatory conditions called CAPS, inflammasome NLRP3 has now been implicated in the pathogenesis of several common diseases including gout and gouty arthritis, Alzheimer disease, diabetes mellitus, silicosis, and some cancers.[7,9,40] It was formerly known as NALP3, PYPAF1, or cryopyrin. Autoproteolytic maturation of caspase-1 zymogens, triggered by microbial ligands, danger-associated molecular patterns (DAMPs), and crystals, leads to secretion of IL-1β and IL-18. Different domains are responsible for the activation of the inflammasome depending on the aggressing agent.[45,46]
- Pyryn: Pyryn, a protein that plays an important role in modulating innate immune responses, is produced by the MEFV gene and usually downregulates inflammation. When defective, it is responsible for recurrent attacks of febrile polyserositis in FMF.[47,48]
- Cryopyrinopathies: Cryopyrinopathies are rare disorders associated with heterozygous mutations with gain-of-function of the gene that encodes NLRP3, which leads to inflammation driven by excessive production of IL-1β.[49] The cryopyrinopathies include familial cold autoinflammatory syndrome (FCAS), Muckle-Wells syndrome (MWS), and chronic infantile, neurologic, cutaneous, and articular (CINCA)/neonatal-onset multisystem inflammatory disease (NOMID) syndrome; initially considered separate entities, however, mutations of the same gene have been found in all 3 so they are now considered representatives in a continuum of subphenotypes.[50]

SUMMARY OF THE AUTOINFLAMMATORY SYNDROMES AND DISEASES

- CAPS: CAPS are inherited autoinflammatory disorders caused by autosomal dominant gain-of-function mutations in the NLRP3 gene on chromosome 1q44.[51] The following entities belong to the CAPS:

o FCAS presents with recurrent episodes of fever, urticaria, articular symptoms, and conjunctivitis that may be triggered by cold. In some families, an association with reactive AA amyloidosis has been described.[52]

o MWS presents with urticaria, remitting fever, remitting coxitis, osteitis, bilateral anterior uveitis, sensorineural hearing loss, and increase in C-reactive protein (CRP) and serum amyloid A (SAA) levels. Amyloidosis is a serious complication affecting about 25% of patients, occasionally with fatal consequences.[49] A report of an 8-year-old girl who responded remarkably to anakinra, with recovering of hearing loss, suggests that early diagnosis and treatment may reduce the long-term consequences of amyloidosis.[53]

o CINCA/NOMID is characterized by the triad of neonatal onset of cutaneous symptoms and signs resembling generalized urticaria, chronic meningitis, and recurrent fever. It presents with a distinctive osteoarthropathy, synovitis mainly of large joints, and overgrowth of epimetaphyseal cartilage, particularly of large bones.[54] The term CINCA is used principally in Europe where it was first described; the term NOMID is more commonly used in the United States. Before the recognition of mutations leading to IL-1β overexpression and the development of targeted therapy, antiinflammatories were used but had limited benefit; treatment with anakinra and rilonacept has shown remarkable success.[49,54,55]

  ■ Adult form: rare. Among 13 patients, 92% had headaches; of those, 77% had features of migraine, 54% had neurosensorial deafness, 69% had myalgias, 46% had papilledema, 15% had optic disc pallor, aseptic meningitis, amyloidosis, and renal failure. It responds to anti-IL-1 therapy.[56]

  ■ Childhood form: cartilage overgrowth eventually causes osseous overgrowth particularly of large bones, deformities that persist beyond skeletal maturity and lead to limb length discrepancy, joint contracture, and early degenerative arthropathy. Blood tests may reveal neutrophilia, anemia, and increased levels of acute phase reactants.[54] Twenty percent of patients die from a variety of complications before reaching adulthood.[49] IL-1 receptor antagonist therapy may result

in dramatic improvement, except of the arthropathy where it is questionable.

• Familial Aicardi-Goutiéres syndrome: Familial Aicardi-Goutiéres syndrome (AGS) is characterized by chilblains, mouth ulcers, chronic unclassified inflammatory skin condition, microcephaly (or normal size head), mild or no mental retardation, spastic paraparesis, and chronic progressive deforming arthropathy of small and large joints with secondary contractures.[57] AGS is an autosomal recessive condition associated with a defect in the 3′-repair exonuclease 1 (TREX1).

• Tumor necrosis factor receptor-associated periodic syndrome: Arthralgia and nonerosive synovitis, nonspecific abdominal and cutaneous abnormalities are among the most common manifestations of tumor necrosis factor receptor-associated periodic syndrome (TRAPS). Chronic erosive joint disease progressing by flare ups and idiopathic recurrent pericarditis were recently added.[58,59] TRAPS was recently reported in a 16 year old girl of short stature with dermatitis, myositis/fasciitis, delayed puberty with amenorrhea, no fever but increased inflammatory parameters on laboratory tests, particularly of amyloid A. Long-term etanercept administration gave her significant clinical improvement, reducing the erythrocyte sedimentation rate and the levels of CRP, IL-6, TNFα, and soluble TNFα receptor 1, but not of IL-12.[60] Formerly known as familial Hibernian fever, it is caused by mutations in the type 1 TNF receptor superfamily member 1A (TNFRSF1A) gene, which may cause aberrant TNF-mediated intracellular signaling and be related to an error in transcription resulting in a defective membrane TNF receptor.[47,61] NF-kappaB and p38 phosphorylation levels of monocytes, lymphocytes, and neutrophils stimulated with TNF are significantly low.[62] For patients who fail with colchicine, etanercept may be a first choice[63,64]; but in a family of 9 patients all carrying a mutation in the TNFRSF1A gene, infliximab failed to cause a response, enhanced antiapoptotic activity and secretion of IL-1β, IL-6, IL-8, IL-12, and the IL-1 receptor was overexpressed; thus caution is advised when prescribing anti-TNFα therapy for these patients.[65]

• Chronic recurrent multifocal osteomyelitis: Chronic recurrent multifocal osteomyelitis (CRMO) involves inflammation with lytic, painful, bone lesions resembling osteomyelitis without an infectious origin; it usually starts during childhood although cases of adult onset have occurred. CRMO is a hereditary, autosomal recessive disease. It is currently treated with antiinflammatory drugs, mostly steroids. Recent studies suggest it may be a disorder of IL-1β regulation, suggesting new therapeutic options.[66]

- Majeed syndrome: CRMO plus dyserythropoietic anemia and an inflammatory neutrophilic dermatoses is known as Majeed syndrome. It is caused by a mutation on the LPIN2 gene, altering the regulation of oxidative stress in macrophages, which leads to tissue infiltration and cell damage. It occurs earlier than typical CRMO and responds well to antiinflammatory agents; it resolves spontaneously in most cases.[8,67]

- Recurrent hydatidiform mole: Recurrent hydatidiform mole is a benign trophoblastic tumor presenting as pregnancy without embryonic development and with cystic degeneration of chorionic villi. It has a strong genetic contribution. Multiple cases have been described within families. The first genetic cause was identified in the NLRP7 protein, similar in structure to NLRP3 and NLRP1, but unlike them, it acts as a negative regulator of IL-1β. It is induced by inflammatory cytokines as part of a negative feedback loop; NLRP7 was also expressed in target organs such as uterus, endometrium, and ovary, therefore dysregulation of inflammatory processes during pregnancy became the new hypothetical mechanism of disease. DNA methylation differences may be the consequence of tissue inflammation.[8]

- Deficiency of IL-1 receptor antagonist: Deficiency of IL-1 receptor antagonist (DIRA) was recently described in a patient with pustular rash, marked osteopenia, lytic bone lesions, respiratory insufficiency, and thrombosis, in whom genetic studies revealed a homozygous deletion on chromosome 2q13, which encompasses several IL-1 family members, including the gene encoding the IL-1-receptor antagonist (IL1-RN). LPS stimulation of mononuclear cells from the patient produced large amounts of proinflammatory cytokines. Treatment with anakinra completely resolved the condition.[68] In the same issue of the New England Journal of Medicine, 9 children from 6 families with neonatal onset of sterile multifocal osteomyelitis, periostitis and pustulosis were reported. All had mutations affecting IL-1RN allowing for unopposed action of IL-1 resulting in life-threatening systemic inflammation with skin and bone involvement.[69]

- Gout: Gout is an arthropathy characterized by increased levels of uric acid (UA) in the blood. The joint most commonly affected is that of the great toe; crystals of UA form and accumulate in the synovial fluids in less than 10% of hyperuricemic patients. Monosodium urate crystal deposition leads to acute inflammation, which resolves spontaneously. UA was identified as a danger signal that triggers the NALP3 inflammasome, activating IL-1, upregulating mediators such as cyclooxygenase, TNF, and IL-8, which in turn cause acute granulocytic inflammation. Colchicine, nonsteroidal antiinflammatory drugs (NSAIDs), corticosteroids, and IL-1 blockers, seem effective in resolving flares. Once the attacks subside, control of UA metabolism is essential; this may be accomplished by diet, xanthine oxidase inhibitors such as allopurinol and febuxostat, and by probenecid-induced uricosuria.[70,71]

- Pseudogout: Pseudogout is an arthritis characterized by sudden painful swelling of 1 or more joints in episodes that last days or weeks. It typically occurs in older adults, most commonly affecting the knees but also the ankles, wrists, and elbows. It is also called calcium pyrophosphate deposition (CPPD) disease, which occurs when pyrophosphate crystals form in the fluid that lubricates joint linings, causing pain and inflammation. The underlying molecular mechanism is related to caspase-1 activating NALP3 resulting in the production of IL-1β and IL-18.[72] Treatment of CPPD arthritis includes ice, rest, joint aspiration, and intra-articular injection of corticosteroids.[73] Anakinra was used successfully in the treatment of resistant disease and in patients with renal failure.[74,75]

- Fibrosing disorders: Fibrosis is a pathologic manifestation in injured organs where there is excessive nonphysiologic synthesis and accumulation of extracellular matrix proteins from activated/differentiated fibroblasts.[76] This results in the replacement of normal tissue components with inflammatory cells and connective tissue scar; it is seen in asthma, lung fibrosis, chronic kidney disease, liver fibrosis, vasculopathies such as atherosclerosis, and skin abnormalities such as keloids, hypertrophic scarring, and scleroderma.[77] External insults such as asbestos, silica, bleomycin, and nephrogenic systemic sclerosis (induced by gadolinium in magnetic resonance contrast) have been identified as causes of organ fibrosis.[8] IL-1 gene complex single nucleotide polymorphism has been associated with severe restrictive lung physiology in systemic sclerosis.[78] NLRP3 inflammasome activation and IL-1β expression have a predominant role in establishing pulmonary inflammation and fibrosis; IL-23 and IL-17A have a similar role.[79,80] IL-1 blockade reduced bleomycin-induced fibrosis in mice and intra-articularly in patients with refractory limited arthrofibrosis after knee surgery.[81,82]

- Type 1 diabetes: Type 1 diabetes is a metabolic condition with hyperglycemia in which destruction of pancreatic islets is evident at an early age; this leads to a marked reduction in insulin production. Most patients have autoantibodies against pancreatic B cells and increased IL-1β production. IL-1 blockade is efficacious in controlling and even reversing antibody-mediated destruction in animal models.[83–85]

- Type 2 diabetes: Type 2 diabetes is a common metabolic condition characterized by insulin resistance and uncontrolled glucose levels. Ultimately, chronic inflammation in the pancreas and adipose tissue causes impaired responsiveness to insulin and results in the development of disease.[5] IL-1 signaling has a role in β-cell dysfunction and destruction via the NF-kappaB and mitogen activation protein kinase pathways leading to endoplasmic reticulum and mitochondrial stresses and apoptosis. Macrophages lacking adenosine triphosphate (ATP)–sensitive potassium channel (K_{ATP}) subunits or ATP binding cassette transporters also activate the inflammasome. Glyburide prevents inflammasome activation in pancreatic cells. IL-1 blockers and IL-1Ra seem efficacious in controlling the inflammatory response, restoring insulin production in dysfunctional islets, and even allowing tissue regeneration.[46,84]

- Schnitzler syndrome: Schnitzler syndrome is characterized by simultaneous occurrence of monoclonal gammopathy, chronic urticaria, and either arthralgia, bone pain, fever of unknown origin, hepatomegaly or splenomegaly, lymphadenopathy, increased erythrocyte sedimentation rate, leukocytosis, thrombosis, and increased bone density. It is nonhereditary. Treatment with IL-Ra significantly inhibits IL-1β expression. Free circulating IL-18 is increased despite low expression in monocytes, suggesting constitutive activation of the inflammasome. Schnitzler syndrome responds well to anakinra.[8,86–88]

- Hereditary periodic fevers: Hereditary periodic fevers is a family of syndromes characterized by recurrent nonspecific systemic manifestations associated with increased acute phase reactants, with negative studies and no evidence of subjacent infection. It includes[89]
  - Mevalonate kinase deficiencies (MKD):
    - Hyperimmunoglobulinemia D periodic fever syndrome (HIDS)
    - Mevalonic aciduria (MA)
  - FMF
  - CAPS
  - TRAPS

- MKD: MKD is divided into 2 syndromes depending on severity: HIDS and the more severe form, MA, are both caused by autosomal recessive mutations in the gene encoding mevalonate kinase (MK), an enzyme leading to cholesterol pathway inactivation. Statins are potent inhibitors of the enzyme directly upstream of MK. Activated fibroblasts from patients with MKD secrete more IL-1β than those from healthy donors.[90] All forms of MKD respond favorably to anti-IL-1 treatments.[91,92]

- HIDS: HIDS is characterized by recurrent inflammatory episodes clinically mimicking FMF. The most frequent signs and symptoms accompanying the febrile attacks include lymphadenopathy, abdominal pain, arthralgia, diarrhea, vomiting, skin lesions, and aphthous ulcers. The age of onset is less than 5 years, the first attack occurring around the age of 6 months (range 0–120 months) with attacks of joint pain of less than 14 days. Educational achievements, employment status, social functioning, general health perception, vitality, and other quality of life issues are affected.[93] The frequency of attacks decreases with age but about half the patients continue to have them about 6 times a year after the age of 20 years. Amyloidosis happens in about 3% of cases and is a severe complication. The median serum IgD level is 400 U/ml, and may be normal in up to 25% of patients. It is a rare hereditary autosomal recessive condition. The biochemical pathway was uncovered by the discovery that HIDS results from mutations in MVK, which encodes an enzyme in the isoprenoid pathway.[48,93] Some demonstrate good clinical responses to anakinra and etanercept, but prolonged febrile episodes with these drugs in a 10-year-old girl were recently reported.[94]

- IL-1 receptor-associated kinase-4 (IRAK-4) deficiency: IRAK-4 deficiency is characterized by recurrent infections by pyogenic bacteria with increased risk for infections with *Streptococcus pneumoniae*. It is a rare hereditary disease of primary immunodeficiency caused by a mutation in the IRAK-4 gene resulting in selective impairment of cellular responses to TLRs other than TLR3 and to most IL-1Rs, including IL-1R, IL-18R, and IL-33R.[95,96]

- Myeloid differentiation-factor 88 (MyD88) deficiency: MyD88 deficiency is a life-threatening, often recurrent, pyogenic bacterial infections (including invasive pneumococci); patients are otherwise healthy, with normal resistance to other microbes. Clinical status improves with age, not due to cellular leakiness in MyD88 deficiency but to compensation and maturation of the adaptive immune system. Autosomal recessive primary immunodeficiency is phenotypically indistinguishable from IRAK-4.[97,98]

- CD: CD and ulcerative colitis (UC) are the 2 most common forms of IBD; clinical and genetic features distinguish them. In CD, the inflammation is typically transmural and discontinuous throughout the gut, whereas in UC it primarily affects the mucosal and submucosal layers of the rectum and colon in a continuous pattern. NOD2 seems to be a genetic discriminating factor as a locus only associated with CD.[8] A mutation inappropriately activates the immune system against intestinal flora. Some anti-TNFα antibodies (infliximab, adalimumab, etanercept) may be efficacious in improving and remitting CD and UC.[99,100]

- Blau syndrome: Blau syndrome is characterized by the clinical triad of granulomatous dermatitis, symmetric polyarthritis, and recurrent uveitis. It is a chronic, autosomal dominant condition and onset occurs before 4 years of age it is caused by mutations in the NOD-2 gene leading to constitutive NF-kappaB activation. The NOD-2 pathway possibly interacts with either the TLR2 or TLR4 pathways.[101] Impaired production of the proinflammatory and antiinflammatory cytokines TNF-α, IL-10, granulocyte-colony stimulating factor G-CSF, and interferon (IFN)-γ may be responsible for the chronic inflammation. IL-1 production by mononuclear cells is not increased, hence it is not surprising that anakinra was ineffective.[40,101]

- Guadeloupe periodic fever: Guadeloupe periodic fever (FCAS2) was first described in 2 families from the Guadeloupe archipelago. Week-long episodic fevers triggered by exposure to cold are associated with arthralgia, myalgia, and other constitutional symptoms. Two affected members of 1 family had sensorineural hearing loss. Although clinically similar to FCAS or MWS, mutational screening of NLRP3 and other known periodic fever genes was negative; because of its similar presentation, it became known as FCAS2.[8]

- Enthesitis: Enthesitis is characterized by inflammation where tendons and ligaments attach onto bones (entheses). It is associated with adjacent osteitis or bone and synovial inflammation. Imaging, histologic, and genetic findings mitigate against the view that in psoriasis the cause is autoimmune and directed against a common autoantigen expressing in the skin and joints. In clinically normal joints, microscopic damage and inflammation may be observed. In distal interphalangeal psoriatic arthritis, inflammation envelops the nail root connected to the subjacent periostium by interdigitating fibers, the extensor, and the collateral tendons. Current thinking is that minor trauma and tissue-related factors have an innate immune drive not involving dysregulation of T-cell function, at least initially.[102] A randomized, placebo-controlled study of etanercept demonstrated statistically significant and clinically relevant benefit in refractory heel enthesitis in patients with ankylosing spondylitis.[103]

- Psoriasis: Psoriasis is a multisystemic disease that primarily affects the skin and the joints, principally characterized by erythematous and scaly plaques. A main cause of cutaneous lesions seems to be dysregulated cytokine production orchestrated by activated Th-1 and Th-17 cells, heavily regulated at transcriptional level.[104] Biological drugs against TNFα, IL-12 and IL-23 are effective in controlling and reducing progression; etanercept, infliximab, adalimumab, and ustekinumab are indicated in psoriasis and psoriatic arthritis that does not respond to conventional treatment.

- Psoriasiform eruptions: Treatment with anti-TNFα agents may cause palmoplantar pustulosis and plaquelike psoriasiform lesions histologically suggesting psoriasis or lichenoid, eczematoid reactions. In a report of 13 patients, MxA, a protein specifically induced by type 1 interferons, was strongly produced and closely associated with recruitment into the skin of CXCR3+ lymphocytes bearing markers of cytotoxic capacity.[105]

- RA: RA is an autoimmune disease that presents at any age, most frequently in women; it often affecting joints symmetrically; the wrists, fingers, knees, feet, and ankles are the sites most commonly involved. Biological agents for RA primarily aim to neutralize circulating and cell-bound proinflammatory cytokines, interfere with the interaction of antigen-presenting and T lymphocytes, eliminate circulating B lymphocytes, or interfere with intracellular signaling in immune-competent cells that cause inflammation.[106]

- Ankylosing spondylitis: Ankylosing spondylitis is a systemic disease manifesting chronic arthritis of the spine and sacroiliac joints, leading to loss of spinal mobility. Extra-articular manifestations include uveitis, aortitis, enthesitis, dactylitis, restrictive lung disease, and consequent pulmonary hypertension. Its susceptibility link to HLA-B27 is one of the strongest known HLA-disease associations. Genetic analyses implicate the IL-1 cluster on chromosome 2q13 as an important susceptibility locus.[8,68] IL-1 is upregulated in spondyloarthropathies, and IL-1 polymorphism in association with ankylosing spondylitis is claimed. IL-1 blockade treatment in patients with ankylosing spondylitis demonstrates a sustained response.[107] Newer long-lasting IL-1Ra monoclonal antibodies should provide a new option.

- Still disease: Autoimmune arthritis that, depending on the age of onset, is classified as idiopathic juvenile arthritis (JIA) or adult-form Still disease (ASD):
  - Pediatric form: JIA is the commonest cause of chronic arthritis in children. Studies of specific genes have been modeled on the premise of shared autoimmunity wherein genetic variants that predispose to other autoimmune phenotypes confer susceptibility to JIA. Genome-wide association studies accelerated the detection of non-HLA susceptibility loci in other autoimmune phenotypes and are likely to uncover novel JIA-associated variants.[108]
  - Systemic JIA is a rare systemic inflammatory disease considered to be a subtype of JIA. Besides arthritis, it is characterized by rash, spiking fevers, serositis, and hepatosplenomegaly. IL-1, IL-6 and IL-18, neutrophils, and monocytes/macrophages (rather than lymphocytes) play a major role in its pathogenesis, distinguishing it from other JIA subtypes. Strongly associated with MAS, systemic JIA should be viewed as an autoinflammatory rather than a classic autoimmune disease. Remarkable improvement has been observed with anti-IL-1 and -IL-6 therapies.[108,109]
  - Adult form: ASD is rare. The diagnosis is solely clinical and often difficult. It must be considered in patients with high spiking fever, transient rash, arthralgia, oligo or polyarticular arthritis, leukocytosis, sore throat, lymphadenopathy and/or splenomegaly, liver dysfunction, and high serum ferritin level.[110]

- SLE: SLE is a disease of unknown cause with female predominance. Clinical criteria as well as immunologic characteristics (eg, autoantibodies) are necessary for diagnosis. Its variable course may be characterized by remissions and relapses. New symptoms like those produced by infection often challenge the differential diagnosis. Patients have 5 times the mortality of the normal population, the main reasons being infection and cardiovascular events rather than disease manifestations.[111] Defective immune regulation and uncontrolled lymphocyte activation as well as expansion of local immune responses, increased antigen-presenting cell maturation, and tissue infiltration by pathogenic cells are all influenced by cytokines and cause organ damage.[112] Deposition of circulating immune complexes do not fully explain the tissue specificity; skin-specific autoinflammatory processes in combination with autoimmune complexes likely play a role in exacerbating or amplifying skin manifestations.[113] IL-6 plays a critical role in the immunopathology, B-cell hyperactivity, and maintenance of the autoinflammatory loop. Blocking IL-6 inhibits anti-dsDNA production in vitro and benefited all lupus models tested.[114]

- Epidermal growth factor receptor (EGFR) antagonist-induced autoinflammatory condition: This condition is characterized by acneiform reactions associated with sterile inflammation, sometimes severe, triggered by pharmacologic inhibition of EGFR signaling in oncologic therapy. The pathogenesis involves the action of IL-1 on the hair follicle.[115]

- Pyogenic arthritis, pyoderma gangrenosum, acne (PAPA) syndrome: PAPA syndrome is characterized by sterile pyogenic arthritis, pyoderma gangrenosum (PG), and acne. The onset of acne coincides with puberty. Sterile skin abscesses may be encountered. PAPA syndrome is inherited as autosomal dominant. The pathogenesis involves alteration of the protein PSTPIP-1 (proline, serine, threonine, phosphatase interactive protein), which co-localizes with pyrin in neutrophils. Mutations in its encoding gene produce hyperphos-phorylated PSTPIP-1, which binds avidly to pyrin, reducing its inhibition of inflammasome activation.[47]

- Periodic fever, aphthous stomatitis, and adenitis (PFAPA) syndrome: PFAPA syndrome starts typically in childhood and is one of the most common causes of periodic fever of unknown origin in that age group.[116] Febrile episodes are intermittent, last 3 to 5 weeks, and are accompanied by oral and pharyngeal aphthous lesions. During attacks, complement (C1QB, C2, SERPING1), IL-1–related (IL-1B, IL-1RN, CASP1, IL18RAP), and IFN-induced (AIM2, IP-10/CXCL10) genes are significantly overexpressed, but T-cell–associated transcripts (CD3, CD8B) are downregulated. Treatment based on evidence of IL-1β activation in a study of 5 patients led to prompt clinical response to IL-1Ra antagonist therapy in all patients.[117]

- PG, acne, and suppurative hidradenitis (PASH) syndrome: Two patients with a clinical presentation similar to, yet distinct from, PAPA syndrome were described recently. Both had PG and acute or remittent acne conglobata, but lacked pyogenic arthritis. Instead, they had suppurative hidradenitis. Mutations in PSTPIP1 exons 1 to 15 were excluded. In the promoter region, increased repetition of the CCTG microsatellite motif was present on 1 allele in both patients. Alterations of the most commonly affected exons of the MEFV, NLRP3, and TNFRSF1A genes were not detectable. One patient was treated with anakinra and responded well, although without complete remission, implying that IL-1β may be pathogenic.[118]

- Atypical hemolytic uremic syndrome (aHUS): Atypical hemolytic uremic syndrome (aHUS) is characterized by Coombs-negative hemolytic anemia, thrombocytopenia, and renal failure. The typical form is caused by Escherichia coli (O157:H7), which produces a vero-toxin similar to the shigga toxin that creates thrombotic microangiopathies leading to erythrocyte fragmentation, platelet consumption, and glomerular hypoperfusion. Except for diarrhea, the clinical symptoms of the typical and atypical variants are practically identical, but aHUS is caused by an inherited mutation in the gene that codes for complement factor H (CFH) and a membrane cofactor protein that binds to complement component 3b (C3b) preventing activation of the complement cascade. Unregulated activity of C3 leads to the production of anaphylatoxins C3a and C5, chemotactans for neutrophilic infiltration and inflammation. Endothelial damage by neutrophils releases thrombin and starts the microangiopathic cascade.[8] Eculizumab, a monoclonal humanized anti-C5 antibody, has shown success in patients with aHUS.[8,119]

- Age-related macular degeneration: Age-related macular degeneration, the leading cause of blindness in developed countries, is caused by a variation on CFH. The substitution of histidine for tyrosine in the Y402H gene causes a 7-fold increase in the risk of developing the disease. Proteins and immune complexes deposit around the macula and retina producing progressive loss of vision.[8] Increased levels of complement-activating molecules including C5a are found in serum. C5a promotes IL-22 and IL-17 expression by CD4+ T cells. The possible inactivation of IL-22 and IL-17 may herald a novel approach.[120]

- Behçet disease: Behçet disease is characterized by chronic inflammatory vasculitis leading to painful ulcerations on the oral mucosa resembling canker sores; genital lesions that may be painful and ulcerate (particularly on the scrotum and vulva); acneiform lesions; tender skin nodules particularly on the legs; uveitis and retinal vasculopathy; arthropathy with swelling and pain mostly in the knees, ankles, elbows, or wrists; inflammation of arteries, including large arteries, and veins, leading to swellings on the arms and legs and thrombotic events; abdominal pain, diarrhea, and bleeding; headaches; fever; disorientation; poor balance; and strokes. Serum soluble cytotoxic lymphocyte antigen 4 (sCTLA4) levels may be low, especially in patients with single nucleotide polymorphisms of the promoter and exon regions on the CTLA4 gene, suggesting that sCTLA may be related to the immunologic abnormalities and clinical expressions.[35] A recent study found that a marked increase in Th-17 cells and a decreased frequency of CD4+ and T-regs in peripheral blood induced by IL-21 correlate with activity. IL-21 and IL-17A–producing T cells were present within the cerebrospinal fluid, brain parenchyma inflammatory infiltrates, and intracerebral blood vessels in patients with active Behçet disease and central nervous system involvement. IL-21 blockade with an IL-21R-Fc restored the Th17 and T-reg homeostasis.[121,122]

- Cherubism: Cherubism is characterized by fibrous and bone hyperplasia of the jaw during infancy. It is a hereditary autosomal dominant disease caused by a mutation on the SH3BP2 gene leading to production of an overly active protein that disrupts critical signaling pathways associated with maintenance of bone tissue and some immune system cells, causing inflammation of the jaw bones and triggering production and activation of osteoclasts.[123]

- Chediak-Higashi syndrome: Chediak-Higashi syndrome is characterized by oculocutaneous albinism, immunodeficiency, and thrombophilia. A defect in microtubule polymerization leads to diminished phagocytic capacity. Autosomal recessive mutation in the lysosomal trafficking regulator (LYST) gene seems to be involved in abnormal membrane fusions. Treatment includes cyclosporine and rituximab for the accelerated phase, followed by allogeneic marrow transplant for the hematologic and immunologic symptoms.[124,125]

- Griscelli syndrome: Griscelli syndrome is characterized by albinism and immunodeficiency, and is usually fatal during infancy. It is a rare autosomal recessive entity. Three types exist, based on genetic and molecular features. A mutation in the RAB27A gene leads to dysfunction of an enzyme involved in exocytosis of cytotoxic vesicles and melanosomas.[126]

- X-Linked lymphoproliferative (XLP) syndrome: XLP syndrome is characterized by severe febrile episodes after exposure to Epstein-Barr virus (fulminating mononucleosis). It is a hereditary immunodeficiency that only affects males due to a mutation in the SH2D1A gene, which affects the CD8 cytotoxic and NK response. Some patients present severe hypogammaglobulinemia and increased risk for hematologic neoplasms.[127]

- Hermansky-Pudlak syndrome: Hermansky-Pudlak syndrome is characterized by oculocutaneous albinism, hemorrhagic diathesis from thrombocytopenia due to platelet storage-pool deficiency and, in some cases, pulmonary fibrosis, granulomatous colitis, and renal failure as a result of cellular accumulation and deposition of ceroid lipofuscin. It is an autosomal recessive syndrome caused by mutations in the HPS1-HPS8 and AP3B1 genes that code for a protein that participates in vesicle formation.[128]

- Familial hemophagocytic lymphohistiocytosis: Familial hemophagocytic lymphohistiocytosis (HLH) is characterized by prolonged fever, splenomegaly, and pancytopenia with evidence of hemophagocytosis (erythrocytes phagocytized by macrophages in bone marrow, spleen, lymph nodes, and cerebrospinal fluid) accompanied by hypertriglyceridemia and hypofibrinogenemia that are reversible with treatment. It is a potentially fatal hereditary disease caused by a mutation of important cytotoxic T-cell and NK function genes, a suppression of CD8+ T cells, which normally deter viral replication during infection that leads to perpetuation of macrophage antigenic activation and decreased macrophage-mediated and cytokine-mediated apoptotic signaling.[8] Initial treatment based on dexamethasone, cyclosporine A, and etoposide is designed to reduce the hypercytokinemia. There are reports of successful treatment with the anti-CD25 antibody daclizumab, the anti-CD52 antibody alemtuzumab, and drugs directed at TNF. Anti-IFN-γ antibody is a promising treatment modality.[129]

- Secondary hemophagocytic lymphohistiocytosis: Secondary hemophagocytic lymphohistiocytosis commonly occurs in infancy and is associated with complications of rheumatic diseases and viral processes. It is clinically similar to primary HLH, and in the dysfunction of NK and cytotoxic T cells. Unlike HLH, the patients have neither a basic immunodeficiency nor a genetic component.[8,129]

- Atherosclerosis: Atherosclerosis is significant contributor to mortality worldwide through complications such as stroke and myocardial infarction. IL-1β plays multiple direct, local roles in the formation and stability of atheroma by eliciting inflammatory responses by macrophages, endothelial cells, and smooth muscle cells. Apolipoprotein E–deficient mice develop accelerated atherosclerotic disease; treatment with an IL-1 receptor antagonist inhibited the formation of atheroma comparable with complete genetic ablation of IL-1β or IL-1R1.[5,130]

- Familial atypical cold urticaria: Lifelong symptoms of familial atypical cold urticaria (FACU) begin in early childhood with pruritus, erythema, and urticaria after exposure to cold. Angioedema with or without syncope occurs in 255 to 75% of patients. Attacks may be triggered by atmospheric conditions, aquatic activities, handling cold objects, or ingesting cold foods and beverages. Skin biopsies demonstrate mast cell infiltrates and postchallenge degranulation.[131] This hereditary autosomal dominant condition thus differs from acquired cold urticaria (ACU) and from FCAS by timing of symptoms and the absence of fever, chills, and joint pains. ACU is usually self-limiting, sporadic, and the cold stimulation test is positive, whereas it is negative in FACU. [This newly described syndrome seems not to be autoinflammatory and is included here for differential purposes only.][131]

- Neutrophilic urticarial dermatosis: Neutrophilic urticarial dermatosis is characterized by an urticarialike rash with pale, flat, or slightly raised nonpruritic macules, papules, and plaques. Skin histology consists of a neutrophilic infiltrate that is perivascular and interstitial, with intense leukocytoclasia but without vasculitis or dermal edema. In a report of 9 patients, 1 had dermographism, 6 had fever, 7 had polyarthritis, and 6 had leukocytosis. Purpura and angioedema are not seen, which differentiates it from neutrophilic urticaria and an associated systemic disease, mainly Schnitzler syndrome, adult-onset Still disease, SLE, and hereditary autoinflammatory fever syndromes, is strongly indicated.[132]

- Nakajo-Nishimura syndrome: Nakajo-Nishimura syndrome is an autosomal recessive inflammatory and wasting disease that usually begins in early infancy with a pernio-like rash. Patients develop periodic high fever and nodular erythemalike eruptions, gradually progressive lipomuscular atrophy on the upper body, mainly the face and upper extremities, characteristic long clubbed fingers with joint contractures. It is caused by a homozygous mutation of the PSMB8 gene, encoding the β5i subunit of the immunoproteasome. Accumulation of ubiquitinated and oxidated proteins as a result of deficiency of proteasome activities cause hyperactivation of p38 MAPK and overproduction of IL-6 and IFNγ-induced protein 10 (IP-10) in patient cells in vitro and in vivo, which may account for the inflammatory response and periodic fever.[133,134]

- Chronic atypical neutrophilic dermatosis with lipodystrophy and elevated temperature (CANDLE) syndrome: CANDLE syndrome is characterized by early-onset recurrent fevers, annular violaceous plaques, persistent violaceous swelling of the eyelids, low weight and height, lipodystrophy, hepatomegaly, and a range of visceral inflammatory manifestations. It is caused by nonsense mutations in the PSMB8 gene. Laboratory abnormalities include chronic anemia and increased levels of acute phase reactants liver enzymes. Histopathology of skin lesions shows atypical mononuclear infiltrates of myeloid lineage and mature neutrophils. Patients express increased levels of IP-10, MCP-1, IL-6, and IL-1Ra. IFN-γ and cytokine blockade may be useful.[135,136]

- Joint contractures, muscular atrophy, microcytic anemia, and panniculitis-associated lipodystrophy (JMP) syndrome: JMP syndrome is characterized by childhood-onset lipodystrophy, muscle atrophy, severe joint contractures, erythematous skin lesions, and microcytic anemia. Variable features include hypergammaglobulinemia, hepatosplenomegaly, seizures, and basal ganglia calcification. It is an autosomal recessive disorder believed to be caused by mutations in the PSMB8 gene, which affects MHC class I antigen-processing resulting in activation of inflammatory cytokine pathways.[137,138]

- Vasculitis: Studies in children suggest that inflammatory disorders such as FMF and other autoinflammatory diseases may predispose to vasculitis, the most common being Henoch-Schonlein purpura and Kawasaki disease (KD).[139] Patients with KD demonstrate increased transcription of IL-1 genes suggesting that it or its receptor may be targets for therapy, particularly for patients resistant to intravenous high-dose immunoglobulin.[140] In patients with ANCA-associated vasculitis, serum IL-17 and IL-23 levels were significantly increased in acute flares, and they remained increased in a proportion of convalescents in whom significant increases in IFN-γ were detected.[141]

- Alopecia areata: Alopecia areata is characterized by a loss of hair in patches (areata), rarely diffuse, with progression in some to total loss of scalp hair (totalis) or to loss of all body hair (universalis).[142] It is hypothesized to be an inflammatory disease with a major genetic component that affects 1% to 2% of the population; perifollicular T-cell infiltrates and local cytokine production play an important part in its pathogenesis. The IL-1 system has major effects on hair growth regulation in vitro, with the inhibitory actions of IL-1α and IL-1β opposed by the receptor antagonist IL-1Ra. Polymorphism of the IL-1Ra gene is associated with more severe clinical outcomes in several chronic inflammatory diseases, including alopecia areata.[143] IL-Ra agonists could be an option for patients who are refractory to conventional therapy.[144]

- Rosacea: Rosacea is a common chronic skin condition affecting the face, characterized by flushing, redness, pustules, and dilated blood vessels. The eyes are often involved; thickening of the skin with enlargement (phymas), especially of the nose, occur in some.[145] Cathelicidin dysfunction emerged as the central factor in the pathogenesis of the inflammation and vascular response.[36,146] Doxycycline reduces production of TNF-α and IL-1β; its antiinflammatory effect is believed to explain its efficacy.[147,148]

- Vitiligo: Vitiligo is characterized by achromic patches on the skin, hair, and mucosa due to autoimmune or autoinflammatory loss of melanocytes from the involved areas. It may be part of a broad, genetically determined diathesis as suggested by familial clustering.[149] It was recently demonstrated that chromosome 17 harbors the gene coding for NALP1. A study has shown various levels of expression of NALP1 gene in patients with vitiligo, higher in those with whole-body involvement. NALP1 at low levels is widely expressed, but at higher levels in immune cells, particularly T cells and Langerhans; different patterns are seen that are consistent with the particular involvement of NALP1 in skin autoimmunity.[150]

- Melanoma: Melanoma is characterized by pigmented melanocytic malignancies that progress from macules to tumors and metastasize readily beyond a certain invasion level. Late-stage human melanoma cells spontaneously secrete active IL-1β via constitutive activation of NALP3 and IL-1R signaling. In contrast, NALP3 functionality in intermediate-stage melanoma cells requires activation of the IL-1R by muramyl dipeptide to secrete IL-1β. In vitro, angiogenesis in melanoma is prevented by inhibitors of caspase-1 and caspase-5 or IL-1 receptor blockade. IL-1 is implicated in the development and progression of human melanoma suggesting that inhibiting the inflammasome pathway or reducing IL-1 activity could be therapeutic.[151,152] New targets for the treatment of metastatic melanoma are emerging; IL-6 and IL-10 blockade are potential strategies.[153] Treatment of in-transit metastatic melanoma with intralesional IL-2 resulted in 76% lesional clearance.[154]

- Alzheimer disease: Neuroinflammation is a complex innate response of neural tissue to diverse stimuli such as pathogens, damaged cells, and irritants. Inflammatory mediators including cytokines, chemokines, and prostaglandins are increased in the cerebrospinal fluid and brain tissue of patients with a history of neuroinflammatory conditions and neurodegenerative disorders such as Alzheimer disease, Parkinson disease, and multiple sclerosis. The microglia and astrocytes express pattern recognition receptors (PRRs), which are always on high alert for pathogens or other inflammatory triggers and participate in the assembly and activation of the inflammasome to produce IL-1β, IL-18, and IL-33, influencing the release of toxins from glial and endothelial cells thus promoting or inhibiting neurodegenerative processes. Modulating the inflammasome may be a plausible strategy for many neuroinflammatory conditions.[155]

- Procalcitonin: Procalcitonin is a laboratory inflammation biomarker of higher sensitivity and specificity than traditional markers (CRP, erythrocyte sedimentation rate, and leukocytosis) to differentiate the causes of fever, particularly in autoimmune, autoinflammatory, and malignant diseases.[156,157]

TREATMENT
Antiinflammatories

Corticosteroids

Corticosteroids are cortisol derivatives that can diffuse across cell membranes to complex with specific cytoplasmic receptors. These complexes enter the nucleus, bind to DNA, and stimulate transcription of mRNA and subsequent synthesis of inhibitory enzymes such as IL-10 and the IL-1 type 2 decoy receptor. Thus, they inhibit early inflammation processes such as edema, fibrin deposition, capillary dilatation, movement of phagocytes into the area, and phagocytic activities. They suppress expression of inflammatory genes encoding T-cell growth factors such as IL-2, IL-4, IL-15, and IL-17 as well as IFN-γ. They reduce expression of genes encoding COX-2, inducible nitric oxide synthase, and intracellular adhesion molecule-1 (ICAM-1) normally induced by IL-1β and TNF-α.[99] Prednisone at a dosage of 1 to 2 mg/kg/d is effective in PFAPA, HIDS, and TRAPS.[98]

Aspirin

Aspirin inhibits COX enzymes COX-1 and COX-2, which synthesize the inflammatory mediators prostaglandins and thromboxane. Synthesis of COX-2 is absent or low in healthy individuals but is upregulated by proinflammatory cytokines such as IL-1 and TNF-α in response to infection or in inflammatory disease.[99] NLRP3 single nucleotide polymorphism may play a role in food-induced anaphylaxis and aspirin-induced asthma in a gain-of-function manner.[158]

NSAIDs

Most NSAIDs work by inhibiting COX-1 and/or COX-2. Specific inhibitors of COX-2 have provided a major advance in the treatment of pain particularly from osteoarthritis or RA; NSAIDs are a central part of the treatment of several autoinflammatory diseases. CRMO responds dramatically to indomethacin.[66,98,99]

Colchicine

Colchicine stops cellular replication inhibiting microtubule formation, arresting the mitotic spindle, and interfering with the metaphase. It has been the treatment of choice for gout but has been partially replaced by NSAIDs. Prophylaxis against frequent recurrent acute CPPD crystal arthritis can be achieved with low-dose oral colchicine.[73] It is also used for certain autoinflammatory diseases; in FMF, pyrin interacts with tubulin and microtubules, suggesting a rationale for the highly efficacious effect of the drug.[8]

Statins

Statins are used to lower cholesterol levels. They are potent inhibitors of 3-hydroxy-3-methylglutaryl-CoA reductase, the enzyme directly upstream of MK. A trial of nearly 18,000 patients evaluated rosuvastatin for cardiovascular events in patients with normal low-density lipoprotein-cholesterol levels. After 1.9 years, CRP decreased by 37% in the treatment group and significantly fewer cardiovascular events occurred, including stroke; mortality was also 20% lower.[159] The anti-inflammatory properties seem independent of their cardioprotective properties. In animal studies, statins induced clinical improvement in several inflammatory conditions. In high doses, they reduce activity in multiple sclerosis, lupus glomerulonephritis, and RA.[99,159]

Glyburide

Glyburide was the first compound identified to prevent cryopyrin activation of IL-1β secretion induced by microbial ligand, DAMP, and crystal. Glyburide binds to K_{ATP} channels in the membrane of pancreatic β cells causing them to depolarize and secrete insulin. Analogues inhibit ATP-induced but not hypothermia-induced IL-1β secretion from monocytes expressing FCAS-associated cryopyrin mutations, suggesting that the inhibition occurs upstream of cryopyrin.[46]

Histone Deacetylase Inhibitors

Histone deacetylase (HDAC) inhibitors are an important class of enzymes that influence gene expression by removing acetyl groups from histones, which leads to chromatin remodeling, and transcriptional suppression of key apoptosis and cell cycle regulatory genes. A novel category of anticancer agents has been developed to counter the actions of HDAC inhibitors by inducing apoptosis, arresting the cell cycle, generating reactive oxygen species, inhibiting angiogenesis, and causing autophagy. HDAC inhibitors exhibit immunosuppressive and antiinflammatory properties reducing cytokine production. Interest in HDAC inhibitors as orally active, safe, antiinflammatory agents is fueled by their ability to reduce disease severity in animal models of inflammatory and autoimmune diseases.[99,160]

Peroxisome Proliferator Activated Receptor Agonists

Peroxisome proliferator activated receptor agonists inhibit arachidonic acid-induced inflammation by enhancing degradation of leukotriene B4, cytokine regulation, and cell adhesion. Thiazolidinedione, used to treat type 2 diabetes mellitus, belongs to the group of drugs with a downstream effect on glucose metabolism. In vitro, they reduce the synthesis and gene expression of TLR2, TLR4, IL-1β, TNF-α, IL-6, and monocyte chemoattractant protein-1 in human monocytes.[99,161]

MicroRNAs

MicroRNAs (miRNAs) are small noncoding RNAs that regulate gene expression by binding to complementary target mRNAs, promoting their decay or inhibiting their translation. miRNAs affect all facets of immune system development, from hematopoiesis to innate and adaptive activation in response to infection.[162] Newer generations of these drugs, synthetically made or encoded by DNA to specifically target overexpressed miRNA, could include small antisense RNAs that antagonize miRNA function.[162]

Anticytokines

Targeting cytokines with monoclonal antibodies has been proved to be effective, particularly in children.[63,163] Therapeutic strategies include (1) cytokine neutralization, (2) cytokine receptor blockade, and (3) antiinflammatory pathway activation.[164]

Kinase Blocking Small Molecules

Glycogen synthase kinase 3 β (GSK3 β) is a serine-threonine kinase originally identified in the conversion of glucose to glycogen. Its inhibition attenuates the activation of NF-kappaB and activates the immunomodulatory transcription factor β-catenin.[165] It induces the secretion of the antiinflammatory cytokine IL-10 and suppresses alloreactive T-cell responses. Combined antiproliferative and antiinflammatory properties of small molecule inhibitors of GSK3 β make them an attractive modality for some inflammatory diseases.[165,166]

Rituximab

Rituximab is a monoclonal antibody against CD20 on B cells. It induces remission of inflammatory processes in mice deficient in the autoimmune regulator (AIRE) gene. It may be useful for patients with autoimmune polyendocrinopathy, candidiasis, and ectodermal dystrophy caused by a similar mutation.[167]

Anakinra

Anakinra is an IL-1 receptor antagonist, effective in the treatment of CAPS. A review of 10 patients treated with anakinra for CINCA/NOMID syndrome, aged 3 months to 20 years, followed for 26 to 42 months, showed the dose required for efficacy to be 1 to 3 mg/kg/d in the 8 oldest and 6 to 10 mg/kg/d for the 2 youngest. Treatment must be initiated before irreversible damage develops because residual nervous system inflammation and deafness persisted in those in whom treatment was delayed; amyloidosis persisted if present at initiation but no lesions developed thereafter.[168] Decreases in febrile attacks in HIDS have been reported.[99] For adults, it is given subcutaneously at 100 mg/d. The German Society of Rheumatology recommends anakinra for (1) RA that fails over 6 months to respond to 2 disease-modifying drugs (DMARDs) 1 of which is methotrexate (MTX), (2) adult-onset and juvenile-onset Still disease that fails to respond to sufficiently glucocorticoids, or if they are inadequate for long-term dosage, or fails with a conventional DMARD, usually MTX.[169]

Rilonacept

Rilonacept is a longer-acting fusion protein for IL-1 blockade. It produces rapid and profound clinical improvement, reduces high sensitivity CRP, and normalizes increased serum amyloid concentrations in CAPS. It is approved by the US Food and Drug Administration as an orphan drug for FCAS and MWS. Its desirable longer half-life makes it useful for those who do not tolerate or have difficulties complying with the daily injections required for anakinra. The main side effects are injection site reactions and increased risk for pulmonary infections.[9,49,169–172]

Canakinumab

Canakinumab is a long-acting, fully humanized, monoclonal antibody specific for IL-1β, blocking its interaction with IL-1R, but does not bind to IL-1α or IL-1Ra. It is indicated for a wide range of autoinflammatory disorders.[51] A randomized, double-blind, placebo-controlled clinical trial on MWS patients showed a complete clinical response in 71% 1 week after initiation and in 97% by week 8. In the randomized withdrawal period, 81% of controls flared compared with 0% of the treatment group.[173]

Gevokizumab

Gevokizumab is a humanized monoclonal antibody that blocks IL-1β; it has a high affinity and a long half-life, allowing for monthly dosing. Clinical trials for types 1 and 2 diabetes mellitus, RA, MWS, FCAS, and Behçet disease are ongoing.[174] In Behçet disease, patients with resistant uveitis and retinal vasculitis induced a rapid-onset and sustained reduction in intraocular inflammation, despite discontinuation of immunosuppressive agents and without the need to increase corticosteroid dosages.[175]

Dermatologist would benefit from knowledge of the expanding list of autoinflammatory diseases and syndromes and the treatments available for them.

REFERENCES

1. Rigante D. The protean visage of systemic autoinflammatory syndromes: a challenge for interprofessional collaboration. Eur Rev Med Pharmacol Sci 2010;14(1):1–18.
2. Ida H, Eguchi K. Autoinflammatory syndrome. Nihon Rinsho 2009;67(3):626–36 [in Japanese].
3. McGonagle D, Savic S, McDermott MF. The NLR network and the immunological disease continuum of adaptive and innate immune-mediated inflammation against self. Semin Immunopathol 2007;29(3):303–13.
4. Theofilopoulos AN, Gonzalez-Quintial R, Lawson BR, et al. Sensors of the innate immune system: their link to rheumatic diseases. Nat Rev Rheumatol 2010;6(3):146–56.
5. Lukens JR, Dixit VD, Kanneganti TD. Inflammasome activation in obesity-related inflammatory

diseases and autoimmunity. Discov Med 2011; 12(62):65–74.

6. Efthimiou P, Flavell RA, Furlan A, et al. Autoinflammatory syndromes and infections: pathogenetic and clinical implications. Clin Exp Rheumatol 2008;26(1 Suppl 48):S53–61.

7. Kanazawa N, Furukawa F. Autoinflammatory syndromes with a dermatological perspective. J Dermatol 2007;34(9):601–18.

8. Masters SL, Simon A, Aksentijevich I, et al. Horror autoinflammaticus: the molecular pathophysiology of autoinflammatory disease. Annu Rev Immunol 2009;27:621–68.

9. Mitroulis I, Skendros P, Ritis K. Targeting IL-1beta in disease; the expanding role of NLRP3 inflammasome. Eur J Intern Med 2010;21(3):157–63.

10. Vereecke L, Beyaert R, van Loo G. The ubiquitin-editing enzyme A20 (TNFAIP3) is a central regulator of immunopathology. Trends Immunol 2009; 30(8):383–91.

11. van der Hilst JC. Recent insights into the pathogenesis of type AA amyloidosis. ScientificWorldJournal 2011;11:641–50.

12. Gadad BS, Britton GB, Rao KS. Targeting oligomers in neurodegenerative disorders: lessons from alpha-synuclein, tau, and amyloid-beta peptide. J Alzheimers Dis 2011;24(Suppl 2):223–32.

13. Fraczek LA, Martin BK. Transcriptional control of genes for soluble complement cascade regulatory proteins. Mol Immunol 2010;48(1–3):9–13.

14. O'Shea JJ, Murray PJ. Cytokine signaling modules in inflammatory responses. Immunity 2008;28(4): 477–87.

15. Jayakar BA, Hashkes PJ. Macrophage activation syndrome: why and what should a gastroenterologist know. J Clin Gastroenterol 2011;45(3):210–4.

16. Gabay C, Lamacchia C, Palmer G. IL-1 pathways in inflammation and human diseases. Nat Rev Rheumatol 2010;6(4):232–41.

17. Henderson C, Goldbach-Mansky R. Monogenic IL-1 mediated autoinflammatory and immunodeficiency syndromes: finding the right balance in response to danger signals. Clin Immunol 2010; 135(2):210–22.

18. Weber A, Wasiliew P, Kracht M. Interleukin-1 (IL-1) pathway. Sci Signal 2010;3(105):cm1.

19. Dinarello CA. Immunological and inflammatory functions of the interleukin-1 family. Annu Rev Immunol 2009;27:519–50.

20. Hauser C, Saurat JH, Schmitt A, et al. Interleukin 1 is present in normal human epidermis. J Immunol 1986;136(9):3317–23.

21. Flores EA, Bistrian BR, Pomposelli JJ, et al. Infusion of tumor necrosis factor/cachectin promotes muscle catabolism in the rat. A synergistic effect with interleukin 1. J Clin Invest 1989;83(5):1614–22.

22. Kelley MJ, Rose AY, Song K, et al. Synergism of TNF and IL-1 in the induction of matrix metalloproteinase-3 in trabecular meshwork. Invest Ophthalmol Vis Sci 2007;48(6):2634–43.

23. Giraldo S, Sanchez J, Felty Q, et al. IL1B (interleukin 1, beta). Atlas Genet Cytogenet Oncol Haematol 2008. Available at: http://AtlasGenetics Oncology.org/Genes/IL1BID40950ch2q13.html. Accessed April 10, 2013.

24. Tamassia N, Castellucci M, Rossato M, et al. Uncovering an IL-10-dependent NF-kappaB recruitment to the IL-1ra promoter that is impaired in STAT3 functionally defective patients. FASEB J 2010;24(5):1365–75.

25. Vannier E, Kaser A, Atkins MB, et al. Elevated circulating levels of soluble interleukin-1 receptor type II during interleukin-2 immunotherapy. Eur Cytokine Netw 1999;10(1):37–42.

26. Yamada H. Current perspectives on the role of IL-17 in autoimmune disease. J Inflamm Res 2010;3:33–44.

27. Sonnenberg GF, Weiner DB. Manipulation of T(H) 17 responses in pulmonary immunity and disease through vaccination. Hum Vaccin 2009; 5(8):510–9.

28. Meng G, Zhang F, Fuss I, et al. A mutation in the Nlrp3 gene causing inflammasome hyperactivation potentiates Th17 cell-dominant immune responses. Immunity 2009;30(6):860–74.

29. Takatori H, Kanno Y, Watford WT, et al. Lymphoid tissue inducer-like cells are an innate source of IL-17 and IL-22. J Exp Med 2009;206(1):35–41.

30. Martinon F, Mayor A, Tschopp J. The inflammasomes: guardians of the body. Annu Rev Immunol 2009;27:229–65.

31. Beutler B. Microbe sensing, positive feedback loops, and the pathogenesis of inflammatory diseases. Immunol Rev 2009;227(1):248–63.

32. Sutmuller R, Garritsen A, Adema GJ. Regulatory T cells and toll-like receptors: regulating the regulators. Ann Rheum Dis 2007;66(Suppl 3): iii91–5.

33. Noh G, Lee JH. Regulatory B cells and allergic diseases. Allergy Asthma Immunol Res 2011;3(3): 168–77.

34. Gray D, Gray M. What are regulatory B cells? Eur J Immunol 2010;40(10):2677–9.

35. Park KS, Baek JA, Do JE, et al. CTLA4 gene polymorphisms and soluble CTLA4 protein in Behcet's disease. Tissue Antigens 2009;74(3):222–7.

36. Peric M, Koglin S, Ruzicka T, et al. Cathelicidins: multifunctional defense molecules of the skin. Dtsch Med Wochenschr 2009;134(1–2): 35–8 [in German].

37. Schauber J, Gallo RL. The vitamin D pathway: a new target for control of the skin's immune response? Exp Dermatol 2008;17(8):633–9.

38. CASP1 caspase 1, apoptosis-related cysteine peptidase [*Homo sapiens* (human)]. National Center for Biotechnology Information. 2013. Available at: http://www.ncbi.nlm.nih.gov/gene/834. Accessed April 10, 2013.

39. Dagenais M, Dupaul-Chicoine J, Saleh M. Function of NOD-like receptors in immunity and disease. Curr Opin Investig Drugs 2010;11(11):1246–55.

40. Martin TM, Zhang Z, Kurz P, et al. The NOD2 defect in Blau syndrome does not result in excess interleukin-1 activity. Arthritis Rheum 2009;60(2):611–8.

41. Lecat A, Piette J, Legrand-Poels S. The protein Nod2: an innate receptor more complex than previously assumed. Biochem Pharmacol 2010;80(12):2021–31.

42. Koonin EV, Aravind L. The NACHT family - a new group of predicted NTPases implicated in apoptosis and MHC transcription activation. Trends Biochem Sci 2000;25(5):223–4.

43. Tschopp J, Martinon F, Burns K. NALPs: a novel protein family involved in inflammation. Nat Rev Mol Cell Biol 2003;4(2):95–104.

44. Wu GQ, Liao YJ, Qin ZQ, et al. PYRIN domain of NALP2 inhibits cell proliferation and tumor growth of human glioblastoma. Plasmid 2010;64(1):41–50.

45. Lamkanfi M, Dixit VM. Inflammasomes: guardians of cytosolic sanctity. Immunol Rev 2009;227(1):95–105.

46. Lamkanfi M, Mueller JL, Vitari AC, et al. Glyburide inhibits the Cryopyrin/Nalp3 inflammasome. J Cell Biol 2009;187(1):61–70.

47. Goldfinger S. The inherited autoinflammatory syndrome: a decade of discovery. Trans Am Clin Climatol Assoc 2009;120:413–8.

48. Ryan JG, Kastner DL. Fevers, genes, and innate immunity. Curr Top Microbiol Immunol 2008;321:169–84.

49. Church LD, Savic S, McDermott MF. Long term management of patients with cryopyrin-associated periodic syndromes (CAPS): focus on rilonacept (IL-1 Trap). Biologics 2008;2(4):733–42.

50. Neven B, Prieur AM, Quartier dit Maire P. Cryopyrinopathies: update on pathogenesis and treatment. Nat Clin Pract Rheumatol 2008;4(9):481–9.

51. Walsh GM. Canakinumab for the treatment of cryopyrin-associated periodic syndromes. Drugs Today (Barc) 2009;45(10):731–5.

52. Alhopuro P, Klimenko T, Aittomaki K. Fever from the cold–familial cold autoinflammatory syndrome. Duodecim 2009;125(5):542–5 [in Finnish].

53. Klein AK, Horneff G. Improvement of sensoneurinal hearing loss in a patient with Muckle-Wells syndrome treated with anakinra. Klin Padiatr 2010;222(4):266–8 [in German].

54. Miyamae T, Inaba Y, Nishimura G, et al. Effect of anakinra on arthropathy in CINCA/NOMID syndrome. Pediatr Rheumatol Online J 2010;8:9.

55. Hedrich CM, Fiebig B, Sallmann S, et al. Good response to IL-1beta blockade by anakinra in a 23-year-old CINCA/NOMID patient without mutations in the CIAS1 gene. Cytokine profiles and functional studies. Scand J Rheumatol 2008;37(5):385–9.

56. Kitley JL, Lachmann HJ, Pinto A, et al. Neurologic manifestations of the cryopyrin-associated periodic syndrome. Neurology 2010;74(16):1267–70.

57. Dale RC, Gornall H, Singh-Grewal D, et al. Familial Aicardi-Goutieres syndrome due to SAMHD1 mutations is associated with chronic arthropathy and contractures. Am J Med Genet 2010;152(4):938–42.

58. Schoindre Y, Feydy A, Giraudet-Lequintrec JS, et al. TNF receptor-associated periodic syndrome (TRAPS): a new cause of joint destruction? Joint Bone Spine 2009;76(5):567–9.

59. Cantarini L, Lucherini OM, Cimaz R, et al. Idiopathic recurrent pericarditis refractory to colchicine treatment can reveal tumor necrosis factor receptor-associated periodic syndrome. Int J Immunopathol Pharmacol 2009;22(4):1051–8.

60. Morbach H, Richl P, Stojanov S, et al. Tumor necrosis factor receptor 1-associated periodic syndrome without fever: cytokine profile before and during etanercept treatment. Rheumatol Int 2009;30(2):207–12.

61. Martorana D, Neri TM. TNF receptor-associated periodic fever syndrome caused by sequence alterations in exonic splicing enhancers: comment on the article by Trubenbach et al. Rheumatol Int 2010;30(9):1269–71.

62. Stjernberg-Salmela S, Ranki A, Karenko L, et al. Low TNF-induced NF-kappaB and p38 phosphorylation levels in leucocytes in tumour necrosis factor receptor-associated periodic syndrome. Rheumatology (Oxford) 2010;49(2):382–90.

63. Roldan R, Ruiz AM, Miranda MD, et al. Anakinra: new therapeutic approach in children with Familial Mediterranean Fever resistant to colchicine. Joint Bone Spine 2008;75(4):504–5.

64. Hoffman HM, Simon A. Recurrent febrile syndromes: what a rheumatologist needs to know. Nat Rev Rheumatol 2009;5(5):249–56.

65. Nedjai B, Hitman GA, Quillinan N, et al. Proinflammatory action of the antiinflammatory drug infliximab in tumor necrosis factor receptor-associated periodic syndrome. Arthritis Rheum 2009;60(2):619–25.

66. Abril JC, Ramirez A. Successful treatment of chronic recurrent multifocal osteomyelitis with indomethacin: a preliminary report of five cases. J Pediatr Orthop 2007;27(5):587–91.

67. Glaser RL, Goldbach-Mansky R. The spectrum of monogenic autoinflammatory syndromes: understanding disease mechanisms and use of targeted

therapies. Curr Allergy Asthma Rep 2008;8(4): 288–98.

68. Reddy S, Jia S, Geoffrey R, et al. An autoinflammatory disease due to homozygous deletion of the IL1RN locus. N Engl J Med 2009;360(23): 2438–44.

69. Aksentijevich I, Masters SL, Ferguson PJ, et al. An autoinflammatory disease with deficiency of the interleukin-1-receptor antagonist. N Engl J Med 2009;360(23):2426–37.

70. Winzer M, Tausche AK, Aringer M. Crystal-induced activation of the inflammasome: gout and pseudogout. Z Rheumatol 2009;68(9):733–9 [in German].

71. Miao ZM, Zhao SH, Yan SL, et al. NALP3 inflammasome functional polymorphisms and gout susceptibility. Cell Cycle 2009;8(1):27–30.

72. Martinon F, Petrilli V, Mayor A, et al. Gout-associated uric acid crystals activate the NALP3 inflammasome. Nature 2006;440(7081):237–41.

73. Richette P, Bardin T. Calcium pyrophosphate deposition disease. Presse Med 2011;40(9 Pt 1):856–64 [in French].

74. McGonagle D, Tan AL, Madden J, et al. Successful treatment of resistant pseudogout with anakinra. Arthritis Rheum 2008;58(2):631–3.

75. Announ N, Palmer G, Guerne PA, et al. Anakinra is a possible alternative in the treatment and prevention of acute attacks of pseudogout in end-stage renal failure. Joint Bone Spine 2009;76(4): 424–6.

76. Ghosh AK, Vaughan DE. Fibrosis: is it a coactivator disease? Front Biosci (Elite Ed) 2012;4: 1556–70.

77. Herzog EL, Bucala R. Fibrocytes in health and disease. Exp Hematol 2010;38(7):548–56.

78. Beretta L, Bertolotti F, Cappiello F, et al. Interleukin-1 gene complex polymorphisms in systemic sclerosis patients with severe restrictive lung physiology. Hum Immunol 2007;68(7):603–9.

79. Gasse P, Riteau N, Vacher R, et al. IL-1 and IL-23 mediate early IL-17A production in pulmonary inflammation leading to late fibrosis. PLoS One 2011;6(8):e23185.

80. Wilson MS, Madala SK, Ramalingam TR, et al. Bleomycin and IL-1beta-mediated pulmonary fibrosis is IL-17A dependent. J Exp Med 2010; 207(3):535–52.

81. Gasse P, Mary C, Guenon I, et al. IL-1R1/MyD88 signaling and the inflammasome are essential in pulmonary inflammation and fibrosis in mice. J Clin Invest 2007;117(12):3786–99.

82. Brown CA, Toth AP, Magnussen B. Clinical benefits of intra-articular anakinra for arthrofibrosis. Orthopedics 2010;33(12):877.

83. Mandrup-Poulsen T, Pociot F, Molvig J, et al. Monokine antagonism is reduced in patients with IDDM. Diabetes 1994;43(10):1242–7.

84. Mandrup-Poulsen T, Pickersgill L, Donath MY. Blockade of interleukin 1 in type 1 diabetes mellitus. Nat Rev Rheumatol 2010;6(3):158–66.

85. Ablamunits V, Henegariu O, Hansen JB, et al. Synergistic reversal of type 1 diabetes in NOD mice with anti-CD3 and interleukin-1 blockade: evidence of improved immune regulation. Diabetes 2012; 61(1):145–54.

86. Eiling E, Schroder JO, Gross WL, et al. The Schnitzler syndrome: chronic urticaria and monoclonal gammopathy–an autoinflammatory syndrome? J Dtsch Dermatol Ges 2008;6(8):626–31.

87. Migliorini P, Del Corso I, Tommasi C, et al. Free circulating interleukin-18 is increased in Schnitzler syndrome: a new autoinflammatory disease? Eur Cytokine Netw 2009;20(3):108–11.

88. Lamprecht P. Adult-onset Still's disease, Schnitzler syndrome, and autoinflammatory syndromes in adulthood. Z Rheumatol 2009;68(9):740–6 [in German].

89. Rigante D. Autoinflammatory syndromes behind the scenes of recurrent fevers in children. Med Sci Monit 2009;15(8):RA179–87.

90. Normand S, Massonnet B, Delwail A, et al. Specific increase in caspase-1 activity and secretion of IL-1 family cytokines: a putative link between mevalonate kinase deficiency and inflammation. Eur Cytokine Netw 2009;20(3):101–7.

91. Bodar EJ, Kuijk LM, Drenth JP, et al. On-demand anakinra treatment is effective in mevalonate kinase deficiency. Ann Rheum Dis 2011;70(12): 2155–8.

92. Korppi M, Van Gijn ME, Antila K. Hyperimmunoglobulinemia D and periodic fever syndrome in children. Review on therapy with biological drugs and case report. Acta Paediatr 2011;100(1):21–5.

93. van der Hilst JC, Bodar EJ, Barron KS, et al. Long-term follow-up, clinical features, and quality of life in a series of 103 patients with hyperimmunoglobulinemia D syndrome. Medicine 2008;87(6):301–10.

94. Shendi HM, Walsh D, Edgar JD. Etanercept and anakinra can prolong febrile episodes in patients with hyperimmunoglobulin D and periodic fever syndrome. Rheumatol Int 2012;32(1):249–51.

95. Picard C, Casanova JL, Puel A. Infectious diseases in patients with IRAK-4, MyD88, NEMO, or Ikappa-Balpha deficiency. Clin Microbiol Rev 2011;24(3): 490–7.

96. Picard C, Puel A, Bonnet M, et al. Pyogenic bacterial infections in humans with IRAK-4 deficiency. Science 2003;299(5615):2076–9.

97. von Bernuth H, Picard C, Jin Z, et al. Pyogenic bacterial infections in humans with MyD88 deficiency. Science 2008;321(5889):691–6.

98. De Sanctis S, Nozzi M, Del Torto M, et al. Autoinflammatory syndromes: diagnosis and management. Ital J Pediatr 2010;36:57.

99. Dinarello CA. Anti-inflammatory agents: present and future. Cell 2010;140(6):935–50.

100. Kuek A, Hazleman BL, Ostor AJ. Immune-mediated inflammatory diseases (IMIDs) and biologic therapy: a medical revolution. Postgrad Med J 2007;83(978):251–60.

101. Son S, Lee J, Woo CW, et al. Altered cytokine profiles of mononuclear cells after stimulation in a patient with Blau syndrome. Rheumatol Int 2010; 30(8):1121–4.

102. McGonagle D. Enthesitis: an autoinflammatory lesion linking nail and joint involvement in psoriatic disease. J Eur Acad Dermatol Venereol 2009; 23(Suppl 1):9–13.

103. Dougados M, Combe B, Braun J, et al. A randomised, multicentre, double-blind, placebo-controlled trial of etanercept in adults with refractory heel enthesitis in spondyloarthritis: the HEEL trial. Ann Rheum Dis 2010;69(8):1430–5.

104. Bak RO, Mikkelsen JG. Regulation of cytokines by small RNAs during skin inflammation. J Biomed Sci 2010;17:53.

105. Seneschal J, Milpied B, Vergier B, et al. Cytokine imbalance with increased production of interferon-alpha in psoriasiform eruptions associated with antitumour necrosis factor-alpha treatments. Br J Dermatol 2009;161(5):1081–8.

106. Kukar M, Petryna O, Efthimiou P. Biological targets in the treatment of rheumatoid arthritis: a comprehensive review of current and in-development biological disease modifying anti-rheumatic drugs. Biologics 2009;3:443–57.

107. Bennett AN, Tan AL, Coates LC, et al. Sustained response to anakinra in ankylosing spondylitis. Rheumatology (Oxford) 2008;47(2):223–4.

108. Angeles-Han S, Prahalad S. The genetics of juvenile idiopathic arthritis: what is new in 2010? Curr Rheumatol Rep 2010;12(2):87–93.

109. Vastert SJ, Kuis W, Grom AA. Systemic JIA: new developments in the understanding of the pathophysiology and therapy. Best Pract Res Clin Rheumatol 2009;23(5):655–64.

110. Haar D, Helin P. Still disease in adults. Ugeskr Laeger 1998;160(21):3062–5 [in Danish].

111. Kleinert S, Feuchtenberger M, Tony HP. Systemic lupus erythematosus. A problem based approach. Internist (Berl) 2010;51(8):1013–26 [quiz: 1027–8]. [in German].

112. Apostolidis SA, Lieberman LA, Kis-Toth K, et al. The dysregulation of cytokine networks in systemic lupus erythematosus. J Interferon Cytokine Res 2011;31(10):769–79.

113. Nishimura H, Strominger JL. Involvement of a tissue-specific autoantibody in skin disorders of murine systemic lupus erythematosus and autoinflammatory diseases. Proc Natl Acad Sci U S A 2006;103(9):3292–7.

114. Tackey E, Lipsky PE, Illei GG. Rationale for interleukin-6 blockade in systemic lupus erythematosus. Lupus 2004;13(5):339–43.

115. Rodeck U. Skin toxicity caused by EGFR antagonists-an autoinflammatory condition triggered by deregulated IL-1 signaling? J Cell Physiol 2009; 218(1):32–4.

116. Caorsi R, Pelagatti MA, Federici S, et al. Periodic fever, apthous stomatitis, pharyngitis and adenitis syndrome. Curr Opin Rheumatol 2010; 22(5):579–84.

117. Stojanov S, Lapidus S, Chitkara P, et al. Periodic fever, aphthous stomatitis, pharyngitis, and adenitis (PFAPA) is a disorder of innate immunity and Th1 activation responsive to IL-1 blockade. Proc Natl Acad Sci U S A 2011;108(17):7148–53.

118. Braun-Falco M, Kovnerystyy O, Lohse P, et al. Pyoderma gangrenosum, acne, and suppurative hidradenitis (PASH)-a new autoinflammatory syndrome distinct from PAPA syndrome. J Am Acad Dermatol 2012;66(3):409–15.

119. Lapeyraque AL, Fremeaux-Bacchi V, Robitaille P. Efficacy of eculizumab in a patient with factor-H-associated atypical hemolytic uremic syndrome. Pediatr Nephrol 2011;26(4):621–4.

120. Liu B, Wei L, Meyerle C, et al. Complement component C5a promotes expression of IL-22 and IL-17 from human T cells and its implication in age-related macular degeneration. J Transl Med 2011;9(1):111.

121. van Daele PL, Kappen JH, van Hagen PM, et al. Managing Behcet's disease: an update on current and emerging treatment options. Ther Clin Risk Manag 2009;5:385–90.

122. Geri G, Terrier B, Rosenzwajg M, et al. Critical role of IL-21 in modulating T(H)17 and regulatory T cells in Behcet disease. J Allergy Clin Immunol 2011; 128(3):655–64.

123. Baskin B, Teebi A, Ray PN. Cherubism 2007 Feb 26 [Updated 2011 Sep 1]. In: Pagon RA, Bird TD, Dolan CR, editors. GeneReviews. Seattle (WA): University of Washington; 1993. Available at: http://www.ncbi.nlm.nih.gov/books/NBK1137/. Accessed July 25, 2011.

124. Introne WJ, Westbroek W, Golas GA, et al. Chediak-Higashi syndrome 2009 Mar 3 [Updated 2012 Feb 16]. In: Pagon RA, Bird TD, Dolan CR, editors. GeneReviews. Seattle (WA): University of Washington; 1993. Available at: http://www.ncbi.nlm.nih.gov/books/NBK5188/. Accessed July 25, 2011.

125. Ogimi C, Tanaka R, Arai T, et al. Rituximab and cyclosporine therapy for accelerated phase Chediak-Higashi syndrome. Pediatr Blood Cancer 2011;57(4):677–80.

126. Van Gele M, Dynoodt P, Lambert J. Griscelli syndrome: a model system to study vesicular trafficking. Pigment Cell Melanoma Res 2009;22(3): 268–82.

127. Rezaei N, Mahmoudi E, Aghamohammadi A, et al. X-linked lymphoproliferative syndrome: a genetic condition typified by the triad of infection, immuno-deficiency and lymphoma. Br J Haematol 2011; 152(1):13–30.

128. Gordillo R, Del Rio M, Thomas DB, et al. Hypertension, chronic kidney disease, and renal pathology in a child with Hermansky-Pudlak syndrome. Int J Nephrol 2011;2011:324916.

129. Tang YM, Xu XJ. Advances in hemophagocytic lymphohistiocytosis: pathogenesis, early diagnosis/differential diagnosis, and treatment. ScientificWorldJournal 2011;11:697–708.

130. Bhaskar V, Yin J, Mirza AM, et al. Monoclonal antibodies targeting IL-1 beta reduce biomarkers of atherosclerosis in vitro and inhibit atherosclerotic plaque formation in Apolipoprotein E-deficient mice. Atherosclerosis 2011;216(2):313–20.

131. Gandhi C, Healy C, Wanderer AA, et al. Familial atypical cold urticaria: description of a new hereditary disease. J Allergy Clin Immunol 2009;124(6): 1245–50.

132. Kieffer C, Cribier B, Lipsker D. Neutrophilic urticarial dermatosis: a variant of neutrophilic urticaria strongly associated with systemic disease. Report of 9 new cases and review of the literature. Medicine 2009;88(1):23–31.

133. Kanazawa N, Arima K, Ida H, et al. Nakajo-Nishimura syndrome. Nihon Rinsho Meneki Gakkai Kaishi 2011;34(5):388–400 [in Japanese].

134. Arima K, Kinoshita A, Mishima H, et al. Proteasome assembly defect due to a proteasome subunit beta type 8 (PSMB8) mutation causes the autoinflammatory disorder, Nakajo-Nishimura syndrome. Proc Natl Acad Sci U S A 2011;108(36):14914–9.

135. Liu Y, Ramot Y, Torrelo A, et al. Mutations in PSMB8 cause CANDLE syndrome with evidence of genetic and phenotypic heterogeneity. Arthritis Rheum 2011;64(3):895–907.

136. Torrelo A, Patel S, Colmenero I, et al. Chronic atypical neutrophilic dermatosis with lipodystrophy and elevated temperature (CANDLE) syndrome. J Am Acad Dermatol 2010;62(3):489–95.

137. Garg A, Hernandez MD, Sousa AB, et al. An autosomal recessive syndrome of joint contractures, muscular atrophy, microcytic anemia, and panniculitis-associated lipodystrophy. J Clin Endocrinol Metab 2010;95(9):E58–63.

138. Agarwal AK, Xing C, DeMartino GN, et al. PSMB8 encoding the beta5i proteasome subunit is mutated in joint contractures, muscle atrophy, microcytic anemia, and panniculitis-induced lipodystrophy syndrome. Am J Hum Genet 2010; 87(6):866–72.

139. O'Neil KM. Progress in pediatric vasculitis. Curr Opin Rheumatol 2009;21(5):538–46.

140. Fury W, Tremoulet AH, Watson VE, et al. Transcript abundance patterns in Kawasaki disease patients with intravenous immunoglobulin resistance. Hum Immunol 2010;71(9):865–73.

141. Nogueira E, Hamour S, Sawant D, et al. Serum IL-17 and IL-23 levels and autoantigen-specific Th17 cells are elevated in patients with ANCA-associated vasculitis. Nephrol Dial Transplant 2010;25(7):2209–17.

142. Barahmani N, de Andrade M, Slusser J, et al. Interleukin-1 receptor antagonist allele 2 and familial alopecia areata. J Invest Dermatol 2002;118(2): 335–7.

143. Tazi-Ahnini R, Cox A, McDonagh AJ, et al. Genetic analysis of the interleukin-1 receptor antagonist and its homologue IL-1L1 in alopecia areata: strong severity association and possible gene interaction. Eur J Immunogenet 2002;29(1):25–30.

144. Abramovits W, Losornio M. Failure of two TNF-alpha blockers to influence the course of alopecia areata. Skinmed 2006;5(4):177–81.

145. van Zuuren EJ, Kramer S, Carter B, et al. Interventions for rosacea. Cochrane Database Syst Rev 2011;(3):CD003262.

146. Schauber J, Gallo RL. Antimicrobial peptides and the skin immune defense system. J Allergy Clin Immunol 2009;124(3 Suppl 2):R13–8.

147. Del Rosso JQ, Webster GF, Jackson M, et al. Two randomized phase III clinical trials evaluating anti-inflammatory dose doxycycline (40-mg doxycycline, USP capsules) administered once daily for treatment of rosacea. J Am Acad Dermatol 2007;56(5):791–802.

148. Cazalis J, Bodet C, Gagnon G, et al. Doxycycline reduces lipopolysaccharide-induced inflammatory mediator secretion in macrophage and ex vivo human whole blood models. J Periodontol 2008; 79(9):1762–8.

149. Spritz RA. The genetics of generalized vitiligo. Curr Dir Autoimmun 2008;10:244–57.

150. Deo SS, Bhagat AR, Shah RN. Genetic variations in nalp1 mRNA expressions in human vitiligo. Indian J Dermatol 2011;56(3):266–71.

151. Okamoto M, Liu W, Luo Y, et al. Constitutively active inflammasome in human melanoma cells mediating autoinflammation via caspase-1 processing and secretion of interleukin-1beta. J Biol Chem 2010; 285(9):6477–88.

152. Spritz RA. The genetics of generalized vitiligo: autoimmune pathways and an inverse relationship with malignant melanoma. Genome Med 2010; 2(10):78.

153. Terai M, Eto M, Young GD, et al. Interleukin 6 mediates production of interleukin 10 in metastatic melanoma. Cancer Immunol Immunother 2011;61(2): 145–55.

154. Boyd KU, Wehrli BM, Temple CL. Intra-lesional interleukin-2 for the treatment of in-transit melanoma. J Surg Oncol 2011;104(7):711–7.

155. Chakraborty S, Kaushik DK, Gupta M, et al. Inflammasome signaling at the heart of central nervous system pathology. J Neurosci Res 2010;88(8): 1615–31.

156. Limper M, de Kruif MD, Duits AJ, et al. The diagnostic role of procalcitonin and other biomarkers in discriminating infectious from non-infectious fever. J Infect 2010;60(6):409–16.

157. Dayer E, Dayer JM, Roux-Lombard P. Primer: the practical use of biological markers of rheumatic and systemic inflammatory diseases. Nat Clin Pract Rheumatol 2007;3(9):512–20.

158. Hitomi Y, Ebisawa M, Tomikawa M, et al. Associations of functional NLRP3 polymorphisms with susceptibility to food-induced anaphylaxis and aspirin-induced asthma. J Allergy Clin Immunol 2009;124(4):779–785.e6.

159. Ridker PM, Macfadyen JG, Nordestgaard BG, et al. Rosuvastatin for primary prevention among individuals with elevated high-sensitivity c-reactive protein and 5% to 10% and 10% to 20% 10-year risk. Implications of the Justification for Use of Statins in Prevention: an Intervention Trial Evaluating Rosuvastatin (JUPITER) trial for "intermediate risk". Circ Cardiovasc Qual Outcomes 2010;3(5): 447–52.

160. Jazirehi AR. Regulation of apoptosis-associated genes by histone deacetylase inhibitors: implications in cancer therapy. Anti Cancer Drugs 2010; 21(9):805–13.

161. Colville-Nash P, Willis D, Papworth J, et al. The peroxisome proliferator-activated receptor alpha activator, Wy14,643, is anti-inflammatory in vivo. Inflammopharmacology 2005;12(5–6):493–504.

162. Davidson-Moncada J, Papavasiliou FN, Tam W. MicroRNAs of the immune system: roles in inflammation and cancer. Ann N Y Acad Sci 2010;1183: 183–94.

163. Link A, Bachmann MF. Immunodrugs: breaking B- but not T-cell tolerance with therapeutic anticytokine vaccines. Immunotherapy 2010;2(4): 561–74.

164. Waykole YP, Doiphode SS, Rakhewar PS, et al. Anticytokine therapy for periodontal diseases: where are we now? J Indian Soc Periodontol 2009;13(2): 64–8.

165. Klamer G, Song E, Ko KH, et al. Using small molecule GSK3beta inhibitors to treat inflammation. Curr Med Chem 2010;17(26):2873–81.

166. Tenor H, Hatzelmann A, Beume R, et al. Pharmacology, clinical efficacy, and tolerability of phosphodiesterase-4 inhibitors: impact of human pharmacokinetics. Handb Exp Pharmacol 2011;(204):85–119.

167. Gavanescu I, Benoist C, Mathis D. B cells are required for Aire-deficient mice to develop multiorgan autoinflammation: a therapeutic approach for APECED patients. Proc Natl Acad Sci U S A 2008;105(35):13009–14.

168. Neven B, Marvillet I, Terrada C, et al. Long-term efficacy of the interleukin-1 receptor antagonist anakinra in ten patients with neonatal-onset multisystem inflammatory disease/chronic infantile neurologic, cutaneous, articular syndrome. Arthritis Rheum 2010;62(1):258–67.

169. Manger B, Gaubitz M, Michels H. Recommendations on therapy using interleukin-1beta-blocking agents. Z Rheumatol 2009;68(9):766–71 [in German].

170. Zhang H. Anti-IL-1beta therapies. Recent Pat DNA Gene Seq 2011;5(2):126–35.

171. McDermott MF. Rilonacept in the treatment of chronic inflammatory disorders. Drugs Today (Barc) 2009;45(6):423–30.

172. Hoffman HM. Rilonacept for the treatment of cryopyrin-associated periodic syndromes (CAPS). Expert Opin Biol Ther 2009;9(4):519–31.

173. ILARIS (Canakinumab) [pakage insert]. Novartis Pharmacueticals; 2009.

174. Geiler J, McDermott MF. Gevokizumab, an anti-IL-1beta mAb for the potential treatment of type 1 and 2 diabetes, rheumatoid arthritis and cardiovascular disease. Curr Opin Mol Ther 2010;12(6):755–69.

175. Gul A, Tugal-Tutkun I, Dinarello CA, et al. Interleukin-1beta-regulating antibody XOMA 052 (gevokizumab) in the treatment of acute exacerbations of resistant uveitis of Behcet's disease: an open-label pilot study. Ann Rheum Dis 2012;71(4):563–6.

Autoinflammatory Diseases in Dermatology
CAPS, TRAPS, HIDS, FMF, Blau, CANDLE

Shivani V. Tripathi, MD, Kieron S. Leslie, DTM&H, FRCP*

KEYWORDS

- Autoinflammatory • Dermatology • CAPS • TRAPS • HIDS • FMF • Blau • CANDLE

KEY POINTS

- CAPS: A spectrum of disease severity that includes fevers, almost daily urticaria, arthralgias, and increases in severity with renal amyloidosis, sensorineural hearing loss, and central nervous system involvement. Gain of function mutation in the *NLRP3* gene.
- TRAPS: An autosomal dominant condition with intermittent fevers lasting 1 to 3 weeks, with centrifugal migratory erythematous rash. Mutations present in gene *TNFRSF1A*.
- HIDS: An autosomal recessive condition with elevated IgD, recurrent fever episodes lasting 3 to 7 days accompanied by an exanthema-like rash, cervical lymphadenopathy, abdominal pain, vomiting, diarrhea, arthralgias, aphthous ulcers, and possible progression to amyloidosis. Mutation present in the *MVK* gene.
- FMF: An autosomal recessive disorder with gene mutation in *MEFV*, characterized by recurrent attacks of fever and polyserositis. The most serious complication is systemic AA amyloidosis. Cutaneous manifestations include erysipelas-like erythema predominately of the lower extremity, ankle, and foot. Colchicine is the mainstay of therapy.
- Blau: An autosomal dominant disorder, also known as early-onset sarcoidosis, defined by the clinical triad of granulomatous dermatitis, symmetric polyarthritis, and recurrent uveitis, with onset in those younger than 4 years with mutations in *CARD15/NOD2*.
- CANDLE: Daily or almost daily fevers starting in infancy, with urticarial rash that is biopsy positive for atypical neutrophils, with residual purpuric pigmentation lasting for weeks. Patients also present with lipodystrophy and low weight and height. Recent finding of a gene mutation in *PSMB8*, but still no definitive treatment to control symptoms.

CRYOPYRIN-ASSOCIATED PERIODIC SYNDROME

Overview

Cryopyrin-associated periodic syndrome (CAPS) (**Fig. 1**) is now the preferred term that encompasses 3 separately described autoinflammatory syndromes (familial cold autoinflammatory syndrome [FCAS], Muckle-Wells syndrome [MWS], and neonatal-onset multisystem inflammatory disease [NOMID]). In practice, a spectrum of disease severity exists for CAPS, with FCAS being the mildest phenotype and NOMID presenting with the most severe with end-organ damage.[1,2]

In the spectrum of CAPS, mutations are present in the *NLRP3* gene, which encodes the

Funding Sources: None.
Conflicts of Interest: Dr Leslie serves as a consultant for Novartis.
Department of Dermatology, University of California San Francisco, 1701 Divisadero Street, Third Floor, San Francisco, CA 94143, USA
* Corresponding author.
E-mail address: lesliek@derm.ucsf.edu

Dermatol Clin 31 (2013) 387–404
http://dx.doi.org/10.1016/j.det.2013.04.005

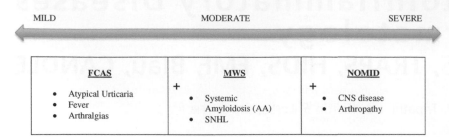

MILD   MODERATE   SEVERE

FCAS		MWS		NOMID
• Atypical Urticaria • Fever • Arthralgias	+	• Systemic Amyloidosis (AA) • SNHL	+	• CNS disease • Arthropathy

Fig. 1. CAPS spectrum of disease. FCAS, familial cold autoinflammatory syndrome; MWS, Muckle-Wells syndrome; NOMID, neonatal onset multisystem inflammatory disease; SNHL, sensorineural hearing loss.

protein cryopyrin. This syndrome is driven by a "gain-of-function mutation" in *NLRP3*, of which there is a total reported 139 mutations. Most mutations have been found in exon 3, although mutations have also been reported in exons 4, 5, and 6, as well as introns 1, 2, 4, 6, and 8.[3] The *NLRP3* gene encodes cryopyrin, which form an oligomeric complex known as an inflammasome, and it is the inflammasome that is involved in the post-translational activation of inflammatory caspases. An inflammasome is a high molecular weight complex that converts inactive pro–caspase-1 to active caspase-1.[4] In general, caspases are thought to be involved as initiators or effectors of apoptosis, but caspase-1 functions as a sub-class of caspases involved in the inflammatory and specifically proinflammatory response.[5] The active form of caspase-1 cleaves inactive cytokine precursors to a secreted and active form, and in CAPS the mutation in *NLRP3* leads to elevated cytokine interleukin (IL)-1β. The elevated IL-1β leads to an inflammatory response with the clinical manifestations of periodic fevers and associated symptoms seen in the spectrum of CAPS.[6]

Diagnosis of CAPS

CAPS encompasses a spectrum of disease severity from mild to severe phenotypes, in which patients present with cold-induced fevers and urticarial-like rash, constitutional symptoms, arthritis, aseptic meningitis, and other types of localized inflammation.[7] The most common initial clinical presentation is an urticarial-like rash starting as early as 2 hours after birth, with most patients presenting before 6 months of age.[8] In addition, patients can present with arthralgias and conjunctival injection, and less commonly they present with constitutional symptoms such as sweating, drowsiness, headache, and thirst.[9]

The rash in CAPS is described as "an atypical urticaria," with minimal or, more likely, absent pruritus in lesions that are subtle figurate

erythematous macules (**Fig. 2**). The rash most frequently follows a circadian rhythm presentation with little to no rash early in the morning, and worsening symptoms and signs as the day progresses. In view of the non-pruritic urticaria and associated joint pains, often the differential includes urticarial vasculitis. However, the rash in CAPS typically resolves within 24 hours without bruising, unlike the lesions in urticarial vasculitis.

With CAPS considered a spectrum, the mildest phenotype, FCAS, typically presents with daily attacks of urticaria, arthralgias, and fever after general exposure to the cold. The disease typically presents in infants and usually before 6 months of age. The moderate form of CAPS, referred to as MWS, also presents with atypical urticarial lesions, cold-induced fevers, arthralgias, and additional features, including systemic amyloidosis, sensorineural hearing loss, and conjunctivitis.[10] The most severe presentation, typically referred to as NOMID, involves neonatal onset of urticarial lesions, end-organ damage, rapidly progressive arthropathy, and central nervous system (CNS) involvement, as well as characteristic facial features of frontal bossing and saddleback nose.[11] The severity of the joint involvement may lead the patient to be misdiagnosed with systemic-onset juvenile idiopathic arthritis (SOJIA); however,

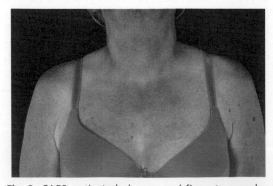

Fig. 2. CAPS: urticated plaques and figurate macules.

SOJIA tends to have a later age of onset. The CNS changes of NOMID include papilledema, chronic aseptic meningitis, headache, vomiting, spastic diplegia, or abnormally high muscle tone and impaired cognitive function.[11,12]

As CAPS progresses in severity from mild to moderate, FCAS to NOMID, high-tone sensorineural hearing loss becomes more frequent. In addition, the severity of hearing loss has been reported as greater in patients with NOMID, with 39% of patients having moderate high-tone hearing loss and 11% having severe high-tone frequency loss, whereas in MWS, 67% had normal hearing and 33% had moderate hearing loss, and none had severe or profound hearing loss at higher frequencies.[13] In addition to hearing loss severity, patients with NOMID present with severe early-onset arthritis, progressing rapidly to deforming arthropathy.[14]

Laboratory Diagnosis and Assessment of CAPS

In CAPS, acute-phase reactants are invariably elevated, such as C-reactive protein (CRP); indeed, CRP is almost never normal irrespective of severity of symptomatology. In addition, serum amyloid A (SAA) levels are usually markedly elevated, but this can be difficult to obtain, as the test is generally not commercially available. Leukocytosis, sometimes as high as 36,000/μL and decreased hematocrit with neutrophilia may be seen on complete blood cell count (CBC). The most serious long term sequelae of CAPS is the development of systemic AA amyloidosis, which most frequently adversely affects the kidneys. Therefore, regular monitoring of renal function should be done with urinalysis to detect for proteinuria.[8]

Physician Orders:

- CBC (showing low hematocrit, slightly elevated neutrophil count, elevated eosinophil count)
- CRP, erythrocyte sedimentation rate (ESR)
- Renal function tests, urinalysis (monitor for proteinuria)
- Cerebrospinal fluid (increased cytokines, elevated opening pressure/increased intracranial pressure) NOMID
- *NLRP3* gene mutation

Histologic examination of the affected skin can support a diagnosis of CAPS, with neutrophilic dermal infiltrate in the reticular dermis, which tends to be peri-eccrine and peri-vascular. The infiltrate tends to be neutrophil predominant versus mast cell predominant.

The characteristic clinical presentation includes an early onset in age, an atypical urticarial rash on trunk and extremities, fever, arthralgias, arthropathy (joint enlargement, endochondral ossification, calcifications, and functional disability), and biopsy findings of a neutrophilic dermal infiltrate. The definitive diagnosis includes these characteristic clinical features in combination with genetic analysis, with gene testing showing mutations in the *NLRP3* gene.

Treatments for CAPS

With the knowledge of increased IL-1 production, targeted therapies have proven to be most effective at controlling symptoms of CAPS and preventing the uncurbed inflammation that leads to amyloidosis. Specifically, anakinra, an IL-1 receptor antagonist, has been shown to be extremely effective at controlling symptoms and signs of disease activity with normalization of inflammatory markers, such as CRP and SAA.[1] Reports have reflected effectiveness in all phenotypes of CAPS and it has recently been approved for the severe phenotypes/NOMID spectrum by the Food and Drug Administration (FDA).[15] Anakinra has a short half-life of 4 to 6 hours, hence requiring daily subcutaneous injections.

Rilonacept, an IL-1 trap, was the first drug that was approved by the FDA for the treatment of CAPS and with a half-life of 8.6 days, it is typically dosed on a weekly schedule with a generally favorable long-term safety profile.[16] Another targeted therapy for CAPS is canakinumab, an IL-1β monoclonal antibody, which is a medication that is FDA approved for CAPS.[17] Because of its half-life of 26 days, its dosing regimen is every 8 weeks. Patients with CAPS on canakinumab showed minimal disease activity during a double-blind randomized control trial with prevention of urticarial rash, minimal levels of CRP, and SAA.[18] There have been no head-to-head studies comparing these 3 agents, although all appear to be extremely effective at controlling the systemic inflammation associated with CAPS.

TUMOR NECROSIS FACTOR RECEPTOR–ASSOCIATED PERIODIC SYNDROME
Overview

Tumor necrosis factor (TNF)-receptor–associated periodic syndrome (TRAPS) is an autosomal dominantly inherited autoinflammatory condition, with recurrent fevers lasting 1 to 3 weeks. Mutations are present in the gene *TNFRSF1A* (TNF receptor Superfamily 1A), located on chromosome 12p13 coding for the 55-kDa TNF 1, which can lead to improper folding and shedding or clearance of TNFR1.[19] One hypothesis on disease pathogenesis includes improper shedding of the TNF receptor leading to increased inflammatory response due to TNF,[20] but other etiologies of pathogenesis include decreased apoptosis, increased nuclear factor kappaB (NF-kB), defective receptor trafficking, and increased reactive oxygen species leading to increased mitogen-activated protein kinase (MAPK) activity.[21] The condition was initially coined familial Hibernian fever by Williamson and colleagues[22] in 1982, when describing an Irish/Scottish family with recurrent fevers, abdominal pain, localized myalgias, and erythematous skin lesions. Recurrent fever, abdominal pain, myalgia, and arthralgia are the most common manifestations of TRAPS, followed by tender erythematous skin lesions, migratory rash with underlying myalgias and arthralgias, chest pain, conjunctivitis, periorbital edema, testicular pain, headaches, lymphadenopathy, and amyloidosis.

Diagnosis of TRAPS

TRAPS is characterized by recurrent fever episodes, which typically last from 1 to 3 weeks, and can occur every 5 to 6 weeks.[23] The intervals between fevers vary, and are longer than those seen in other hereditary systemic autoinflammatory diseases, although variability in frequency and presentation is perhaps the greatest in TRAPS. Recurrent inflammatory episodes occur either spontaneously or after minor triggers, such as local injury, minor infection, stress, exercise, or hormonal changes. The median age of onset of TRAPS is 3 years old, with a range from 2 weeks to 53 years of age; therefore, TRAPS may not be diagnosed until adolescence or adulthood.

Initially, an individual will present with muscle cramps or myalgias that migrate in a centrifugal pattern. Myalgia is nearly always present in patients with TRAPS, and is usually a harbinger of an attack, and typically presents in conjunction with fever. Affected muscles can be tender and warm to palpation, and can be followed by overlying skin manifestations. Abdominal symptoms include cramping and nausea, with vomiting present in 92% of patients. In addition, genitourinary symptoms, such as scrotal pain and testicular pain, have also been reported. Ocular manifestations, including periorbital edema/pain and conjunctivitis, are common and uveitis and pulmonary symptoms of pleuritis are seen in 32% of patients.[24]

The most common dermatologic manifestation is a centrifugal migratory erythematous rash (**Figs. 3** and **4**), overlying an area affected by myalgia, which can be painful and warm to the touch.[25] In 1997, McDermott and colleagues[26] reported cutaneous manifestations in 69% of individuals followed with TRAPS, which included erythematous patches and indurated lesions. In an evaluation of 25 patients with TRAPS, cutaneous manifestations were present in 84% of patients, which lasted from a range of 4 to 21 days, with a mean duration of 13 days, with lesions, including large annular patches, erythematous dermal macules and patches, and generalized erythematous reticulated patches and plaques ranging in size from 1 to 28 cm. Migration of the lesions to a distal extremity was also a distinctive feature.[27] In this review of patients with TRAPS, 44% presented with ocular symptoms, including conjunctival pain and redness and/or periorbital edema.

Histology showed perivascular lymphocytes and monocytes, and no biopsy specimens showed granulomatous or leukocytoclastic vasculitis.

Laboratory assessment of TRAPS

TRAPS typically presents with marked elevation of inflammatory markers during inflammatory episodes, specifically ESR, CRP, fibrinogen, and haptoglobin, although an acute phase response may be seen even when the patient is asymptomatic. In addition, CBC may show neutrophil leukocytosis, thrombocytosis, and normochromic and hypochromic anemia. In addition, levels of soluble TNF receptor can be measured using commercially

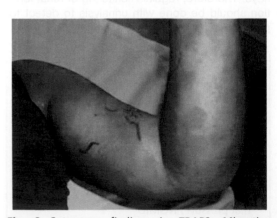

Fig. 3. Cutaneous findings in TRAPS. Migrating erythematous macular rash during an inflammatory attack in a patient with TRAPS. (*From* van der Hilst JCH, van der Meer JWM, Drenth JPH. Autoinflammatory fever syndromes. In: Rich R, Fleisher T, Shearer E, et al. editors. Clinical Immunology: Principles and Practice. third edition. Philadelphia: Elsevier/Mosby; 2008; with permission.)

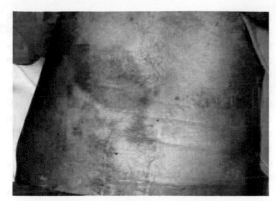

Fig. 4. Cutaneous findings in TRAPS. Migratory, erythematous macular rash on the abdomen and chest of a patient with TRAPS. The rash extends from the midline to the right lateral chest wall. Notice the surgical scars from previous exploratory laparotomies. (*From* Brydges S, Athreya B, Kasther DL. Periodic Fever Syndromes in Children. In: Cassidy JT, Petty RE, editors. Textbook of Pediatric Rheumatology. fifth edition. Philadelphia: Elsevier Saunders; 2005; with permission.)

available enzyme-linked immunosorbent assays (ELISAs), showing low serum levels of soluble TNF receptor (<1 ng/mL) in patients with TRAPS. Plasma concentrations of soluble tumor necrosis factor receptor superfamily 1A (sTNFRSF1A) were measured.[28] However, the relationship between defects in sTNFRSF1A (the TNF Receptor Superfamily) shedding and plasma concentration of this receptor was inconsistent and may not be a predictor of disease severity.[28] A more reliable predictor of disease severity is the degree of elevation of acute-phase reactants, as TNFRSF1A measurements can vary substantially based on degree of inflammatory activity. Another acute-phase reactant, SAA, is increased by stimulation from cytokines, including TNF-α, and with significant sustained elevation amyloid deposition may occur in various organs leading to AA amyloidosis.[29] To monitor for the development of systemic amyloidosis, regular urinalysis for proteinuria is imperative in a patient with TRAPS, as this progression can be seen in up to 14% of patients.

Physician Orders:

- ESR, CRP, haptoglobin, fibrinogen, ferritin
- CBC (showing low hematocrit, slightly elevated neutrophil count, elevated eosinophil count)
- Renal function tests, urinalysis (monitor for proteinuria)
- *TNFRSF1A gene mutation*

Treatment for TRAPS

Providing patients with effective therapy has been challenging, although symptomatic relief may be seen with high-dose nonsteroidal anti-inflammatory drugs (NSAIDs). During an attack, patients typically require prednisone, typically useful in dosages greater than 20 mg per day,[25] although, because there can be side effects with long-term use of high doses of corticosteroids, a short course of steroid started at 1 mg/kg per day tapered over a course of 7 to 10 days during an attack can be used.[23] Patients typically fail to respond to treatment with colchicine, and this lack of response can help to differentiate TRAPS from other conditions that do respond to colchicine (such as FMF).[30] With the various proposed methods of pathogenesis, various and diverging responses to treatment exist after lack of response to NSAIDs and prednisone. TNF-α blockade with etanercept has shown symptomatic improvement and reduction in acute-phase reactants.[27] Notably, there has been a paradoxic reaction in patients with other TNF-α inhibitors, infliximab or adalimumab, with an increase in proinflammatory cytokines,[31] so these treatments are less in favor. However, not all patients will respond to etanercept, and in those individuals with TRAPS, anakinra has been show to prevent short-term and long-term relapses.[32,33] Canakinumab, which is a monoclonal antibody to IL-1β, has also showed amelioration of inflammation severity in patients not responding to etanercept. Treatment with canakinumab brought resolution of clinical manifestations and in normalizing markers of inflammation as well.[34]

HYPERIMMUNOGLOBULINEMIA D SYNDROME
Overview

Hyperimmunoglobulinemia D syndrome (HIDS) is a rare autosomal recessively inherited autoinflammatory disease characterized by recurrent fevers and elevated polyclonal immunoglobulin D (IgD).[35] Mutations in the *MVK* gene encoding mevalonate kinase, an enzyme involved in the biosynthesis of cholesterol and isoprenoids, leads to a spectrum of clinical manifestations collectively termed mevalonate kinase deficiency (MKD), which includes recurrent febrile attacks seen in HIDS to a more severe phenotype, mevalonic aciduria (MA). The severe phenotype of MA includes the febrile attacks of HIDS and also includes psychomotor retardation, facial dysmorphia, cataracts, and failure to thrive.[36] For MA, most mutations occur in cluster in the C-terminal region of the protein,[37] whereas most patients with HIDS are compound heterozygotes for a missense mutation in the *MVK* gene, with more than 80% of patients presenting with the V3371 mutation.[38] Thus, the genotype and phenotype correlate such that patients with MA have no mevalonate kinase activity and have a severe phenotype, whereas patients with HIDS may have residual enzyme activity of up to 5% to 15% and a less severe phenotype, reflecting the phenotypic differences seen in HIDS versus MA.[39]

Diagnosis of HIDS

In addition to recurrent fevers and an elevated serum polyclonal IgD level, associated episodes typically occur with lymphadenopathy, abdominal pain, arthralgias, vomiting and diarrhea, and aphthous ulcers.[40] For a febrile episode of HIDS, typical provocations can include vaccinations, infections, minor trauma, or surgery and other physical or emotional stress, although an episode can occur without any trigger at all with the mean age of initial attack occurring at 6 months of age (range 0–120 months). In HIDS, the febrile attacks and other symptoms of abdominal pain start in infancy, and can occur with or without triggers with episodes lasting between 3 and 7 days, with periods of 4 to 6 weeks between attacks, and, as the patient ages, the frequency of attacks can decrease and the severity of attacks may decrease as well.[41] Data obtained from 103 patients with HIDS showed that febrile episodes can be accompanied by presence of lymphadenopathy, splenomegaly, arthralgias, abdominal pain, aphthous ulcers, and cutaneous lesions, and long-term complications were rare, although an infrequent complication was amyloidosis (2.9%).[40] Lymphadenopathy, reported in 90% of patients, is a defining feature of HIDS, which typically involves cervical lymph nodes and can include axillary and inguinal localization as well.

The combination of early onset of febrile attacks lasting for days that are initially separated by approximately a month, along with abdominal pain, vomiting, and diarrhea, can also be accompanied by joint and cutaneous symptoms (**Fig. 5**). In an analysis of 35 patients with HIDS, 79% of patients had skin lesions during a febrile episode with the most common lesions being erythematous macules followed by papules, typically 0.5 to 2.0 cm, but some patients also presented with urticarial lesions, annular erythema, and palpable purpura. Patients tended to present with a consistent pattern during subsequent attacks, with lesions localized primarily to trunk

and extremities lasting for the length of the attack (5–10 days), but resolving between febrile attacks.[42] However, the histopathology on cutaneous lesions in patients with HIDS was more variable, with findings ranging from mainly vasculitis, varying numbers of polymorphonuclear neutrophils (PMNs), and sometimes Sweet syndrome–like, and rarely a deep vasculitis picture on biopsy. However, almost all biopsy specimens showed perivascular inflammatory infiltrates composed of a variable number of lymphocytes and PMNs.[42]

In addition to fever, abdominal pain is a characteristic feature, with accompanying diarrhea and vomiting that can resemble an acute abdomen. There are reports of patients undergoing exploratory surgery for concerns of appendicitis. In some reports, finding that adhesions were present suggested sterile peritonitis as the cause of the abdominal pain.[43]

The definitive diagnosis of HIDS requires either a mutation in both alleles of the *MVK* gene or the finding of reduced function of the MVK enzyme. Most patients are compound heterozygous for missense mutations in the *MVK* gene, resulting in reduced activity of the MVK enzyme. In addition, the *MVK* gene reveals a mutation, and urinary mevalonic acid can also be slightly elevated, although usually not to the extent of the more severe MA.

Laboratory Assessment of HIDS

At the start of an attack, along with fevers, patients may have elevated acute-phase reactants: ESR,

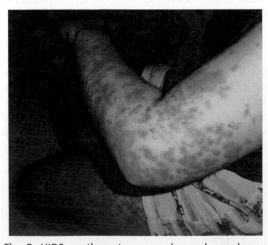

Fig. 5. HIDS: erythematous macules and papules on trunk and extremities. (*From* Brydges S, Athreya B, Kasther DL. Periodic Fever Syndromes in Children. In: Cassidy JT, Petty RE, editors. Textbook of Pediatric Rheumatology. fifth edition. Philadelphia: Elsevier Saunders; 2005; with permission.)

CRP, and SAA.[44] During an attack, acute-phase reactants increase, with CRP reported at a median of 163 (range, 36–404 mg/L), as well as leukocytosis. Between attacks, there was occasionally an increase in these inflammatory markers, although less than during the attack.

Normal serum IgD (in those without HIDS) measured by radioimmunoassay varies in the literature, ranging between 0.2 and 121.0 mg/L, with mean reported at different levels from 25 mg/L to 50 mg/L.[45] In HIDS, patients typically have 3 times the normal range, with the median IgD concentration in patients elevated to 400 U/mL (range of <0.8–5300 IU/mL), with patients typically having consistently elevated IgD levels of higher than 60 mg/L.[40] This was not universally present in patients, as in 22% of patients the highest concentration of IgD was less than 60 mg/L; therefore, a low IgD level does not exclude the diagnosis of HIDS. In addition to elevated IgD, there is also possible concomitant elevation of serum IgA, which tends to increase with IgD as a patient ages.[46,47] Also, patients with HIDS tended to have slightly elevated levels of mevalonic acid in urine, with a median value of 17 mmol/mol creatinine (normal <1) with a range from 2.8 to 10,000, and usually these numbers normalized, but the values were rarely as elevated as in patients with MA. So checking urinary mevalonic acid levels can assist in a diagnosis of HIDS, but detecting the *MVK* gene mutation is the definitive test.[36]

Physician Orders:

- CBC (showing leukocytosis)
- CRP, ESR
- SAA
- IgD
- Urinary mevalonic acid
- *MVK* gene mutation

Treatment of HIDS

There is not a currently established treatment for HIDS, and the available experience comes from a variety of case reports. The goals of management are to reduce duration of attack, avoid unnecessary surgical intervention, as patients can present with abdominal pain that mimics an acute abdomen, and prevent progression to systemic amyloidosis. Typically colchicine is ineffective although NSAIDS may reduce fever and pain. Other forms of management include statins and

biologic treatments. Because mevalonate is the product of HMG-CoA reductase, and mevalonate buildup is present in HIDS, it is thought that the use of an HMG-CoA inhibitor, such as simvastatin, might reduce the mevalonate production and reduce the mevalonate overload due to mevalonate kinase deficiency.[48] Six patients with HIDS were followed for 2 treatment periods with either simvastatin, 80 mg per day, or placebo for 24 weeks, separated by a 4-week washout period in a double-blind fashion. Simvastatin resulted in a drop in urinary mevalonic acid concentration in all patients and decreased the number of febrile days in 5 of 6 patients.

Etanercept (TNF-α inhibitor) and anakinra (IL-1 receptor antagonist) have been used in the treatment of HIDS as well. In a prospective observational study, 2 patients with MA started continuous treatment with anakinra (1–2 mg/kg per day) and 9 patients with HIDS chose between continuous treatment and on-demand treatment (starting at first symptoms of attack, 100 mg per day or 1 mg/kg per day for 5–7 days). Eight patients with HIDS preferred on-demand treatment from the start. This induced a clinical response ($\geq$50% reduction in duration) in 8 of 12 treated attacks without a change in attack frequency.[49]

Treatment with etanercept has produced variable responses, in one case report a patient on etanercept at a dosage of 0.8 mg/kg per week had great improvement of both attacks and acute-phase response but with persistent massive hepatosplenomegaly.[50] In a follow-up study of 103 patients with HIDS, multiple medications were tried, including prednisone, statins, colchicine, antibiotics, etanercept, anakinra, thalidomide, and cyclosporine. A favorable response was seen only in the following medications: 11 of 45 on prednisone, 2 of 18 on statins, 4 of 13 on etanercept, and 4 of 11 on anakinra.[40] However, in a recent case report, both etanercept and anakinra prolonged or failed to improve an attack in HIDS.[51,52] Thus, HIDS still requires clinical trials for more definitive methods of treatment.

FAMILIAL MEDITERRANEAN FEVER
Overview

Familial Mediterranean fever (FMF) is an autosomal recessive disorder caused by mutations in the marenostrin-encoding fever (*MEFV*) gene, located on chromosome 16p13.3, which encodes for the protein pyrin (marenostrin), that presents with recurrent attacks of fever lasting 24 to 72 hours and serositis.[53] Pyrin is part of the inflammasome complex and acts as an inhibitor of the nucleotide-binding domain leucine-rich repeat-containing receptors, pyrin domain containing 3 (NLRP3) inflammasome. Mutations lead to dysregulated activation of NLRP3 inflammasome, overproduction of IL-1β, leading to inappropriate neutrophil activation, and systemic inflammation.[54]

Mutations in *MEFV* include 4 conservative missense mutations (M680I, M694V, M694I, V726A), clustered in exon 10, which, together with mutation E148Q, in exon 2, account for the vast majority of FMF chromosomes identified in patients.[55,56] It has been established that the phenotypic variability of the disease is, at least partly, due to allelic heterogeneity. Mutation M694V is associated with a severe phenotype and amyloidosis, and mutation V726A with a milder form of the disease.[57] In addition, homozygosity for the M694V mutation leads to a particularly severe disease phenotype with higher levels of acute phase reactants and progression to amyloidosis.[58] Disease-causing mutations result in a gain of function in pyrin, but that disease expression is dependent on the amount of mutated protein produced, explains why even in the heterozygous state patients with FMF present with clinical disease.[59]

Patients present with fever (96%), sterile peritonitis (91%), pleuritis (51%), and arthritis (45%).[60] The classic skin manifestation is erysipelas-like erythema (ELE), with lesions typically present on the lower extremities (**Figs. 6** and **7**). Rarely is ELE the first manifestation of FMF, although it is present in a range of 5% to 30% of patients at some point in their disease.[61] In addition, ELE is typically seen in more severe gene mutations; patients with the

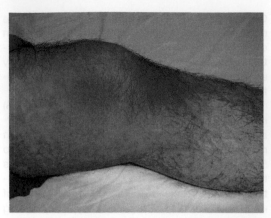

Fig. 7. ELE of FMF: erythematous plaques on the lower extremity. (*Courtesy of* Aydin Fatma, MD. Professor in Dermatology. Ondokuz Mayis University, School of Medicine, Department of Dermatology, Samsun, Turkey.)

M694V/M694V genotype were found to have an earlier age of onset, higher frequency of joint involvement, and higher frequency of ELE.[62]

This disease is considered the most common periodic fever syndrome, and typically presents among patients of eastern Mediterranean origin, especially Sephardic Jewish, Armenian, Turkish, and Arab individuals. Turkey seems to have the highest reported cases of FMF, with prevalence ranging from 1:400 to 1:1000,[63] followed by Israel (1:1000) and Armenia (1:500), although cases have also been reported in France, Germany, Italy, Spain, Australia, and the United States.[53]

Diagnosis of FMF

In FMF, individuals typically present with their first febrile attack before 20 years of age, and also present with fevers and subsequent sterile peritonitis, pleuritis, and arthritis that typically persists for a short period of time, from a few hours to 3 to 4 days. In two-thirds of patients, the initial attack manifests in the first decade, and 90% were affected by the end of the second decade. The Tel Hashomer criteria provide criteria for a diagnosis of FMF,[64] which include fever and one or more of the major signs, or fever and 2 minor signs. The major signs include fever, abdominal pain, chest pain, skin eruption (ELE), and joint pain, such as recurrent monoarthritis. Minor signs include laboratory values of elevated ESR, leukocytosis, and elevated serum concentration of fibrinogen.

Attacks present with fever and serositis; commonly peritonitis, pleuritis, and/or synovitis, and rarely are the cutaneous manifestations seen in the initial attack. The attacks are typically short-lived and resolve spontaneously. The peritonitis

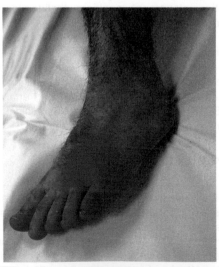

Fig. 6. ELE of FMF: erythematous plaques on the foot. (*Courtesy of* Aydin Fatma, MD. Professor in Dermatology. Ondokuz Mayis University, School of Medicine, Department of Dermatology, Samsun, Turkey.)

seen in FMF presents with abdominal pain and distention, loss of bowel signs, and imaging that may reveal air fluid levels. This presentation may be confused with an acute abdomen; however, within 6 to 12 hours symptoms begin to improve and by 48 hours symptoms have typically resolved.[65]

The dermatologic manifestations include ELE with hot, tender, and swollen erythematous patches from 15 to 50 cm on the lower extremities. Typically, involvement is unilateral. Although ELE is the associated pathognomonic cutaneous manifestation, there are reports of septal and lobular panniculitis accompanying FMF.[66] Other cutaneous manifestations described are Henoch-Schonlein purpura (HSP) in 5% to 7% of children with FMF, polyarteritis nodosa in fewer than 1% of patients, and episodic purpuric lesions. Other cutaneous manifestations include urticaria,[67] subcutaneous nodules,[68] and herpes simplex labialis.[69] Histopathology in ELE lesions of FMF have been reported to show moderate perivascular infiltrate in the papillary dermis consisting of eosinophils, neutrophils, and mononuclear cells. In addition, extravasation of erythrocytes can be seen around blood vessels of the superficial vascular plexus and dilation of the lymphatic capillaries. The reticular dermis shows marked edema and sparse lymphocytic infiltrate.[66] Definitive diagnosis of FMF includes a combination of clinical presentation along with evidence of mutation in the MEFV gene (**Figs. 6** and **7**).

Laboratory Assessment of FMF

In diagnosis and monitoring of FMF, common findings include leukocytosis with a left shift, an elevated ESR, and elevated haptoglobin, fibrinogen, SAA, and CRP. Renal function should be monitored with an evaluation for proteinuria to determine if there is any progression to systemic AA amyloidosis. Levels of both CRP and SAA are typically elevated in patients with FMF, even during attack-free periods. Patients with FMF can also have elevated levels of homocysteine and lipoprotein, which are typically not ordered in diagnosis but are reflective of an inflammatory process.[70]

Physician Orders:
- CBC (showing leukocytosis)
- CRP, ESR, haptoglobin, fibrinogen
- SAA
- UA
- *MEFV* mutation

Treatment of FMF

The treatment of choice for patients with FMF is colchicine, with doses typically ranging from 1.5 to 2.0 mg per day, and has been shown to prevent the deposition of amyloid in organs. Treatment with colchicine 1 mg per day prevents renal amyloidosis even if the FMF attacks do not respond to the drug. In addition, in patients who already have renal amyloidosis, treatment with colchicine has been shown to prevent proteinuria and worsening of disease.[71,72] In patients resistant to colchicine, there have been a few reports of the successful use of thalidomide[73,74]; many reports of success with etanercept[75] and other anti-TNF agents (infliximab, adalimumab, golimumab),[76,77] especially in patients with more severe disease manifestations, such as proteinuria and sacroiliitis; few reports of sulfasalazine[78] (dosed 50 mg/kg per day); and emerging reports of success with anakinra (100 mg per day).[79,80]

BLAU SYNDROME
Overview

Blau is an inherited chronic autoinflammatory autosomal dominant disorder defined by the clinical triad of granulomatous dermatitis, symmetric polyarthritis, and recurrent uveitis with onset in patients younger than 4 years.[81] The syndrome is defined by missense mutations in the region encoding the nucleotide-binding domain of the caspase recruitment domain gene (CARD15/NOD2).[82]

For 2 different granulomatous diseases, Crohn disease and Blau syndrome, 2 distinct alterations of CARD15/NOD2 are present: Crohn disease–associated variants predominantly reside in the C-terminal leucine-rich repeats (LRRs), whereas Blau syndrome–associated mutations occur in the NACHT domain. In NOD2, the NACHT domain displays ATPase activity that is critical for inflammatory signaling responses, specifically signaling of NF-kB, with mutation increasing autoinflammatory processing in Blau syndrome.[83] In contrast, the LRR domain involvement in Crohn disease is responsible for recognition of bacterial polysaccharides. Thus, mutations in different regions of CARD15 are responsible for proteins that manifest in different functions, and thus there are distinct phenotypic manifestations.[84]

Blau syndrome and early-onset sarcoidosis (EOS) are thought to be the same condition, with the differentiating factor being that Blau is the familial manifestation and EOS is the sporadic manifestation of the disease. Children with EOS present with the clinical manifestations of dermatitis, systemic polyarthritis, and recurrent uveitis, although mutations are sporadic in *CARD15/NOD2* for EOS rather than inherited, such as in Blau, they share a common genetic etiology.[85]

Typically, patients with Blau initially present with arthritis and skin manifestations. The joint manifestations include symmetric polyarthritis of the hands and feet with boggy joint swelling, erythema, warmth, and tenderness.[86] Granulomatous involvement can include the conjunctiva, lacrimal gland, retina, and optic nerve.[87] Less frequent symptoms include persistent or intermittent fever, granulomatous arteritis with cranial neuropathies, renal lesions, liver granulomas, and malignant hypertension.

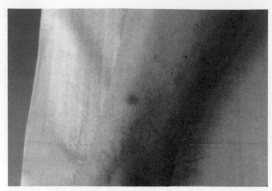

Fig. 9. BLAU cutaneous manifestation: reddish-brown papules on the extremity. (*Courtesy of* Dr Leonardo Punzi, University of Padova, Padova, Italy.)

Diagnosis of BLAU

Blau syndrome is characterized by early onset, typically between ages 2 and 4 years, with median age manifestation at 26.5 months.[86] Most patients present before 4 to 5 years of age, usually with arthritis and skin manifestations, and later with ocular manifestations, usually between 7 and 12 years of age.[88]

The typical dermatologic presentation is pinpoint yellowish to reddish-brown papules that can become confluent (**Figs. 8 and 9**). The dermatitis can present intermittently and subside during a period of years, leaving pitted scars at sites of previous papules. Skin biopsy shows non-caseating granulomas predominately composed of periodic acid-Schiff–positive histiocytes and multinucleated giant cells.[89] In a child with granulomatous dermatitis, mutational analysis of *NOD2/CARD15* should be done to confirm diagnosis. Granulomatous skin lesions typically include 2 main eruptions that affect the trunk

and extremities symmetrically: (1) a papulonodular tender brownish rash and (2) subcutaneous nodules.[85] In the differential of the lesions of Blau syndrome is lichen scrofulosorum (LS), a cutaneous manifestation of tuberculosis or a hypersensitive immunologic skin reaction to an occult internal focus of tuberculosis, which presents also with small yellow to red-brown papules.[90] On pathology, LS shows superficial granuloma in the vicinity of a hair follicle composed of epitheliod cells, Langerhans cells, and lymphoid cells at the periphery. In addition to pathology coinciding with LS, patients have a positive purified protein derivative/Mantoux test.[91] Ocular involvement, which typically presents later, tends to be more severe and includes recurrent anterior or panuveitis along with ocular pain, photophobia, and blurred vision.[87,88]

Arthritis can be severe, with deformities leading to periarticular swelling and joint space narrowing that leads to erosive changes and flexion contractures of the fingers and toes, known as camptodactyly, and decreased motion of large joints.[92] In a child presenting with generalized papules, histopathologic study is required for clarification. The early onset of granulomatous dermatitis should prompt eye and joint examination at regular intervals; the definitive diagnosis of Blau is made with evidence of mutation in the *NOD2* gene.

Laboratory Assessment of Blau

In addition, serum lipids, antinuclear antibody (ANA) and rheumatoid factor, as well as chest radiograph should be done to rule out other causes of granulomatous disease. For monitoring Blau, rather than regular laboratory evaluation, regular eye examinations, and joint radiographs should be performed if symptoms arise.[93]

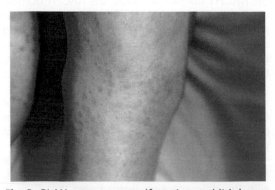

Fig. 8. BLAU cutaneous manifestation: reddish-brown papules becoming confluent on the extremity. (*Courtesy of* Dr Leonardo Punzi, University of Padova, Padova, Italy.)

Physician Orders:

- CBC (showing leukocytosis)
- ANA, rheumatoid factor
- Radiographs (chest and joint)
- **CARD15/NOD2 mutation**

Treatments for Blau

For the triad of granulomatous rash, arthritis, and ocular involvement, initially a low-dose glucocorticoid is generally satisfactory during the quiescent stage, with higher doses required in the acute stages. However, because the disease is typically progressive, specifically with worsening ocular involvement, treatment requires step-up to biologic agents; the same applies for worsening arthritis and uveitis, macular edema, and other ocular disease. If prolonged periods of glucocorticoids, with dosages greater than prednisone 10 mg per day required for a patient, then immunosuppressive agents, such as methotrexate, cyclosporine A, mycophenolate mofetil, canakinumab, and anakinra may be tried.[94,95]

In a case report of a child with progressive ocular involvement which progressed and thus failed oral prednisone, i.v. methylprednisone, methotrexate, infliximab, adalimumab, mycophenolate mofetil, abatacept subsequently responded to canakinumab which was well tolerated and led to rapid quiescence of uveitis.[95] Thus, response to an IL-1 blocker suggests that pathogenesis of Blau syndrome could be mediated by IL-1, including canakinumab, as well as other biologic agents may prove beneficial in patients with progressive disease that is unresponsive to more conventional treatments. Ocular symptoms lead to the most significant morbidity and mortality due to noncaseating epitheliod granulomas leading to uveitis, photophobia, blurred vision, and multifocal choroiditis, as well as secondary glaucoma and cataracts with visual impairment blindness. As a result, once Blau syndrome is diagnosed, many patients will require long-term immunosuppressive therapy or systemic corticosteroids.

CANDLE
Overview

Chronic atypical neutrophilic dermatosis with lipodystrophy and elevated temperature (CANDLE) is an autoinflammatory syndrome recently described in children. The patients described presented with symptoms in the first few years of life, most with daily or almost daily fevers higher than 38.5°C by 6 months of age, with poor response to NSAIDs.[96]

In addition, patients present with characteristic annular violaceous plaques on the trunk and additional areas that become purpuric lasting for weeks, which may resolve with residual hyperpigmentation.[96–98] The initial 4 patients described all had swollen eyelids and thick lips, progressive lipodystrophy, and arthralgias without arthritis.[96] All 10 patients described in the literature are of low weight and height.[96–98] Of the first 4 patients described, 2 were sisters of non-consanguineous parents. This and other presentations suggest an inherited component to CANDLE and a recent genomic analysis of 9 patients showed mutations in *PSMB8* (proteasome subunit B type 8), with 5 being previously reported and 4 being new patients. Similarly, homozygosity mapping in an autosomal-recessive autoinflammatory syndrome characterized by joint contractures, muscle atrophy, microcytic anemia, and panniculitis-induced lipodystrophy (also known as JMP syndrome) seen in adults showed mutation in *PSMB8*.[99] With the inclusion of CANDLE into the list of disorders related to a mutation in *PSMB8*, the nature of this novel autoinflammatory syndrome is expanded.

Diagnosis of CANDLE

The characteristic clinical findings present in infancy are the dermatologic manifestations of annular violaceous plaques (**Figs. 10** and **11**), almost daily temperatures higher than 38.5°C, violaceous eyelid swelling, low weight and height, and progressive lipodystrophy. Along with characteristic findings on skin biopsy, all can help to support the diagnosis. Histopathology of lesional skin shows atypical mononuclear infiltrates of myeloid lineage and mature neutrophils. In the initial 4 patients, repeated skin biopsies showed dense perivascular and interstitial infiltrate involving the papillary and reticular dermis. These atypical cells

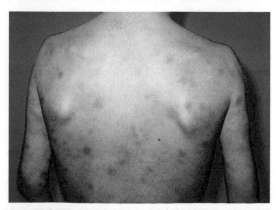

Fig. 10. CANDLE: annular violaceous plaques on trunk and extremities-posterior view. (*Courtesy of* Dr Antonio Torrelo, Madrid, Spain.)

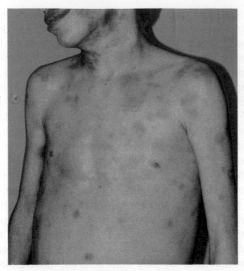

Fig. 11. CANDLE: annular violaceous plaques on trunk and extremities-anterior view. (*Courtesy of Dr Antonio Torrelo, Madrid, Spain.*)

were mainly composed of mononuclear cells, with large, vesicular, elongated or kidney-shaped nuclei, a single inconspicuous nucleolus, and scant eosinophilic cytoplasm, giving the impression of an atypical myeloid lineage cell interstitial infiltrate, resembling leukemia. The myeloid lineage was confirmed with immunohistochemistry staining with myeloperoxidase, lysozyme, Mac387, CD68 (KP1), and CD45. The atypical myeloid cells were intermixed in the specimens with mature neutrophils.

In addition to the clinical findings and biopsy confirmation, there are laboratory abnormalities of elevated aspartate aminotransferase, alanine aminotransferase, hypochromic anemia, and elevated acute-phase reactants. Along with the data on genetic analyses revealing that mutations in *PSMB8* cause CANDLE syndrome, there is a recently identified dysregulation of the interferon (IFN) signaling pathway; all 9 studied patients showed high, although variable, levels of IFNγ-inducible protein 10 (IP-10).[98] Other variable clinical features include hypertrichosis, acanthosis nigricans, and alopecia areata in the diagnosis of CANDLE.[96,97]

Differential of CANDLE

Many of the features seen in CANDLE resemble the CAPS severe variant of NOMID, FMF, TRAPS, and HIDS. Unique to CANDLE is the combination of early-onset violaceous plaques with residual purpuric pigmentation, early-onset almost daily recurrent fevers higher than 38.5°C, gradual and persistent eyelid swelling, lipodystrophy, and

recurrent annular violaceous plaques with interstitial infiltrates of immature myeloid cells and neutrophils. In addition, these patients did not have gene mutations in *MEFV, TNFRSF1A,* and *NLRP3.* Lipodystrophy is a unique feature of CANDLE. Although lipodystrophy is also present, such as acquired partial lipodystrophy (due to lamin B2 mutations), congenital generalized lipodystrophy (due to mutations in the *AGPAT2* gene), leprechaunism (due to mutations in the *INSR* gene), and familial partial lipodystrophy (mutations in the *lamin A/C and PPAR-γ genes*), these conditions do not present with CANDLE's cutaneous manifestations and recurrent fevers. Sweet syndrome (acute febrile neutrophilic dermatosis) typically presents with fever and cutaneous plaques, but it is rare in neonates and its chronic course can be associated with myelodysplastic syndrome; bone marrow biopsy and cytogenetic studies are normal in patients with CANDLE.

Other cutaneous eruptions in the differential include leukemia cutis. Although skin biopsies in CANDLE show atypical myeloid cells with some maturation into neutrophils, leukemia cutis lacks the latter and rather shows atypical mitoses. Typically leukemia cutis eventually goes on to develop into overt leukemia. Other annular eruptions that can be ruled out by the unique presentation of CANDLE include annular erythema of infancy, erythema annulare centrifugum, familial annular erythema, erythema chronicum migrans of Lyme disease, eosinophilic cellulitis, neonatal lupus erythematosus, annular urticaria, erythema multiforme, and erythema gyratum repens.

Laboratory Assessment of CANDLE

Typically the diagnosis of CANDLE is on clinical and histopathological grounds, but laboratory analysis can help to support the diagnosis, as the documented patients present with hypochromic anemia, so a CBC with differential is helpful. In addition, with the recurring fevers, patients will have elevated acute phase reactants: ESR and CRP. Patients also present with transaminitis, so liver function tests can help with a diagnosis as well. Few patients present with elevated triglycerides and increased platelet counts.[96]

Physician Orders:
- CBC (hypochromic anemia)
- ESR, CRP
- Liver function tests
- *PSMB8* mutation

Table 1
Autoinflammatory diseases and dermatology

	CAPS	TRAPS	FMF	HIDS	Blau	CANDLE
Gene	*NLRP3 gene*	*TNFRSF1A*	*MEFV*	*MVK gene*	*CARD15/NOD2*	*PSMB8*
Gene Product	Cryopyrin	TNFRSF1A	Pyrin	Mevalonate Kinase	a	b
Inheritance	AD	AD	AR	AR	AD	
Fevers	Fevers daily	Fevers 1–3 wk	Fevers 24–72 h	Fevers 3–7 d, period of 4–6 wk between attacks		Daily fevers
Clinical	FCAS: Fevers, arthralgias MWS: + SNHL, AA NOMID: + CNS +Arthropathy	Recurrent fever, abdominal pain, myalgia, arthralgia	Fever, sterile pleuritis arthritis Peritonitis	Initial attack- mean age of 6 mo (0–120 mo) Cervical LN, abdominal pain, vomiting, diarrhea, arthralgias, aphthous ulcers	Granulomatous rash Arthritis Ocular involvement	Neutrophilic Dermatosis Lipodystrophy Arthralgia Daily fevers
Typical cutaneous findings	Atypical urticaria	Centrifugal migratory erythematous patches and plaques with underlying myalgia/ arthralgias	ELE	Erythematous macules and papules, 0.5–2 cm localized to trunk and extremities	Pinhead-sized, lichenoid, yellow to brown papules in clusters	Annular violaceous plaques

Abbreviations: AD, autosomal dominant; AR, autosomal recessive; CANDLE, chronic atypical neutrophilic dermatosis with lipodystrophy and elevated temperature; CAPS, cryopyrin-associated periodic syndrome; *CARD15/NOD2*, caspase recruitment domain-containing protein 15/nucleotide-binding oligomerization domain-containing protein 2; CNS, central nervous system; ELE, erysipelas like erythema; FCAS, familial cold autoinflammatory syndrome; FMF, familial Mediterranean fever; HIDS, hyperimmunoglobulinemia D syndrome; LN, lymphadenopathy; MWS, Muckle-Wells syndrome; NOMID, neonatal onset multisystem inflammatory syndrome; *PSMB8*, Proteasome subunit, beta type, 8; SAA, systemic amyloidosis; SNHL, sensorineural hearing loss; TRAPS, tumor necrosis factor (TNF) receptor-associated periodic syndrome.
a caspase recruitment domain containing protein 15 nucleotide-binding oligomerization domain-containing protein 2.
b Proteasome subunit, beta type, 8.

Treatment of CANDLE

For the reported patients, the responses to treatment with steroid-sparing agents were inconsistent and most patients required high-dose prednisone (1–2 mg/kg per day), but patients with CANDLE would rebound after tapering (0.5/mg/kg per day). TNF-α inhibitors provided only temporary relief in some patients but led to flares in others. Methotrexate in combination with calcineurin inhibitors allowed for a lower level of steroid administration, although patients who presented with skin and joint flares with fever required additional administration of biologic agents. Anti–IL-1 therapy did not reduce the requirement for steroids, and IL-6 blocking agents did not reduce clinical symptoms of cutaneous eruptions or improve fatigue, but did normalize the ESR and CRP and the anemia. Still, there is no definitive treatment for CANDLE and the partial treatment along with the continued need for steroids along with blocking IL-1, TNF blockers, and IL-6R inhibitors points to the need for further information on the disease pathogenesis of CANDLE.[96–98] Currently, clinical trials are in process for blockers of IFN and, with the identification of mutations in *PSMB8* as the cause of CANDLE syndrome and the dysregulation of the IFN signaling pathway, there is movement forward in understanding the pathogenesis and hence targets for CANDLE.[98]

SUMMARY

Familiarity and recognition of cutaneous manifestations of autoinflammatory diseases is imperative in their diagnosis and management (**Table 1**). When considering the differential for the autoinflammatory diseases reviewed in this article (CAPS, TRAPS, HIDS, FMF, Blau, and CANDLE), one must exclude more common diseases as possible etiologies, such as autoimmune disease (adult-onset Still disease, Behcet disease, and infection, specifically sarcoidosis, tuberculosis, HIV, syphilis, and so forth). When considering one autoinflammatory condition, others should be included in the differential as well (ie, in FMF vs TRAPS, cutaneous manifestations may help to differentiate the two). A definitive diagnosis depends not only on clinical, cutaneous, histopathology, and laboratory findings, but is solidified with the finding of a relevant genetic mutation for a given syndrome. Although these diseases are rare, patients can be severely affected from cutaneous manifestations, febrile attacks, and end-organ damage, such as systemic amyloidosis compromising renal function. As more is understood about clinical presentation and pathogenesis, treatment options for these conditions have been increasing as well. The spectrum includes systemic steroid and colchicine to more trials of biologic agents, specifically targets to IL-1 and TNF blockers. Although our clinical understanding of cutaneous presentation and systemic presentation of disease continues to increase in clarity, we continue to work toward improvement in understanding these conditions from a genetic to clinical presentation and to define treatment options that specifically address each autoinflammatory disease.

REFERENCES

1. Leslie KS, Lachmann HJ, Bruning E, et al. Phenotype, genotype, and sustained response to anakinra in 22 patients with autoinflammatory disease associated with CIAS-1/NALP3 mutations. Arch Dermatol 2006;142(12):1591–7.
2. Kilcline C, Shinkai K, Bree A, et al. Neonatal-onset multisystem inflammatory disorder: the emerging role of pyrin genes in autoinflammatory diseases. Arch Dermatol 2005;141(2):248–53.
3. Infevers [Internet] [cited 2013 Feb 23]. Available at: http://fmf.igh.cnrs.fr/ISSAID/infevers/. Accessed January 15, 2013.
4. Agostini L, Martinon F, Burns K, et al. NALP3 forms an IL-1beta-processing inflammasome with increased activity in Muckle-Wells autoinflammatory disorder. Immunity 2004;20(3):319–25.
5. Bauernfeind F, Ablasser A, Bartok E, et al. Inflammasomes: current understanding and open questions. Cell Mol Life Sci 2011;68(5):765–83.
6. Yu JR, Leslie KS. Cryopyrin-associated periodic syndrome: an update on diagnosis and treatment response. Curr Allergy Asthma Rep 2011;11(1):12–20.
7. Masters SL, Lobito AA, Chae J, et al. Recent advances in the molecular pathogenesis of hereditary recurrent fevers. Curr Opin Allergy Clin Immunol 2006;6(6):428–33.
8. Chang C. The pathogenesis of neonatal autoimmune and autoinflammatory diseases: a comprehensive review. J Autoimmun 2013;41:100–10.
9. Koné-Paut I, Piram M. Targeting interleukin-1β in CAPS (cryopyrin-associated periodic) syndromes: what did we learn? Autoimmun Rev 2012;12(1):77–80.
10. Muckle TJ, Wells M. Urticaria, deafness, and amyloidosis: a new heredo-familial syndrome. Q J Med 1962;31:235–48.
11. Goldbach-Mansky R. Current status of understanding the pathogenesis and management of patients with NOMID/CINCA. Curr Rheumatol Rep 2011;13(2):123–31.
12. Torbiak RP, Dent PB, Cockshott WP. NOMID—a neonatal syndrome of multisystem inflammation. Skeletal Radiol 1989;18(5):359–64.

13. Ahmadi N, Brewer CC, Zalewski C, et al. Cryopyrin-associated periodic syndromes: otolaryngologic and audiologic manifestations. Otolaryngol Head Neck Surg 2011;145(2):295–302.

14. Prieur AM, Griscelli C, Lampert F, et al. A chronic, infantile, neurological, cutaneous and articular (CINCA) syndrome. A specific entity analysed in 30 patients. Scand J Rheumatol Suppl 1987;66: 57–68.

15. Sibley CH, Plass N, Snow J, et al. Sustained response and prevention of damage progression in patients with neonatal-onset multisystem inflammatory disease treated with anakinra: a cohort study to determine three- and five-year outcomes. Arthritis Rheum 2012;64(7):2375–86.

16. Hoffman HM, Throne ML, Amar NJ, et al. Long-term efficacy and safety profile of rilonacept in the treatment of cryopryin-associated periodic syndromes: results of a 72-week open-label extension study. Clin Ther 2012;34(10):2091–103.

17. Yokota S, Kikuchi M, Nozawa T, et al. An approach to the patients with cryopyrin-associated periodic syndrome (CAPS): a new biologic response modifier, canakinumab. Nihon Rinsho Meneki Gakkai Kaishi 2012;35(1):23–9 [in Japanese].

18. Lachmann HJ, Lowe P, Felix SD, et al. In vivo regulation of interleukin 1beta in patients with cryopyrin-associated periodic syndromes. J Exp Med 2009; 206(5):1029–36.

19. McDermott MF, Aksentijevich I, Galon J, et al. Germline mutations in the extracellular domains of the 55 kDa TNF receptor, TNFR1, define a family of dominantly inherited autoinflammatory syndromes. Cell 1999;97(1):133–44.

20. Aksentijevich I, Galon J, Soares M, et al. The tumor-necrosis-factor receptor-associated periodic syndrome: new mutations in TNFRSF1A, ancestral origins, genotype-phenotype studies, and evidence for further genetic heterogeneity of periodic fevers. Am J Hum Genet 2001;69(2):301–14.

21. Savic S, Dickie LJ, Battellino M, et al. Familial Mediterranean fever and related periodic fever syndromes/autoinflammatory diseases. Curr Opin Rheumatol 2012;24(1):103–12.

22. Williamson LM, Hull D, Mehta R, et al. Familial Hibernian fever. Q J Med 1982;51(204):469–80.

23. Hull KM, Drewe E, Aksentijevich I, et al. The TNF receptor-associated periodic syndrome (TRAPS): emerging concepts of an autoinflammatory disorder. Medicine (Baltimore) 2002;81(5):349–68.

24. Jesus AA, Oliveira JB, Aksentijevich I, et al. TNF receptor-associated periodic syndrome (TRAPS): description of a novel TNFRSF1A mutation and response to etanercept. Eur J Pediatr 2008; 167(12):1421–5.

25. Schmaltz R, Vogt T, Reichrath J. Skin manifestations in tumor necrosis factor receptor-associated periodic syndrome (TRAPS). Dermatoendocrinol 2010;2(1):26–9.

26. McDermott EM, Smillie DM, Powell RJ. Clinical spectrum of familial Hibernian fever: a 14-year follow-up study of the index case and extended family. Mayo Clin Proc 1997;72(9):806–17.

27. Toro JR, Aksentijevich I, Hull K, et al. Tumor necrosis factor receptor-associated periodic syndrome: a novel syndrome with cutaneous manifestations. Arch Dermatol 2000;136(12):1487–94.

28. Aganna E, Hammond L, Hawkins PN, et al. Heterogeneity among patients with tumor necrosis factor receptor-associated periodic syndrome phenotypes. Arthritis Rheum 2003;48(9):2632–44.

29. Cantarini L, Lucherini OM, Muscari I, et al. Tumour necrosis factor receptor-associated periodic syndrome (TRAPS): state of the art and future perspectives. Autoimmun Rev 2012;12(1): 38–43.

30. Cantarini L, Lucherini OM, Cimaz R, et al. Idiopathic recurrent pericarditis refractory to colchicine treatment can reveal tumor necrosis factor receptor-associated periodic syndrome. Int J Immunopathol Pharmacol 2009;22(4):1051–8.

31. Nedjai B, Quillinan N, Coughlan RJ, et al. Lessons from anti-TNF biologics: infliximab failure in a TRAPS family with the T50M mutation in TNFRSF1A. Adv Exp Med Biol 2011;691:409–19.

32. Obici L, Meini A, Cattalini M, et al. Favourable and sustained response to anakinra in tumour necrosis factor receptor-associated periodic syndrome (TRAPS) with or without AA amyloidosis. Ann Rheum Dis 2011;70(8):1511–2.

33. Gattorno M, Federici S, Pelagatti MA, et al. Diagnosis and management of autoinflammatory diseases in childhood. J Clin Immunol 2008; 28(Suppl 1):S73–83.

34. Brizi MG, Galeazzi M, Lucherini OM, et al. Successful treatment of tumor necrosis factor receptor-associated periodic syndrome with canakinumab. Ann Intern Med 2012;156(12):907–8.

35. Van der Meer JW, Vossen JM, Radl J, et al. Hyperimmunoglobulinaemia D and periodic fever: a new syndrome. Lancet 1984;1(8386):1087–90.

36. Bader-Meunier B, Florkin B, Sibilia J, et al. Mevalonate kinase deficiency: a survey of 50 patients. Pediatrics 2011;128(1):e152–9.

37. Houten SM, Koster J, Romeijn GJ, et al. Organization of the mevalonate kinase (MVK) gene and identification of novel mutations causing mevalonic aciduria and hyperimmunoglobulinaemia D and periodic fever syndrome. Eur J Hum Genet 2001; 9(4):253–9.

38. Cuisset L, Drenth JP, Simon A, et al. Molecular analysis of MVK mutations and enzymatic activity in hyper-IgD and periodic fever syndrome. Eur J Hum Genet 2001;9(4):260–6.

39. Hoffmann GF, Charpentier C, Mayatepek E, et al. Clinical and biochemical phenotype in 11 patients with mevalonic aciduria. Pediatrics 1993;91(5): 915–21.

40. Van der Hilst JC, Bodar EJ, Barron KS, et al. Long-term follow-up, clinical features, and quality of life in a series of 103 patients with hyperimmunoglobulinemia D syndrome. Medicine (Baltimore) 2008; 87(6):301–10.

41. Drenth JP, Van der Meer JW. Hereditary periodic fever. N Engl J Med 2001;345(24):1748–57.

42. Drenth JP, Boom BW, Toonstra J, et al. Cutaneous manifestations and histologic findings in the hyper-immunoglobulinemia D syndrome. International Hyper IgD Study Group. Arch Dermatol 1994; 130(1):59–65.

43. Korppi M, Van Gijn ME, Antila K. Hyperimmuno-globulinemia D and periodic fever syndrome in children. Review on therapy with biological drugs and case report. Acta Paediatr 2011;100(1): 21–5.

44. Simon A, Bijzet J, Voorbij HA, et al. Effect of in-flammatory attacks in the classical type hyper-IgD syndrome on immunoglobulin D, cholesterol and parameters of the acute phase response. J Intern Med 2004;256(3):247–53.

45. Vladutiu AO. Immunoglobulin D: properties, mea-surement, and clinical relevance. Clin Diagn Lab Immunol 2000;7(2):131–40.

46. Stankovic K, Grateau G. Auto inflammatory syn-dromes: diagnosis and treatment. Joint Bone Spine 2007;74(6):544–50.

47. Klasen IS, Göertz JH, Van de Wiel GA, et al. Hyper-immunoglobulin A in the hyperimmunoglobulin-emia D syndrome. Clin Diagn Lab Immunol 2001; 8(1):58–61.

48. Simon A, Drewe E, Van der Meer JW, et al. Simvastatin treatment for inflammatory attacks of the hyperimmunoglobulinemia D and periodic fe-ver syndrome. Clin Pharmacol Ther 2004;75(5): 476–83.

49. Bodar EJ, Kuijk LM, Drenth JP, et al. On-demand anakinra treatment is effective in mevalonate kinase deficiency. Ann Rheum Dis 2011;70(12): 2155–8.

50. Topaloğlu R, Ayaz NA, Waterham HR, et al. Hyper-immunoglobulinemia D and periodic fever syn-drome; treatment with etanercept and follow-up. Clin Rheumatol 2008;27(10):1317–20.

51. Shendi HM, Walsh D, Edgar JD. Etanercept and anakinra can prolong febrile episodes in patients with hyperimmunoglobulin D and periodic fever syndrome. Rheumatol Int 2012;32(1):249–51.

52. Marchetti F, Barbi E, Tommasini A, et al. Inefficacy of etanercept in a child with hyper-IgD syndrome and periodic fever. Clin Exp Rheumatol 2004; 22(6):791–2.

53. Ben-Chetrit E, Touitou I. Familial Mediterranean fever in the world. Arthritis Rheum 2009;61(10):1447–53.

54. Hesker PR, Nguyen M, Kovarova M, et al. Genetic loss of murine pyrin, the Familial Mediterranean Fever protein, increases interleukin-1β levels. PLoS One 2012;7(11):e51105.

55. Gershoni-Baruch R, Brik R, Shinawi M, et al. The differential contribution of MEFV mutant alleles to the clinical profile of familial Mediterranean fever. Eur J Hum Genet 2002;10(2):145–9.

56. Gershoni-Baruch R, Shinawi M, Leah K, et al. Familial Mediterranean fever: prevalence, pene-trance and genetic drift. Eur J Hum Genet 2001; 9(8):634–7.

57. Dewalle M, Domingo C, Rozenbaum M, et al. Phenotype-genotype correlation in Jewish patients suffering from familial Mediterranean fever (FMF). Eur J Hum Genet 1998;6(1):95–7.

58. Padeh S, Shinar Y, Pras E, et al. Clinical and diag-nostic value of genetic testing in 216 Israeli children with familial Mediterranean fever. J Rheumatol 2003; 30(1):185–90.

59. Chae JJ, Cho YH, Lee GS, et al. Gain-of-function pyrin mutations induce NLRP3 protein-independent interleukin-1β activation and severe autoinflammation in mice. Immunity 2011;34(5): 755–68.

60. Samuels J, Aksentijevich I, Torosyan Y, et al. Familial Mediterranean fever at the millennium. Clinical spectrum, ancient mutations, and a sur-vey of 100 American referrals to the National In-stitutes of Health. Medicine (Baltimore) 1998; 77(4):268–97.

61. Lidar M, Doron A, Barzilai A, et al. Erysipelas-like erythema as the presenting feature of familial Med-iterranean fever. J Eur Acad Dermatol Venereol 2012. [Epub ahead of print].

62. Shinar Y, Livneh A, Langevitz P, et al. Genotype-phenotype assessment of common genotypes among patients with familial Mediterranean fever. J Rheumatol 2000;27(7):1703–7.

63. Onen F. Familial Mediterranean fever. Rheumatol Int 2006;26(6):489–96.

64. Livneh A, Langevitz P, Zemer D, et al. Criteria for the diagnosis of familial Mediterranean fever. Arthritis Rheum 1997;40(10):1879–85.

65. Sohar E, Gafni J, Pras M, et al. Familial Mediterra-nean fever. A survey of 470 cases and review of the literature. Am J Med 1967;43(2):227–53.

66. Radakovic S, Holzer G, Tanew A. Erysipelas-like erythema as a cutaneous sign of familial Mediterra-nean fever: a case report and review of the histo-pathologic findings. J Am Acad Dermatol 2013; 68(2):e61–3.

67. Baumal A, Kantor I. Urticaria and dermographism with Mediterranean fever. Report of a case. Arch Dermatol 1961;84:630–2.

68. Azizi E, Fisher BK. Cutaneous manifestations of familial Mediterranean fever. Arch Dermatol 1976; 112(3):364–6.

69. Siegal S. Familial paroxysmal polyserositis. Analysis of fifty cases. Am J Med 1964;36:893–918.

70. Ben-Zvi I, Livneh A. Chronic inflammation in FMF: markers, risk factors, outcomes and therapy. Nat Rev Rheumatol 2011;7(2):105–12.

71. Zemer D, Livneh A, Langevitz P. Reversal of the nephrotic syndrome by colchicine in amyloidosis of familial Mediterranean fever. Ann Intern Med 1992;116(5):426.

72. Sevoyan MK, Sarkisian TF, Beglaryan AA, et al. Prevention of amyloidosis in familial Mediterranean fever with colchicine: a case-control study in Armenia. Med Princ Pract 2009;18(6):441–6.

73. Seyahi E, Ozdogan H, Masatlioglu S, et al. Successful treatment of familial Mediterranean fever attacks with thalidomide in a colchicine resistant patient. Clin Exp Rheumatol 2002;20(4 Suppl 26):S43–4.

74. Seyahi E, Ozdogan H, Celik S, et al. Treatment options in colchicine resistant familial Mediterranean fever patients: thalidomide and etanercept as adjunctive agents. Clin Exp Rheumatol 2006; 24(5 Suppl 42):S99–103.

75. Takada K, Aksentijevich I, Mahadevan V, et al. Favorable preliminary experience with etanercept in two patients with the hyperimmunoglobulinemia D and periodic fever syndrome. Arthritis Rheum 2003;48(9):2645–51.

76. Ozgocmen S, Akgul O. Anti-TNF agents in familial Mediterranean fever: report of three cases and review of the literature. Mod Rheumatol 2011; 21(6):684–90.

77. Erten S, Erten SF, Altunoglu A. Successful treatment with anti-tumor necrosis factor (anti-TNF)-alpha of proteinuria in a patient with familial Mediterranean fever (FMF) resistant to colchicine: anti-TNF drugs and FMF. Rheumatol Int 2012;32(4):1095–7.

78. Bakkaloglu SA, Aksu T, Goker B, et al. Sulphasalazine treatment in protracted familial Mediterranean fever arthritis. Eur J Pediatr 2009;168(8):1017–9.

79. Kuijk LM, Govers AM, Frenkel J, et al. Effective treatment of a colchicine-resistant familial Mediterranean fever patient with anakinra. Ann Rheum Dis 2007;66(11):1545–6.

80. Meinzer U, Quartier P, Alexandra JF, et al. Interleukin-1 targeting drugs in familial Mediterranean fever: a case series and a review of the literature. Semin Arthritis Rheum 2011;41(2):265–71.

81. Blau EB. Familial granulomatous arthritis, iritis, and rash. J Pediatr 1985;107(5):689–93.

82. Miceli-Richard C, Lesage S, Rybojad M, et al. CARD15 mutations in Blau syndrome. Nat Genet 2001;29(1):19–20.

83. Tigno-Aranjuez JT, Abbott DW. Ubiquitination and phosphorylation in the regulation of NOD2 signaling and NOD2-mediated disease. Biochim Biophys Acta 2012;1823(11):2022–8.

84. Wang X, Kuivaniemi H, Bonavita G, et al. CARD15 mutations in familial granulomatosis syndromes: a study of the original Blau syndrome kindred and other families with large-vessel arteritis and cranial neuropathy. Arthritis Rheum 2002;46(11):3041–5.

85. Kanazawa N, Okafuji I, Kambe N, et al. Early-onset sarcoidosis and CARD15 mutations with constitutive nuclear factor-kappaB activation: common genetic etiology with Blau syndrome. Blood 2005; 105(3):1195–7.

86. Rosé CD, Wouters CH, Meiorin S, et al. Pediatric granulomatous arthritis: an international registry. Arthritis Rheum 2006;54(10):3337–44.

87. Latkany P. Blau syndrome. Ophthalmology 2004; 111(4):853 [author reply: 853–4].

88. Kurokawa T, Kikuchi T, Ohta K, et al. Ocular manifestations in Blau syndrome associated with a CARD15/Nod2 mutation. Ophthalmology 2003; 110(10):2040–4.

89. Stoevesandt J, Morbach H, Martin TM, et al. Sporadic Blau syndrome with onset of widespread granulomatous dermatitis in the newborn period. Pediatr Dermatol 2010;27(1):69–73.

90. Thami GP, Kaur S, Kanwar AJ, et al. Lichen scrofulosorum: a rare manifestation of a common disease. Pediatr Dermatol 2002;19(2):122–6.

91. Park YM, Hong JK, Cho SH, et al. Concomitant lichen scrofulosorum and erythema induratum. J Am Acad Dermatol 1998;38(5):841–3.

92. Raphael SA, Blau EB, Zhang WH, et al. Analysis of a large kindred with Blau syndrome for HLA, autoimmunity, and sarcoidosis. Am J Dis Child 1993; 147(8):842–8.

93. Punzi L, Gava A, Galozzi P, et al. Miscellaneous non-inflammatory musculoskeletal conditions. Blau syndrome. Best Pract Res Clin Rheumatol 2011;25(5):703–14.

94. Aróstegui JI, Arnal C, Merino R, et al. NOD2 gene-associated pediatric granulomatous arthritis: clinical diversity, novel and recurrent mutations, and evidence of clinical improvement with interleukin-1 blockade in a Spanish cohort. Arthritis Rheum 2007;56(11):3805–13.

95. Simonini G, Xu Z, Caputo R, et al. Clinical and transcriptional response to the long-acting interleukin-1 blocker canakinumab in Blau syndrome-related uveitis. Arthritis Rheum 2013;65(2):513–8.

96. Torrelo A, Patel S, Colmenero I, et al. Chronic atypical neutrophilic dermatosis with lipodystrophy and elevated temperature (CANDLE) syndrome. J Am Acad Dermatol 2010;62(3):489–95.

97. Ramot Y, Czarnowicki T, Maly A, et al. Chronic atypical neutrophilic dermatosis with lipodystrophy and elevated temperature syndrome: a case report. Pediatr Dermatol 2011;28(5):538–41.

98. Liu Y, Ramot Y, Torrelo A, et al. Mutations in proteasome subunit β type 8 cause chronic atypical neutrophilic dermatosis with lipodystrophy and elevated temperature with evidence of genetic and phenotypic heterogeneity. Arthritis Rheum 2012;64(3):895–907.

99. Agarwal AK, Xing C, DeMartino GN, et al. PSMB8 encoding the β5i proteasome subunit is mutated in joint contractures, muscle atrophy, microcytic anemia, and panniculitis-induced lipodystrophy syndrome. Am J Hum Genet 2010; 87(6):866–72.

Autoinflammatory Pustular Neutrophilic Diseases

Haley B. Naik, MD, Edward W. Cowen, MD, MHSc*

KEYWORDS

- Pustular psoriasis • Palmoplantar pustulosis • Subcorneal pustular dermatosis
- Deficiency of IL-1 receptor antagonist (DIRA) • PAPA syndrome • SAPHO syndrome

KEY POINTS

- Deficiency of the interleukin 1 (IL-1) receptor antagonist (DIRA) is an autosomal-recessive autoinflammatory disease characterized by perinatal-onset pustular dermatosis resembling pustular psoriasis, multifocal aseptic osteomyelitis, and periostitis. It can be effectively treated with IL-1 receptor antagonists.
- Pyogenic arthritis, pyoderma gangrenosum, and acne compose PAPA syndrome, an autosomal-dominant autoinflammatory syndrome caused by mutations in the *PSTPIP1* gene.
- Synovitis, acne, pustulosis, hyperostosis, and osteitis compose the autoinflammatory syndrome known as SAPHO. Chronic recurrent multifocal osteomyelitis is likely a subtype of SAPHO that predominantly affects children.
- Pustular psoriasis constitutes a spectrum of inflammatory pustular dermatoses ranging from localized acrodermatitis continua of Hallopeau and palmoplantar pustulosis to generalized disorders including von Zumbusch pustular psoriasis and impetigo herpetiformis.
- The clinical similarities between defined autoinflammatory diseases with neutrophilic pustules and pustular psoriasis provides potential new mechanisms of treatment with biological agents targeting autoinflammatory pathways.

DEFICIENCY OF THE INTERLEUKIN 1 RECEPTOR ANTAGONIST

In 2009, Goldbach-Mansky and colleagues described an autosomal-recessive autoinflammatory disorder known as deficiency of the interleukin 1 (IL-1) receptor antagonist (DIRA) (Fig. 1).[1–6] DIRA is caused by homozygous loss of function mutations in *IL1RN*, the gene encoding the IL-1 receptor antagonist. Mutations lead to unopposed IL-1 signaling and resultant uncontrolled life-threatening systemic inflammation. Heterozygous carriers of loss of function mutations in *IL1RN* seem to be asymptomatic.[1–6] Fewer than 20 cases from the United States, Canada, the Netherlands, Brazil, and Puerto Rico have been described. First-generation mutations in these distinct geographic populations are believed to be founder mutations. The allele frequencies of the founder mutations in Newfoundland and Puerto Rico are estimated at 0.2% and 1.3%, respectively.

DIRA is characterized by perinatal-onset pustular dermatitis resembling pustular psoriasis, multifocal aseptic osteomyelitis, periostitis, leukocytosis, and increased acute-phase reactants. Affected individuals present between birth and 2.5 weeks of age with fetal distress, pustular rash, joint swelling, oral lesions, and pain with

Disclosures: None.
Dermatology Branch, Center for Cancer Research, National Cancer Institute, National Institutes of Health, Building 10, Room 12N238, 10 Center Drive, MSC 1908, Bethesda, MD 20892-1908, USA
* Corresponding author.
E-mail address: cowene@mail.nih.gov

Dermatol Clin 31 (2013) 405–425
http://dx.doi.org/10.1016/j.det.2013.04.001
0733-8635/13/$ – see front matter Published by Elsevier Inc.

derm.theclinics.com

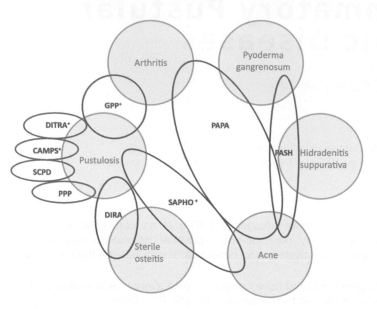

Fig. 1. Overlapping clinical features of pustular dermatoses. CAMPS, CARD 14-mediated pustular psoriasis; DIRA, deficiency of IL-1 receptor antagonist; DITRA, deficiency of the IL-36 receptor antagonist; GPP, generalized pustular psoriasis; PAPA, pyogenic arthritis, pyoderma gangrenosum, and acne; PASH, pyoderma, acne, and suppurative hidradenitis; PPP, palmoplantar pustulosis; SAPHO, synovitis, acne, pustulosis, hyperostosis, and osteitis; SCPD, subcorneal pustular dermatosis. '+' denotes presence of associated fevers.

movement. Premature birth is sometimes noted. Fever is typically absent. Cutaneous eruptions range from discrete crops of pustules to generalized pustulosis (**Fig. 2**). Ichthyosiform changes can be seen. Nail changes include pitting and onychomadesis. Respiratory insufficiency and thrombotic events have also been reported. Bony changes include epiphyseal ballooning of long bones, anterior rib-end widening, periosteal elevation of long bones, and multifocal osteolytic lesions. Less commonly, widening of the clavicles, metaphyseal erosions, and osteolytic skull lesions can be seen.[2] Mortality secondary to multiorgan failure in the setting of severe inflammatory response and pulmonary hemosiderosis

with progressive interstitial fibrosis has been reported. Laboratory abnormalities include leukocytosis and marked increase of serum erythrocyte sedimentation rate and C-reactive protein levels. Cutaneous histopathology is characterized by epidermal acanthosis and hyperkeratosis and extensive neutrophilic infiltration of epidermis and dermis by neutrophils and pustule formation.[1]

The differential diagnosis of DIRA includes bacterial osteomyelitis, infantile cortical hyperostosis, infantile pustular psoriasis, and chronic recurrent multifocal osteomyelitis (CRMO). Genetic sequencing is required for definitive diagnosis. DIRA can be effectively treated with the IL-1 receptor antagonist anakinra,[1,5,7] suggesting a potentially important role for IL-1 antagonism in the management of diseases with pustular phenotype. Individuals with less deleterious mutations have also been managed with corticosteroids and acitretin.[2] Given the severity of disease and availability of effective therapy, the key to successful management and reduced morbidity and mortality is early recognition of this condition and early implementation of anti-IL-1 therapy, before the development of irreversible bony lesions, respiratory disease, or other life-threatening events.

DEFICIENCY OF THE IL-36 RECEPTOR ANTAGONIST, A MONOGENIC FORM OF PUSTULAR PSORIASIS

Although most patients with pustular psoriasis lack a family history of similar disease, several familial cases have been reported, leading to a potential insight into common pathways of

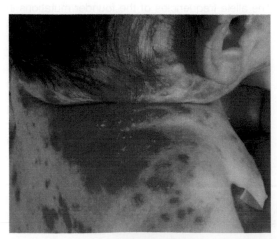

Fig. 2. DIRA. Bright red plaques studded with crops of pustules in an infant. (*Courtesy of* Raphaela Goldbach-Mansky.)

pustular skin disease.[8–15] In 2011, Marrakchi and colleagues[13] identified inactivating mutations in the IL-36 receptor antagonist (*IL-36RN*) gene in 9 Tunisian families with an autosomal-recessive form of generalized pustular psoriasis (GPP). This disease, known as deficiency of the IL-36 receptor antagonist (DITRA), was also reported in a second group of 5 individuals from the United Kingdom who did not have a family history of GPP,[14] as well as in 1 Japanese adult male.[16] IL-36 is an IL-1 family cytokine that binds to the IL-36 receptor, enabling the recruitment of the IL-1 receptor accessory protein and subsequent signal transduction involving nuclear factor kappa-light-chain-enhancer of activated B cells (NFκB) and mitogen-activated protein (MAP) kinases. The IL-36 receptor antagonist is encoded on chromosome 2 and competitively binds the IL-36 receptor, thereby providing negative feedback to IL-36 signaling.[13,14] Deficiency of the IL-36 receptor antagonist leads to an exaggerated inflammatory response, analogous to that resulting from IL-1 receptor antagonist deficiency in patients with DIRA, and further implicates the relevance of these pathways in pustular disease pathogenesis.

DITRA is characterized by sudden-onset, recurrent, and severe GPP, high-grade fever, asthenia, neutrophilia, and increased inflammatory markers. Although disease onset occurs during childhood in most cases, adult onset has also been described. Death caused by septicemia has been reported in 5 cases.[13] Concomitant psoriasis vulgaris, palmoplantar pustulosis (PPP), or psoriatic arthritis have not been reported, supporting the assertion that *IL36RN* mutations are responsible for a specific subtype of GPP. Histopathologic studies have shown spongiform pustules, acanthosis with elongation of rete ridges, and parakeratosis in the stratum corneum, consistent with histopathology of pustular psoriasis.[13] The differential diagnosis of DITRA includes GPP and acute generalized exanthematous pustulosis (AGEP). Acitretin, topical and oral steroids, adalimumab, and phototherapy have been used with varying degrees of success in patients with DITRA.[13]

CARD14-MEDIATED PUSTULAR PSORIASIS

De novo mutations in caspase recruitment domain family member 14 (*CARD14*) have also been described in a monogenic form of childhood GPP called CARD14-mediated pustular psoriasis (CAMPS).[9,10] *CARD14* mutations have also been previously implicated in plaque-type psoriasis and pityriasis rubra pilaris (PRP).[9,10,17] CARD14 activates NFκB. Activating missense mutations in *CARD14* upregulate NFκB, subsequently increasing the transcription of psoriasis-associated chemokines and cytokines, including IL-8, chemokine (C-C motif) ligand 20, and IL-36.[10]

CAMPS is characterized by childhood-onset generalized pustulosis, fevers, palmoplantar keratoderma, and nail pitting. Psoriatic arthritis has not been described in CAMPS, although it has been reported in CARD14-associated plaque psoriasis and PRP.[9,10] Poor response to methotrexate, cyclosporine, infliximab, and anakinra have been reported; however, 1 case of CAMPS has been successfully managed with IL-12/IL-23 antagonist ustekinumab.[18]

PYOGENIC ARTHRITIS, PYODERMA GANGRENOSUM, AND ACNE SYNDROME

The syndrome of pyogenic arthritis, pyoderma gangrenosum, and acne (PAPA) was coined by Lindor and colleagues in 1997,[19] although it was first described in 1975 in a patient with "streaking leukocyte factor."[20] This rare autosomal-dominant autoinflammatory syndrome is caused by mutations in the gene encoding CD2-binding protein 1, also known as proline-serine-threonine-phosphatase-interacting protein 1 (*PSTPIP1*). Mutations in *PSTPIP1* lead to hyperphosphorylation of the protein and subsequent increased binding affinity to pyrin, thereby causing dysregulation of IL-1β production.[21–24] Genotype analyses of families have shown variable penetrance, including genetic carriers without symptoms and others with typical PAPA syndrome features within the same family.[25]

Clinically, PAPA syndrome is characterized by aseptic inflammation of the skin and joints. Painful, recurrent, sterile monoarticular arthritis with prominent neutrophilic infiltrate usually occurs in the first decade of life and may be the presenting sign of disease. Elbows, knees, and ankles are most often involved, and the natural history of persistent disease leads to significant joint destruction. Skin involvement is variable. Pathergy is a commonly observed phenomenon and pustule formation followed by ulceration may be induced early in life following vaccination or minimal trauma (**Fig. 3**). Severe nodulocystic acne and pyoderma gangrenosum tend to develop around puberty and may persist into adulthood.[19,20,26–32] Cystic acne persisting until the seventh decade of life has been reported.[19] Hidradenitis suppurativa has also been reported in a few cases, but is not a consistent clinical feature.[19] Other dermatologic manifestations described in the setting of PAPA include rosacea and psoriasis.[30] Sulfonamide-induced pancytopenia has also been reported in 23% to 40% of patients with PAPA, although the

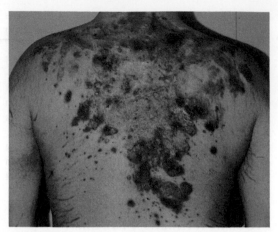

Fig. 3. PAPA syndrome. Cribiform pyoderma gangrenosum ulcers in the setting of severe scarring from acne conglobata.

significance of these observations is not well understood.[19,32]

Laboratory findings in PAPA syndrome reflect a systemic inflammatory state with leukocytosis and increased acute-phase reactants, but are otherwise nondiagnostic. Increases in IL-1β and tumor necrosis factor α (TNF-α) production in peripheral blood leukocytes have been observed. Infectious processes, vasculopathy, coagulopathy, and autoimmune disease should be ruled out in the evaluation of patients. Histopathology of cystic acne lesions reveals distended follicles, with cystic spaces and follicular openings filled with keratinaceous debris and numerous bacteria. Ruptured cystic contents induce a brisk neutrophilic inflammatory infiltrate surrounding expanded follicles. Histopathology of pyoderma gangrenosum is similar to that seen with pyoderma gangrenosum in other settings. Early lesions show a neutrophilic vascular infiltrate. Actively expanding lesions show neutrophilic infiltrates with leukocytoclasia. Marked tissue necrosis with surrounding mononuclear cell infiltrates is seen in ulcers. Synovial fluid aspirations show sterile neutrophil-predominant infiltrate.[30]

The differential diagnosis for articular manifestations of PAPA syndrome includes monoarticular septic arthritis and, in children, CRMO. The presence of both severe acne and pyoderma gangrenosum, or the presence of PAPA findings in family members, should prompt consideration of PAPA syndrome, synovitis, acne, pustulosis, hyperostosis, osteitis (SAPHO) syndrome, and pyoderma gangrenosum secondary to underlying inflammatory bowel disease. Pyoderma, acne, and suppurative hidradenitis (PASH) syndrome is a recently described autoinflammatory disorder that may also be considered in the differential

diagnosis of PAPA syndrome.[33] Although mutations in *PSTPIP1* were not found in the 2 reported patients with PASH, heterozygous repetition of the CCTG microsatellite motif in the *PSTPIP1* promoter were detected. The significance of these findings is unknown. In contrast to PAPA syndrome, joint involvement was not reported in the 2 reported patients with PASH.

Medications targeting IL-1 and TNF-α have been most successful in managing the manifestations of PAPA syndrome. The most consistent responses have been observed with the TNF-α antagonists etanercept, adalimumab, and infliximab.[27,34–36] Response to the anti-IL-1 agent, anakinra, has been more variable,[26,28,34] but seems to be more effective in the management of joint manifestations rather than cutaneous disease.[28] Joint disease is also responsive to corticosteroids; however, acne may be exacerbated with systemic therapy. Joint effusions may also be surgically managed with drainage or intra-articular steroid injection. Combination therapy with anakinra and anti-TNF-α agents is associated with increased risk of infection, and should be undertaken with caution. Topical and systemic retinoids have been effective in combination with biological agents for the management of cystic acne. Patients should be counseled regarding the pathergic component of disease, and advised to avoid trauma to the integument.

SAPHO SYNDROME

Since the 1960s, associations between pustular dermatologic manifestations and osteoarticular manifestations have been reported under various designations, including pustulotic arthro-osteitis, sternocostoclavicular hyperostosis, acne-associated spondyloarthropathy, acquired hyperostosis syndrome, and CRMO. In 1987, Chamot and colleagues[37] proposed a unifying syndrome known as SAPHO syndrome. The prevalence of this rare syndrome is estimated to be fewer than 4 in 10,000, with a female predilection. SAPHO can present at any age; however, onset is most common in children and young adults. A similar condition first described in 1972, known as CRMO, is now largely believed to represent a subset of SAPHO that predominates in the pediatric population.[38] CRMO, congenital dyserythropoietic anemia, and Sweets syndrome are features of Majeed syndrome, a rare autosomal-recessive disorder reported in 3 Middle Eastern families.[39–41] Other associated findings of Majeed syndrome include fevers and growth failure. Mutations in the *LPIN2* gene, which encodes lipin 2, are implicated in Majeed syndrome.[42] Lipin 2 is a protein that plays a role in lipid metabolism; however, lipid abnormalities have not been reported in patients with Majeed syndrome. The genetic basis of SAPHO/CRMO is still unknown.

Osteoarticular manifestations are the hallmark of SAPHO syndrome, and occur regardless of the presence of dermatologic manifestations.[37] The most commonly involved areas include the anterior chest wall (65%–90%), followed by the spine (30%), particularly the thoracic spine. Sacroileitis may also occur, and mandibular lesions can be seen in up to 10% of adults.[43,44] Long bone involvement is rare in adults, but involvement of the tibia and femur is common in children.[45,46] Synovitis distant from sites of bony involvement is seen in up to 30% of adults but is rarely noted in children.[46] Surrounding soft tissue swelling and erythema can also develop, and morning stiffness is common. The essential features of SAPHO syndrome, including osteitis, hyperostosis, and PPP, can also be seen in CRMO; however, bony involvement in CRMO frequently affects the metaphyses of tubular bones, a feature not typically seen in SAPHO.[47]

Dermatologic manifestations of SAPHO may occur concurrently, before or after osteoarticular disease, and are more frequent in adults than in children.[48–50] Seventy percent of children and 15% of adults never show cutaneous disease. Cutaneous lesions consist of neutrophilic pustular dermatoses. PPP is most common, affecting up to 60% of patients who develop dermatologic manifestations.[48] Acne conglobata and acne fulminans occur in approximately 25% of patients, with a notable male predominance.[48] Similarly, hidradenitis suppurativa may also be seen and predominates in men.[51,52] Rarely, pyoderma gangrenosum and Sweet syndrome may occur.[53–55] Although systemic manifestations are uncommon in SAPHO syndrome, fever and moderate increases in acute-phase reactants may occur, and up to 10% of patients with SAPHO syndrome develop inflammatory bowel disease, most commonly after the onset of SAPHO symptoms.[46,48,53,56] Histopathology of SAPHO-associated PPP is identical to that of PPP.

The differential diagnosis for the osteoarticular manifestations of SAPHO syndrome includes bacterial osteomyelitis, primary bone tumors, metastatic disease, and eosinophilic granuloma. SAPHO syndrome should be considered in patients with PPP or nodulocystic acne in conjunction with a history of bony pain, particularly anterior chest wall pain. Dermatologic and osteoarticular findings should also be evaluated in patients with inflammatory bowel disease. Many individual signs and symptoms of SAPHO syndrome are nonspecific, and therefore it is a diagnosis of exclusion. Although validated diagnostic criteria do not exist, inclusion criteria for diagnosis have been proposed (**Table 1**).[57] The presence of 1 of the 4 listed

Table 1
Inclusion and exclusion criteria for SAPHO syndrome

Inclusion criteria	Osteoarticular manifestations of acne conglobata, acne fulminans, or hidradenitis suppurativa (ie, inflammatory synovitis, anterior chest wall hyperostosis or osteitis, hyperostosis or osteitis at another site, or spondylitis or spondylodiscitis)
	Osteoarticular manifestations of PPP (ie, inflammatory synovitis, hyperostosis ± osteitis, or spondylitis or spondylodiscitis)
	Hyperostosis (of the anterior chest wall, limbs or spine) with or without dermatosis
	CRMO involving the axial or peripheral skeleton with or without dermatosis
Exclusion criteria	Septic osteomyelitis
	Infectious chest wall arthritis
	Infectious PPP
	Palmoplantar keratoderma
	Diffuse idiopathic skeletal hyperostosis, except for fortuitous association
	Osteoarticular manifestations of retinoid therapy
Other reported features	Possible association with psoriasis vulgaris
	Possible association with an inflammatory enterocolopathy
	Features of ankylosing spondylitis
	Presence of low-virulence bacterial infections

The presence of 1 of the 4 inclusion criteria is sufficient for diagnosis of SAPHO syndrome.
Data from Benhamou CL, Chamot AM, Kahn MF. Synovitis-acne-pustulosis hyperostosis-osteomyelitis syndrome (SAPHO). A new syndrome among the spondyloarthropathies? Clin Exp Rheumatol 1988;6(2):109–12.

Table 2
Proposed criteria for CRMO and nonbacterial osteitis

Major Diagnostic Criteria	Minor Diagnostic Criteria
1. Radiologically proved osteolytic/sclerotic bone lesion 2. Multifocal bone lesions 3. PPP or psoriasis 4. Sterile bone biopsy with signs of inflammation or fibrosis, sclerosis	1. Normal blood count and good general state of health 2. C-reactive protein and erythrocyte sedimentation rate mildly to moderately increased 3. Observation time longer than 6 mo 4. Hyperostosis 5. Associated with other autoimmune diseases apart from PPP or psoriasis 6. Grade I or II relatives with autoimmune or autoinflammatory disease, or with nonbacterial osteitis

Two major criteria or 1 major and 3 minor criteria is sufficient for a diagnosis of CRMO.

Adapted from Jansson A, Renner ED, Ramser J, et al. Classification of non-bacterial osteitis: retrospective study of clinical, immunologic and genetic aspects in 89 patients. Rheumatology (Oxford) 2007;46(1):154–60; with permission.

inclusion criteria is sufficient for diagnosis of SAPHO syndrome. Diagnostic criteria have also been established for CRMO and nonbacterial osteitis (**Table 2**). The diagnosis of Majeed syndrome can be established by genetic evaluation performed in the setting of CRMO, anemia, and inflammatory neutrophilic dermatosis.

Although the disease course is highly variable between individuals, the prognoses for SAPHO syndrome and CRMO are good, and disabling complications are rare.[48,53] Peripheral arthritis may lead to erosive joint disease in adults. Adults may also suffer from bony deformities and limb length discrepancies. CRMO is generally considered to be a self-limiting condition, with healing of sclerotic bone lesions and normalization of bone within 5 years of disease remission.[58]

The pathogenesis of SAPHO is poorly understood, and a variety of therapies have been used with variable benefit. Nonsteroidal antiinflammatory agents and intra-articular corticosteroids have been useful in the management of joint inflammation.[37,48] Bisphosphonates may achieve pain relief and sustained remission of bony disease, presumably as a result of inhibition of bone resorption and antiinflammatory properties; however, responses are variable.[59–63] Systemic corticosteroids in combination with disease-modifying antirheumatic drugs (DMARDs) such as methotrexate and azathioprine have been used with some benefit for the management of bony and cutaneous disease.[48,56] Anti-TNF-α agents, including etanercept, adalimumab and infliximab, have shown promise in the management of bone disease in SAPHO syndrome, with generally rapid improvement in bone pain as early as after the first treatment.[64–67] TNF-α blockade has also been beneficial for the management of pustular dermatoses associated with SAPHO

syndrome. However, the development of SAPHO syndrome was reported in a patient with inflammatory bowel disease treated with infliximab.[68] In addition, the paradoxical induction of pustular skin diseases in patients treated with anti-TNF-α agents is a well-known phenomenon.[69] In 6 of 7 patients with SAPHO, improvement in cutaneous and bony manifestations was reported with the IL-1 antagonist anakinra, suggesting a potential targeted therapy for this syndrome.[70,71]

PUSTULAR PSORIASIS AND CLINICAL VARIANTS
Overview

Genetic advances in monogenic pustular diseases such as DIRA and DITRA have implicated IL-1 family proteins in the development of pustular disease and have led to the successful use of targeted IL-1–blocking agents for these conditions. These insights may provide clues to the pathogenesis of other pustular dermatoses that are believed to have a polygenic cause, such as pustular psoriasis and its variants, and to the potential application of similar targeted therapies for these recalcitrant skin conditions.

Pustular psoriasis is characterized by noninfective macroscopic pustules. In 85% of patients, typical plaque psoriasis precedes the appearance of GPP.[72] Twenty-five percent of children with pustular psoriasis have a family history of psoriasis, suggesting a strong genetic component. In adults, pustular psoriasis is less common than plaque-type psoriasis, with an estimated prevalence of 0.1% in the general population and a female predominance (female-to-male ratio 3:2).[73,74] However, in children, a male predominance is seen (male-to-female ratio 3:2). Male children have an earlier age of disease onset

(3.5 months of age), compared with females (8 years of age).[75] Although pustular psoriasis has long been believed to be a variant of psoriasis, pustular psoriasis and its variants have distinct HLA susceptibility loci, which suggests that these 2 categories of disease may be genetically distinct.[76,77] Whereas skin manifestations of psoriasis vulgaris are associated with HLA-Cw6, HLA-DRB1*0701/2, HLA-B13, HLA-B17, and HLA-B37,[78] these alleles are not associated with GPP, acrodermatitis continua of Hallopeau (ACH), or PPP.[77,79] Peripheral psoriatic arthritis alone has been associated with HLA-B27, however, this allele is most strongly associated with radiographic sacroileitis.[80] HLA-B27 is also associated with GPP and ACH in the setting of axial arthritis,[77,81] as well as PPP in the context of SAPHO syndrome[54,82] and reactive arthritis, which is characterized by uveitis, urethritis, and spondyloarthritis.[83]

In 1968, Baker and Ryan described 2 distinct clinical presentations of pustular psoriasis.[73,84] The first group was characterized by onset of plaque psoriasis before age 40 years. Individuals developed pustular psoriasis after exposure to a precipitating factor (**Box 1**), and lesions tended to resolve, with a return to more classic plaque-type psoriasis after treatment. In contrast, the second group was characterized by disease onset later in life, with a peak incidence between ages 41 and 60 years.[73] Initial psoriatic lesions in this group tended to occur in atypical distributions, such as the flexural areas, palmoplantar surfaces, or the fingertips. These lesions were followed shortly thereafter by pustular lesions that progressed rapidly, often with accompanying systemic manifestations, including fever and leukocytosis. A significant subset of this group presented with pustular psoriasis without antecedent plaque disease. External precipitating factors were less common in this group, and individuals typically had significant morbidity and mortality attributable to both the aggressiveness of the disease and the advanced age of some patients. Baker and Ryan also noted that localized and generalized forms of pustular psoriasis could overlap with one another over time.[73]

Pustular psoriasis can also be divided into 2 phenotypic categories: localized and generalized disease. Other more specific classification systems have been proposed, however, one system has not been uniformly used.[73,84,85]

GPP

GPP consists of von Zumbusch-type GPP and annular pustular psoriasis (APP). In pregnant

---

> **Box 1**
> **Precipitants of pustular psoriasis**
>
> Infection (most notably streptococcal infection, vaccines[a])
>
> Drugs
>
> - Corticosteroids
> - Nonsteroidal antiinflammatory drugs (aspirin, phenylbutazone, oxyphenbutazone)
> - Salicylates (aspirin[a])
> - Penicillin
> - Sulfonamides
> - Lithium
> - Morphine
> - Topical coal tar
> - Pyrogallol
> - Topical chrysarobin
> - Potassium iodide
> - Progestins
> - Arsenicals
> - Hydroxychloroquine
> - Anti-TNF-α agents
>
> Pregnancy
>
> Menstruation
>
> Stress
>
> Surgery
>
> Alcohol
>
> Sunlight, sunburn
>
> Exertion
>
> Seasonal variation
>
> Birch pollen[a]
>
> Milk
>
> Pork
>
> [a] Denotes precipitant associated with juvenile GPP.

---

women, von Zumbusch-type GPP is called impetigo herpetiformis. Subcorneal pustular dermatosis (SCPD) is a controversial variant of pustular psoriasis characterized by superficial pustules forming annular and gyrate patterns.

von Zumbusch-type GPP

In 1910, Leo Ritter von Zumbusch described a fulminant variant of GPP characterized by sudden-onset, inflamed plaques studded with sterile pustules.[86] Clinical diagnostic criteria for GPP have been proposed (**Table 3**).[87]

Table 3
Diagnostic criteria for GPP
All 5 criteria must be met for diagnosis.
1. Systemic symptoms such as fever and general malaise are present
2. Multiple, isolated, noninfectious pustules are present in the flushed skin all over the body or over a wide area
3. Kogoj spongiform pustules are histopathologically confirmed
4. Some of the following laboratory test results are obtained during the clinical course
a. Leukocytosis and shift to the left
b. Precipitated erythrocyte sedimentation rate, positive C-reactive protein, and high antistreptolysin O antibody levels
c. Increases in IgG or IgA
d. Hypoproteinemia, hypocalcemia, and so forth
5. Recurrence of the above-listed clinical and histologic findings

Adapted from Umezawa Y, Ozawa A, Kawasima T, et al. Therapeutic guidelines for the treatment of generalized pustular psoriasis (GPP) based on a proposed classification of disease severity. Arch Dermatol Res 2003;295(Suppl 1): S43–54; with permission.

The first manifestations of von Zumbusch-type GPP are typically fever and leukocytosis for 1 to 2 days, followed by skin edema and erythema.[88] Pustules appear shortly thereafter within erythematous plaques in crops that coalesce into lakes of pus. Generalized erythroderma may occur. Skin pain, burning, diaphoresis, and pruritus are common symptoms. Systemic findings, including malaise, fatigue, anorexia, and arthritis parallel skin disease in adults. Arthritis develops in approximately one-third of patients, often involving the distal interphalangeal joints but may also involve the sacroiliac and other joints.[73] Joint disease is uncommon in children with pustular psoriasis.[89,90] Nail findings typical of psoriasis, including hypertrophy, thickening, subungual pustulation, nail pitting, and onycholysis, are commonly seen in von Zumbusch-type GPP.[11,89–91] Although cutaneous infections are uncommon, pulmonary infections, pyogenic abscesses, and cystitis may occur.[88]

Oral findings in von Zumbusch-type GPP include migratory arcuate and circinate plaques on the dorsal tongue consistent with geographic tongue. Similar findings may occur on the buccal mucosa.[92,93] Some speculate that these oral manifestations may represent a *forme fruste* of pustular psoriasis,[92] whereas others believe that

oral mucosal manifestations are a harbinger of GPP.[91,94] The most commonly reported ocular manifestation is purulent sterile conjunctivitis[11,12,95,96]; however, iridocyclitis,[12] corneal ulceration,[12] and corneal exfoliation[97] may develop.

Leukocytosis is the most common laboratory abnormality in von Zumbusch-type GPP. Decreased serum calcium concentration is a result of hypoalbuminemia.[73,98] Ionized calcium is typically normal, and patients are therefore not symptomatic. Increased alkaline phosphatase, transaminase, and bilirubin levels may also be seen.[73,95] Absolute hypovolemia secondary to fluid losses may lead to prerenal azotemia.[91,98] Gram-positive septicemia and herpes simplex virus conjunctivitis have been reported in juvenile cases.[75] Mortality in patients with von Zumbusch-type GPP is most commonly caused by cardiac failure, sepsis, or acute respiratory distress syndrome.[84,99–102]

The course of von Zumbusch-type GPP is episodic, and symptoms may recur several times a year or only upon exposure to precipitants. Cutaneous and systemic symptoms may spontaneously remit or may require prolonged therapy to induce remission. Despite the significant morbidity associated with acute episodes of von Zumbusch-type GPP in children, the prognosis of affected patients is generally good. Conservative topical management with corticosteroids and topical calcipotriol, or narrow-band UV-B in combination with topical therapy, is the preferred first-line therapy for management of von Zumbusch-type GPP in children, and resolution with supportive conservative topical management can usually be achieved in this patient population.[103] Second-line agents include cyclosporine, methotrexate, and systemic retinoids.[104] Methotrexate 0.2 mg/kg/wk has been shown to be effective in the management of von Zumbusch-type GPP in children.[105–107] Etanercept has also been used safely for von Zumbusch-type GPP in children, and may be considered for recalcitrant disease.[108]

In adults, systemic retinoids are considered by some to be first-line therapy for von Zumbusch-type GPP.[87,109–111] Isotretinoin may be preferred to acitretin in women with von Zumbusch-type GPP of childbearing age given its short half-life; however, it may be less efficacious than acitretin.[112] Response is typically seen within several days to weeks. Methotrexate, cyclosporine, and infliximab are alternative options.[113,114] Given the rapid response after cyclosporine and infliximab treatment, many clinicians now consider these first-line agents for the management of von Zumbusch-type GPP. Care should be exercised with methotrexate use in elderly patients and individuals with hepatic disease, and methotrexate and cyclosporine must be used with caution in patients with renal dysfunction. Psoralen plus ultraviolet A (PUVA) has also been combined with acitretin for management of von Zumbusch-type GPP.[110]

Although systemic corticosteroid taper may induce a flare of pustular disease, judicious use of corticosteroids in the setting of disease flare may be helpful for acute management. Corticosteroids are best used in combination with steroid-sparing agents such as biologics or DMARDs and require slow tapering.[87] Adalimumab, etanercept, and alefacept have been used with some success in the management of GPP, but are considered second-line agents for von Zumbusch-type GPP.[115,116] The IL-1 antagonist anakinra and IL-12/IL-23 antagonist ustekinumab have been used in isolated cases, but have not been systematically studied in this population.[117,118]

Impetigo herpetiformis

Impetigo herpetiformis refers to the development of von Zumbusch-type GPP during pregnancy. A personal or family history of psoriasis may be present in these patients.[91,119,120] Disease onset is typically in the third trimester, although it may occur earlier in pregnancy, and both cutaneous and systemic symptoms resolve gradually after delivery or termination of pregnancy.[15,91,120–122] Recurrence may occur with subsequent pregnancy, ovulation, or oral contraceptive use, suggesting a role for progesterone in disease precipitation.[15,91,120,121,123,124] In addition, von Zumbusch-type GPP has been reported in the setting of progesterone challenge.[95]

Like von Zumbusch-type GPP, cutaneous and systemic findings of impetigo herpetiformis are abrupt in onset. However, unlike von Zumbusch-type GPP, early involvement of the flexural surfaces and healing with hyperpigmentation are common in impetigo herpetiformis.[91,120,122,125] Erosive and circinate plaques involving the tongue, buccal mucosa, and esophagus may occur. Subungual pustules may result in onycholysis.[126] Symptomatic hypocalcemia is common and necessitates close monitoring of mother and fetus. Fetal mortality as high as 89% has been reported.[15] Placental insufficiency is the most frequently cited cause for fetal mortality.[15,122]

First-line therapy for impetigo herpetiformis includes topical calcipotriol, topical and oral corticosteroids, and cyclosporine. Cyclosporine is pregnancy category C according to the US Food and Drug Administration (FDA) classification, however, it has been used in the setting of acute disease flares with significant systemic manifestations.[111,127,128] Narrow-band UV-B in combination

with topical steroids and cyclosporine has also been used during pregnancy.[129] Biologics including etanercept, adalimumab, and infliximab are FDA pregnancy category B, and data for their use in this clinical scenario are limited. Infliximab has been used successfully for impetigo herpetiformis in the postpartum period.[130] Topical and systemic retinoids and methotrexate are FDA pregnancy category X and thus contraindicated in pregnancy. Patients treated in the postpartum period with these agents should be advised not to breastfeed while receiving therapy.[131–134] PUVA has been used with success in 1 case but is not advisable given fetal exposure to psoralens.[135]

APP

APP, also known as erythema circine recidivants, is a rare variant of GPP with a recurrent course but good overall prognosis.[136] Although APP does not have a predilection for childhood, it is the most frequent presentation of pustular psoriasis in childhood, with mean age of onset of 11 years in children.[136,137] Adult-onset APP typically presents during the sixth or seventh decades of life and seems to have a greater predilection for women than men.[73,93]

APP onset is not typically preceded or followed by plaque psoriasis. Unlike von Zumbusch-type GPP and impetigo herpetiformis, APP has a less severe course, characterized by diffuse, slowly migrating, annular, and gyrate erythematous plaques with sterile pustules along the advancing edges involving the trunk, neck, and extremities (Fig. 4).[73,138] Polyarthritis can develop. Pruritus may be present; however, other systemic symptoms and laboratory abnormalities, including leukocytosis, hypocalcemia, and increased acute-phase reactants are typically absent in both

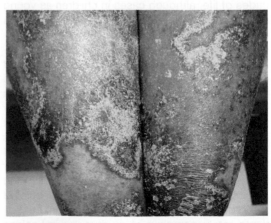

Fig. 4. APP. Gyrate plaques of APP notable for central sparing and erythematous border studded with pustules and yellow crusting. (*Courtesy of* Jeffrey Callen.)

children and adults.[84] Recurrent courses may occur over decades, but episodes are typically less severe than seen in von Zumbusch-type GPP. Features of von Zumbusch-type GPP and APP may overlap within the same patient.

Given the subacute nature of APP, some patients with mild disease respond well to topical corticosteroids and warm water compresses, whereas others may require systemic therapy. Acitretin,[139] dapsone,[138,140,141] and methotrexate have been successful in patients requiring systemic therapy. Low-dose methotrexate has been used with success in the pediatric setting.[105] Success with systemic retinoids has also been reported, but must be used with care in the pediatric population.[142,143]

SCPD

SCPD, or Sneddon-Wilkinson disease, was first described by Sneddon and Wilkinson in 1956.[144] Since SCPD was first described, controversy has ensued regarding its classification.[145–148] Some experts contend that SCPD is not a distinct entity but rather part of the spectrum of psoriasis and pustular psoriasis, resembling the annular pattern of pustular psoriasis.[145] In a review of 103 patients, Baker and Ryan reported 10 patients with APP, some of whom showed subcorneal pustules resembling SCPD. One longitudinal study reported that 10 of 23 patients with SCPD progressed to clinical and histopathologic evidence of pustular psoriasis or plaque psoriasis 3 to 40 years after initial diagnosis of SCPD.[149] Four of these 10 patients had a family history of psoriasis or pustular psoriasis. These data suggest that SCPD and pustular psoriasis may be closely related conditions.

This rare disorder is more common in females than males (female-to-male ratio 4:1). Onset typically occurs between the fifth and seventh decades of life, although cases in children as young as 3 months have been reported.[150–153] SCPD is clinically characterized by abrupt onset of superficial flaccid pustules distributed in the flexural surfaces, including the axillae, groin, and inframammary folds, which progress over 24 to 48 hours to form annular and gyrate patterns in a generalized distribution. Pustules are typically seen in the setting of normal-appearing skin, but may be found in the setting of erythematous skin. The disease course is chronic, characterized by exacerbations and remissions, sometimes for many years (**Fig. 5**). Acral skin, face, nails, and mucosal surfaces are rarely involved. Associated symptoms include irritation and skin pain, but patients rarely complain of pruritus.[144,154] Lesions heal with hyperpigmentation without scarring. SCPD has been associated with pyoderma

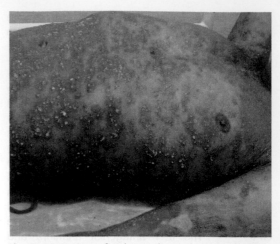

Fig. 5. SCPD. Superficial pustules and scale collarettes in annular and gyrate patterns overlying a relatively noninflammatory background.

gangrenosum,[155,156] inflammatory bowel disease,[148,149,157] and IgA monoclonal gammopathy, including IgA myeloma.[155,158,159] Infectious precipitants, including urinary tract infections and upper respiratory infections, have also been described.[160] Systemic manifestations including fever, malaise, fatigue, and arthralgias are rare in SCPD.[149] In the first reported cases in children, fever and leukocytosis were noted, but subsequent case reports have indicated that there is no difference in clinicopathologic features and prognosis of SPCD between adults and children.[152,153]

Histopathologically, SCPD is characterized by accumulation of subcorneal neutrophils atop fairly normal-appearing epidermis, in which spongiosis and acantholysis are absent.[144] In contrast to pustular psoriasis, neutrophils may migrate through the epidermis, but do not form spongiform pustules. Spongiosis, microabscesses, acanthosis, and regular elongation of rete ridges are not observed. SCPD can be differentiated from pemphigus and benign familial pemphigus by the lack of acantholysis, although acantholysis can be seen in older lesions.[161] Bacteria and fungal elements are absent. Direct and indirect immunofluorescence studies are negative. Flexural distribution, subcorneal (rather than subepidermal) pustules, and lack of pruritus distinguish SPCD from dermatitis herpetiformis.

Cases clinically resembling SCPD but showing IgA deposition in the skin and circulating IgA antibodies have been reported and called IgA pemphigus, intraepidermal IgA pustulosis, intraepidermal neutrophilic IgA dermatosis, and intercellular IgA dermatosis. Controversy exists over whether these cases represent a subgroup of SCPD or are a distinct entity.[162] Clinically, IgA pemphigus frequently involves the scalp and face, which may aid in distinguishing this condition from SCPD. Further confusing matters, some reports have noted that IgA deposits may not be seen by immunofluorescence early in disease onset, and multiple skin biopsies may be required to make a diagnosis of IgA pemphigus.[163] Serum and urine protein electrophoresis are prudent components of the evaluation of patients with SCPD.

Most but not all patients with SCPD respond to sulfones, presumably because of their ability to inhibit neutrophil chemotaxis. Dapsone should be used with caution and requires close monitoring given hematologic adverse effects. In addition to dapsone, other antineutrophilic drugs, including colchicine, sulfapyridine, and sulfamethoxypyrazine, have also been used with variable success.[149,152,164] Topical steroids have also been used successfully as monotherapy or in combination with dapsone.[165] Variable results have been reported with oral retinoids.[166,167] Broad-band and narrow-band UV-B, PUVA, and re-PUVA have been reported to be successful in the management of SCPD, although PUVA was found ineffective in one case.[124,159,168–170] Recalcitrant disease has been managed successfully with infliximab.[171,172]

Localized Pustular Psoriasis

Localized pustular psoriasis can be debilitating because of the sites affected, but unlike GPP, it is not commonly associated with systemic symptoms. This group of diseases includes ACH, PPP, and palmoplantar pustular psoriasis.

ACH

In 1890, Francois Henri Hallopeau[173] described a painful acral pustular condition characterized by sterile pustules involving the distal fingers and, less often, the toes. This rare and often disabling condition, termed ACH or dermatitis repens, is most common in middle-aged women.[174] Disease onset often occurs after localized trauma or infection involving a single digit.[174] Pustules develop, with hyperemia involving the distal aspect of 1 or 2 digits, and progress proximally. Pustulation may involve the nail bed and nail matrix, leading to onychodystrophy, destruction of the nail plate, and anonychia. Inflammatory paronychia is common. ACH may progress to involve the hands, forearms, and feet. Skin atrophy, dermal sclerosis, osteolysis of the distal phalanges, and arthropathy of the interphalangeal joints are seen in prolonged, refractory, or untreated cases.[175] ACH has a chronic relapsing course, with intermittent episodes of acute postulation, which is frequently refractory to therapy. Spontaneous remission is uncommon. In rare instances, syndactyly and involvement of the nasal tip may occur.[176] In the setting of long-standing disease, most often in elderly individuals, subsequent episodes of generalized pustular eruption have been reported.[84,177]

ACH is often refractory to therapy. Attempts to treat with numerous different topical, systemic, and biological agents have met with mixed results (**Box 2**).

PPP and palmoplantar pustular psoriasis

PPP is a painful, debilitating inflammatory skin condition characterized by crops of sterile pustules

---

Box 2
Potential therapies for ACH
Systemic antimicrobials[176,177]
Tetracyclines
Azithromycin
Dapsone
Topical medications[176,177,209]
Topical steroids
Calcipotriol
Tazarotene
Betamethasone
Topical 5-fluorouracil
Topical tacrolimus
Phototherapy[176,209–211]
Narrow-band UV-B
Psoralen UV-A
Grenz rays
Immunomodulators[176,209,211]
Prednisone
Acitretin
Hydroxycarbamide
Colchicine
Methotrexate
Cyclosporine
Biological agents
Adalimumab[a]: 6 cases[211–215]
Infliximab: 2 cases[211,216,217]
Etanercept[b]: 5 cases[211,218–222]
Ustekinumab: 1 case[211]
Anakinra: 1 case[211]
[a] Some patients treated in combination with topical steroids and cyclosporine.
[b] Some patients treated in combination with topical steroids or acitretin.

localized to the palms and soles. Disease onset tends to occur between ages 30 and 50 years, with a female predilection (female-to-male ratio 3:2). A higher prevalence of smoking is noted in patients with PPP than in patients with other dermatoses, and a higher prevalence of PPP is noted in smokers compared with nonsmokers.[178–181] Other precipitating factors include trauma, stress, warm weather, and upper respiratory infection.[182]

Most cases of PPP are chronic, however, acute cases of PPP after febrile illness with sudden onset (24–48 hours) and rapid resolution (2–3 weeks) have been reported and seem to portend a favorable prognosis.[183] Whereas acute PPP may last several days to weeks, chronic PPP may last several decades, with periods of resolution lasting less than 1 year in most patients.[182]

PPP is characterized by pustules in a background of normal-appearing or inflamed skin on the palmar or plantar surfaces (**Fig. 6**).[182] PPP can be disabling secondary to painful fissures, pruritus, and burning sensation of the skin. Nail dystrophy from subungual pustulation can progress to nail destruction, and onycholysis may occur in one-third of patients.[184,185] Both arthritis and arthralgias have also been reported in the setting of PPP.[186,187] Aseptic osteitis of the sternoclavicular joint has been reported in association with PPP in the context of SAPHO syndrome.[37] An increased prevalence of antithyroid antibodies and thyroid disease is noted in patients with PPP.[188,189]

Approximately 10% to 20% of patients with PPP have plaque psoriasis on other parts of the body, a clinical distinction called palmoplantar pustular psoriasis. The dorsal surfaces of the hands and feet may also be involved in these cases. The relationship between PPP and palmoplantar pustular psoriasis is controversial: whereas some clinicians speculate that both conditions lie on a spectrum of pustular psoriasis, others assert that they are distinct entities. Similarities in histopathology, neutrophil dysfunction, and chemokines profiles have been reported in PPP and psoriasis, suggesting a common pathogenic mechanism[190]; however, as mentioned earlier, genetic predisposing factors differ between PPP and psoriasis.[191]

Disease clearance can be achieved with medium-potency topical corticosteroids under hydrocolloid dressing occlusion, however, recurrence is common following cessation of therapy.[192] PUVA has been reported to induce clearance in approximately 40% of people with PPP.[193] Acitretin has been shown to improve disease in about two-thirds of people with PPP, but may require continued treatment to avoid recurrent symptoms.[194,195] Low-dose cyclosporine (1–2.5 mg/kg/d) has led to moderate objective improvement in about two-thirds of patients with PPP within 1 month.[196,197] Tetracycline antibiotics also produced objective improvement in about one-half of patients with PPP, however, complete clearance is rarely seen.[198,199] There are no randomized controlled trials supporting the use of methotrexate, although one uncontrolled prospective study showed benefit in one-third of treated patients, who primarily represented individuals with evidence of psoriasis at other sites.[200]

Studies of biological agents in PPP have resulted in conflicting data. A placebo-controlled trial of etanercept in 15 patients did not show a statistical benefit.[201] Adalimumab was associated with improvement in cutaneous and articular disease in a single patient.[202] Sequential therapy with adalimumab and infliximab was effective in the management of refractory PPP in 1 case.[203] Caution must be exercised with the administration of TNF-α inhibitors because paradoxical induction of psoriasis, pustulosis, and PPP have been reported with these agents.[204,205] More recently, ustekinumab resulted in disease clearance in 6 of 9 patients with PPP.[111]

Acropustulosis of infancy

Acropustulosis of infancy (AI) is one of the most common forms of pustular psoriasis presenting in childhood.[75,136,206] This condition predominates in male children of African descent; however, it may occur in both sexes and in all races.[207,208] One series reported acropustulosis in 4.7% of patients with juvenile psoriasis, with approximately two-thirds of cases occurring in children younger than 5 years.[206]

AI is characterized by intermittent crops of intensely pruritic vesiculopustules occurring on the acral surfaces. Vesiculopustules do not coalesce. Disease onset typically occurs before 10 months of age, and lesions tend to persist for

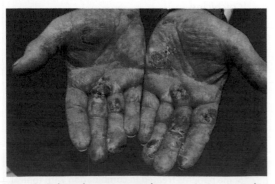

Fig. 6. Palmoplantar pustular psoriasis. Pustules, scaling, and painful erosions with overlying hemorrhagic crust on the palmar surfaces. (*Courtesy of* Kristina Callis-Duffin.)

about 2 years, resolving by age 3 years.[207,208] Although AI spontaneously remits, potent topical steroids are useful for disease management. Pustular lesions show a striking response to sulfones, particularly dapsone,[208] however, the risks of methemoglobinemia and other hematologic adverse events may outweigh its benefit for a self-limited condition.

Histopathology of Pustular Psoriasis and Variants

Neutrophils are the predominant feature on histopathologic examination of pustular psoriasis and its variants in both children and adults. The epidermis is notable for variable hyperplasia, absent granular layer, parakeratosis, suprapapillary thinning, intracorneal aggregates of neutrophils (Munro microabscesses), and epidermal spongiosis with neutrophils (spongiform pustules of Kogoj). Prominent and dilated vessels are noted in the superficial dermis, with sparse mononuclear cell infiltrate and scattered neutrophils in the dermis.[161] Special stains for bacteria or fungal elements are negative. In APP, subcorneal pustules may be observed.[136] In SCPD, subcorneal neutrophils accumulate atop normal-appearing epidermis, in which spongiosis, spongiform pustules, microabscesses, acanthosis, and acantholysis are absent.[144] In PPP, eosinophils and mast

Table 4
Differential diagnosis of pustular psoriasis and its variants

Condition	Differential Diagnosis
von Zumbusch-type GPP Impetigo herpetiformis	Acute generalized exanthematous pustulosis SCPD Diffuse impetigo Folliculitis Miliary tuberculosis Tinea corporis Cutaneous candidiasis Generalized seborrheic dermatitis Reactive arthritis Generalized seborrheic dermatitis Reactive arthritis Childhood bullous dermatosis[a] Miliaria pustulosa[a] Staphylococcal scalded skin syndrome[a]
Annular pustular psoriasis	Erythema annular centrifugum Erythema gyratum repens Tinea corporis Granuloma annulare Urticaria Erythema multiforme Erythema chronicum migrans Subcutaneous lupus erythematosus Annular erythema of infancy[a]
SCPD	IgA pemphigus APP Dermatitis herpetiformis Tinea corporis
Acrodermatitis of Hallopeau	Herpetic whitlow Tinea manuum or pedis Dyshidrotic eczema Bacterial or fungal paronychia Secondarily infected malignancy Secondarily infected contact dermatitis
PPP Palmoplantar pustular psoriasis	Tinea mannum/pedis/unguium Dyshidrotic eczema Contact dermatitis Bacterial or fungal infection

[a] Consider especially in children.

cells may be seen surrounding pustules in the upper dermis, and the normal spiral columnar architecture of eccrine ducts is absent.[182] In AI, both neutrophils and eosinophils may be seen within intraepidermal vesicles both on histopathology and smear.[208]

Differential Diagnosis of Pustular Psoriasis and Variants

The differential diagnosis for GPP includes AGEP, SCPD, reactive arthritis, and cutaneous infections, including impetigo, folliculitis, miliary tuberculosis, and generalized candidiasis. In addition, tinea corporis and gyrate erythemas should be considered in the differential diagnosis of APP. In children, childhood bullous dermatosis, miliaria pustulosa, staphylococcal scalded skin syndrome, and generalized seborrheic dermatitis should also be considered. IgA pemphigus, pemphigus foliaceus, and dermatitis herpetiformis should be considered on the differential for SCPD (Table 4).

The differential diagnosis of acral pustulosis includes cutaneous fungal infection, bacterid eruption, and dyshidrotic eczema. If pustulosis is limited to the digits, herpetic whitlow, secondarily infected malignancy, and chronic bacterial, fungal, or viral paronychia should also be considered. In children, acral pustular eruptions should prompt skin examination for scabies.

SUMMARY

Pustular psoriasis and its variants share several overlapping cutaneous, systemic, and osteoarticular features. The classification of these diseases will continue to evolve over the coming years as underlying biological pathways are elucidated, allowing differentiation based on shared mechanisms of disease rather than clinical similarities alone. Recent genetic insights into several rare monogenic forms of pustular disease have already revealed new autoinflammatory pathways and highlight the potential for new targeted interventions for these challenging conditions.

REFERENCES

1. Aksentijevich I, Masters SL, Ferguson PJ, et al. An autoinflammatory disease with deficiency of the interleukin-1-receptor antagonist. N Engl J Med 2009;360(23):2426–37.
2. Jesus AA, Osman M, Silva CA, et al. A novel mutation of IL1RN in the deficiency of interleukin-1 receptor antagonist syndrome: description of two unrelated cases from Brazil. Arthritis Rheum 2011;63(12):4007–17.
3. Levenson D. New inherited immune disorder revealed. Am J Med Genet A 2009;149(9):fm V–fm VI.
4. Minkis K, Aksentijevich I, Goldbach-Mansky R, et al. Interleukin 1 receptor antagonist deficiency presenting as infantile pustulosis mimicking infantile pustular psoriasis. Arch Dermatol 2012;148(6):747–52.
5. Reddy S, Jia S, Geoffrey R, et al. An autoinflammatory disease due to homozygous deletion of the IL1RN locus. N Engl J Med 2009;360(23):2438–44.
6. Stenerson M, Dufendach K, Aksentijevich I, et al. The first reported case of compound heterozygous IL1RN mutations causing deficiency of the interleukin-1 receptor antagonist. Arthritis Rheum 2011;63(12):4018–22.
7. Schnellbacher C, Ciocca G, Menendez R, et al. Deficiency of interleukin-1 receptor antagonist responsive to anakinra. Pediatr Dermatol 2012. [Epub ahead of print].
8. Hubler WR Jr. Lingual lesions of generalized pustular psoriasis. Report of five cases and a review of the literature. J Am Acad Dermatol 1984;11(6):1069–76.
9. Jordan CT, Cao L, Roberson ED, et al. Rare and common variants in CARD14, encoding an epidermal regulator of NF-kappaB, in psoriasis. Am J Hum Genet 2012;90(5):796–808.
10. Jordan CT, Cao L, Roberson ED, et al. PSORS2 is due to mutations in CARD14. Am J Hum Genet 2012;90(5):784–95.
11. Landry M, Muller SA. Generalized pustular psoriasis. Observations on the course of the disease in a familial occurrence. Arch Dermatol 1972;105(5):711–6.
12. Lindgren S, Groth O. Generalized pustular psoriasis. A report on thirteen patients. Acta Derm Venereol 1976;56(2):139–47.
13. Marrakchi S, Guigue P, Renshaw BR, et al. Interleukin-36-receptor antagonist deficiency and generalized pustular psoriasis. N Engl J Med 2011;365(7):620–8.
14. Onoufriadis A, Simpson MA, Pink AE, et al. Mutations in IL36RN/IL1F5 are associated with the severe episodic inflammatory skin disease known as generalized pustular psoriasis. Am J Hum Genet 2011;89(3):432–7.
15. Oumeish OY, Farraj SE, Bataineh AS. Some aspects of impetigo herpetiformis. Arch Dermatol 1982;118(2):103–5.
16. Sugiura K, Takeichi T, Kono M, et al. A novel IL36RN/IL1F5 homozygous nonsense mutation, p. Arg10X, in a Japanese patient with adult-onset generalized pustular psoriasis. Br J Dermatol 2012;167(3):699–701.
17. Fuchs-Telem D, Sarig O, van Steensel MA, et al. Familial pityriasis rubra pilaris is caused by mutations in CARD14. Am J Hum Genet 2012;91(1):163–70.

18. Habal NC, Chen Y, Jordan C, et al. Pathogenesis study of infantile-onset, severe pustular psoriasis reveals a de novo mutation in CARD14 causing psoriasis which responds clinically to IL-12/23 blocking treatment with ustekinumab [abstract]. Arthritis Rheum 2011;63(Suppl 10):310.

19. Lindor NM, Arsenault TM, Solomon H, et al. A new autosomal dominant disorder of pyogenic sterile arthritis, pyoderma gangrenosum, and acne: PAPA syndrome. Mayo Clin Proc 1997;72(7):611–5.

20. Jacobs JC, Goetzl EJ. "Streaking leukocyte factor," arthritis, and pyoderma gangrenosum. Pediatrics 1975;56(4):570–8.

21. Waite AL, Schaner P, Richards N, et al. Pyrin modulates the intracellular distribution of PSTPIP1. PLoS One 2009;4(7):e6147.

22. Demidowich AP, Freeman AF, Kuhns DB, et al. Brief report: genotype, phenotype, and clinical course in five patients with PAPA syndrome (pyogenic sterile arthritis, pyoderma gangrenosum, and acne). Arthritis Rheum 2012;64(6):2022–7.

23. Shoham NG, Centola M, Mansfield E, et al. Pyrin binds the PSTPIP1/CD2BP1 protein, defining familial Mediterranean fever and PAPA syndrome as disorders in the same pathway. Proc Natl Acad Sci U S A 2003;100(23):13501–6.

24. Yu JW, Fernandes-Alnemri T, Datta P, et al. Pyrin activates the ASC pyroptosome in response to engagement by autoinflammatory PSTPIP1 mutants. Mol Cell 2007;28(2):214–27.

25. Schellevis MA, Stoffels M, Hoppenreijs EP, et al. Variable expression and treatment of PAPA syndrome. Ann Rheum Dis 2011;70(6):1168–70.

26. Brenner M, Ruzicka T, Plewig G, et al. Targeted treatment of pyoderma gangrenosum in PAPA (pyogenic arthritis, pyoderma gangrenosum and acne) syndrome with the recombinant human interleukin-1 receptor antagonist anakinra. Br J Dermatol 2009;161(5):1199–201.

27. Cortis E, De Benedetti F, Insalaco A, et al. Abnormal production of tumor necrosis factor (TNF)–alpha and clinical efficacy of the TNF inhibitor etanercept in a patient with PAPA syndrome [corrected]. J Pediatr 2004;145(6):851.

28. Dierselhuis MP, Frenkel J, Wulffraat NM, et al. Anakinra for flares of pyogenic arthritis in PAPA syndrome. Rheumatology (Oxford) 2005;44(3):406–8.

29. Hong JB, Su YN, Chiu HC. Pyogenic arthritis, pyoderma gangrenosum, and acne syndrome (PAPA syndrome): report of a sporadic case without an identifiable mutation in the CD2BP1 gene. J Am Acad Dermatol 2009;61(3):533.

30. Tallon B, Corkill M. Peculiarities of PAPA syndrome. Rheumatology 2006;45(9):1140–3.

31. Wise CA, Gillum JD, Seidman CE, et al. Mutations in CD2BP1 disrupt binding to PTP PEST and are responsible for PAPA syndrome, an autoinflammatory disorder. Hum Mol Genet 2002;11(8):961–9.

32. Yeon HB, Lindor NM, Seidman J, et al. Pyogenic arthritis, pyoderma gangrenosum, and acne syndrome maps to chromosome 15q. Am J Hum Genet 2000;66(4):1443.

33. Braun-Falco M, Kovnerystyy O, Lohse P, et al. Pyoderma gangrenosum, acne, and suppurative hidradenitis (PASH)–a new autoinflammatory syndrome distinct from PAPA syndrome. J Am Acad Dermatol 2012;66(3):409–15.

34. Smith EJ, Allantaz F, Bennett L, et al. Clinical, molecular, and genetic characteristics of PAPA syndrome: a review. Curr Genomics 2010;11(7):519.

35. Stichweh DS, Punaro M, Pascual V. Dramatic improvement of pyoderma gangrenosum with infliximab in a patient with PAPA syndrome. Pediatr Dermatol 2005;22(3):262–5.

36. Tofteland ND, Shaver TS. Clinical efficacy of etanercept for treatment of PAPA syndrome. J Clin Rheumatol 2010;16(5):244–5.

37. Chamot AM, Benhamou CL, Kahn MF, et al. Acne-pustulosis-hyperostosis-osteitis syndrome. Results of a national survey. 85 cases. Rev Rhum Mal Osteoartic 1987;54(3):187–96.

38. Giedion A, Holthusen W, Masel LF, et al. Subacute and chronic "symmetrical" osteomyelitis. Ann Radiol (Paris) 1972;15(3):329–42.

39. Majeed HA, Al-Tarawna M, El-Shanti H, et al. The syndrome of chronic recurrent multifocal osteomyelitis and congenital dyserythropoietic anaemia. Report of a new family and a review. Eur J Pediatr 2001;160(12):705–10.

40. Majeed HA, El-Shanti H, Al-Rimawi H, et al. On mice and men: an autosomal recessive syndrome of chronic recurrent multifocal osteomyelitis and congenital dyserythropoietic anemia. J Pediatr 2000;137(3):441–2.

41. Majeed HA, Kalaawi M, Mohanty D, et al. Congenital dyserythropoietic anemia and chronic recurrent multifocal osteomyelitis in three related children and the association with Sweet syndrome in two siblings. J Pediatr 1989;115(5 Pt 1):730–4.

42. Ferguson PJ, Chen S, Tayeh MK, et al. Homozygous mutations in LPIN2 are responsible for the syndrome of chronic recurrent multifocal osteomyelitis and congenital dyserythropoietic anaemia (Majeed syndrome). J Med Genet 2005;42(7):551–7.

43. Depasquale R, Kumar N, Lalam RK, et al. SAPHO: what radiologists should know. Clin Radiol 2012;67(3):195–206.

44. Earwaker JW, Cotten A. SAPHO: syndrome or concept? Imaging findings. Skeletal Radiol 2003;32(6):311–27.

45. Beretta-Piccoli BC, Sauvain MJ, Gal I, et al. Synovitis, acne, pustulosis, hyperostosis, osteitis (SAPHO)

syndrome in childhood: a report of ten cases and review of the literature. Eur J Pediatr 2000;159(8): 594–601.

46. Huber AM, Lam PY, Duffy CM, et al. Chronic recurrent multifocal osteomyelitis: clinical outcomes after more than five years of follow-up. J Pediatr 2002;141(2):198–203.

47. Khanna G, Sato TS, Ferguson P. Imaging of chronic recurrent multifocal osteomyelitis. Radiographics 2009;29(4):1159–77.

48. Hayem G, Bouchaud-Chabot A, Benali K, et al. SAPHO syndrome: a long-term follow-up study of 120 cases. Semin Arthritis Rheum 1999 Dec; 29(3):159–71.

49. Kahn MF, Bouvier M, Palazzo E, et al. Sternoclavicular pustulotic osteitis (SAPHO). 20-year interval between skin and bone lesions. J Rheumatol 1991;18(7):1104–8.

50. Sonozaki H, Mitsui H, Miyanaga Y, et al. Clinical features of 53 cases with pustulotic arthro-osteitis. Ann Rheum Dis 1981;40(6):547–53.

51. Bhalla R, Sequeira W. Arthritis associated with hidradenitis suppurativa. Ann Rheum Dis 1994; 53(1):64–6.

52. Rosner IA, Burg CG, Wisnieski JJ, et al. The clinical spectrum of the arthropathy associated with hidradenitis suppurativa and acne conglobata. J Rheumatol 1993;20(4):684–7.

53. Colina M, Govoni M, Orzincolo C, et al. Clinical and radiologic evolution of synovitis, acne, pustulosis, hyperostosis, and osteitis syndrome: a single center study of a cohort of 71 subjects. Arthritis Rheum 2009;61(6):813–21.

54. Kahn MF, Bouchon JP, Chamot AM, et al. Chronic enterocolopathies and SAPHO syndrome. 8 cases. Rev Rhum Mal Osteoartic 1992;59(2):91–4.

55. Yamasaki O, Iwatsuki K, Kaneko F. A case of SAPHO syndrome with pyoderma gangrenosum and inflammatory bowel disease masquerading as Behcet's disease. Adv Exp Med Biol 2003;528: 339–41.

56. Jansson A, Renner ED, Ramser J, et al. Classification of non-bacterial osteitis: retrospective study of clinical, immunological and genetic aspects in 89 patients. Rheumatology (Oxford) 2007;46(1):154–60.

57. Benhamou CL, Chamot AM, Kahn MF. Synovitis-acne-pustulosis hyperostosis-osteomyelitis syndrome (SAPHO). A new syndrome among the spondyloarthropathies? Clin Exp Rheumatol 1988; 6(2):109–12.

58. Jurik AG, Helmig O, Ternowitz T, et al. Chronic recurrent multifocal osteomyelitis: a follow-up study. J Pediatr Orthop 1988;8(1):49–58.

59. Amital H, Applbaum Y, Aamar S, et al. SAPHO syndrome treated with pamidronate: an open-label study of 10 patients. Rheumatology 2004;43(5): 658–61.

60. Guignard S, Job-Deslandre C, Sayag-Boukris V, et al. Pamidronate treatment in SAPHO syndrome. Joint Bone Spine 2002;69(4):392–6.

61. Solau-Gervais E, Soubrier M, Gerot I, et al. The usefulness of bone remodelling markers in predicting the efficacy of pamidronate treatment in SAPHO syndrome. Rheumatology (Oxford) 2006; 45(3):339–42.

62. Colina M, La Corte R, Trotta F. Sustained remission of SAPHO syndrome with pamidronate: a follow-up of fourteen cases and a review of the literature. Clin Exp Rheumatol 2009;27(1):112.

63. Kopterides P, Pikazis D, Koufos C. Successful treatment of SAPHO syndrome with zoledronic acid. Arthritis Rheum 2004;50(9):2970–3.

64. Abdelghani KB, Dran DG, Gottenberg JE, et al. Tumor necrosis factor-α blockers in SAPHO syndrome. J Rheumatol 2010;37(8):1699–704.

65. Aieska De Souza M, Solomon GE, Strober BE. SAPHO syndrome associated with hidradenitis suppurativa successfully treated with infliximab and methotrexate. Bull NYU Hosp Jt Dis 2011; 69(2):185–7.

66. Castellví I, Bonet M, Narváez JA, et al. Successful treatment of SAPHO syndrome with adalimumab: a case report. Clin Rheumatol 2010; 29(10):1205–7.

67. Vilar-Alejo J, Dehesa L, de la Rosa-del Rey P, et al. SAPHO syndrome with unusual cutaneous manifestations treated successfully with etanercept. Acta Derm Venereol 2010;90(5):531.

68. Van Den Eynde M, Lecluyse K, Chioccioli C, et al. Crohn's disease and the SAPHO syndrome during treatment with infliximab: a case report and review of literature. Gastroenterol Clin Biol 2007;31(6–7): 607–10.

69. Sfikakis P, Iliopoulos A, Elezoglou A, et al. Psoriasis induced by anti–tumor necrosis factor therapy: a paradoxical adverse reaction. Arthritis Rheum 2005;52(8):2513–8.

70. Colina M, Pizzirani C, Khodeir M, et al. Dysregulation of P2X7 receptor-inflammasome axis in SAPHO syndrome: successful treatment with anakinra. Rheumatology 2010;49(7):1416–8.

71. Wendling D, Prati C, Aubin F. Anakinra treatment of SAPHO syndrome: short-term results of an open study. Ann Rheum Dis 2012;71(6): 1098–100.

72. Koch F. Zur Frage der Identität von Impetigo herpetiformis, Psoriasis pustulosa und Psoriasis vulgaris. Hautarzt 1952;3:165–8 [in German].

73. Baker H, Ryan TJ. Generalized pustular psoriasis. A clinical and epidemiological study of 104 cases. Br J Dermatol 1968;80(12):771–93.

74. De Oliveira ST, Maragno L, Arnone M, et al. Generalized pustular psoriasis in childhood. Pediatr Dermatol 2010;27(4):349–54.

75. Zelickson BD, Muller SA. Generalized pustular psoriasis in childhood. Report of thirteen cases. J Am Acad Dermatol 1991;24(2 Pt 1):186–94.

76. Ward JM, Barnes RM. HLA antigens in persistent palmoplantar pustulosis and its relationship to psoriasis. Br J Dermatol 2006;99(5):477–83.

77. Zachariae H, Overgaard Petersen H, Kissmeyer Nielsen F, et al. HL-A antigens in pustular psoriasis. Dermatologica 1977;154(2):73–7.

78. Brenner W, Gschnait F, Mayr WR. HLA B13, B17, B37 and Cw6 in psoriasis vulgaris: association with the age of onset. Arch Dermatol Res 1978; 262(3):337–9.

79. Karvonen J, Tiilikainen A, Lassus A. HL-A antigens in patients with persistent palmoplantar pustulosis and pustular psoriasis. Ann Clin Res 1975;7(2): 112–5.

80. Woodrow JC, Ilchysyn A. HLA antigens in psoriasis and psoriatic arthritis. J Med Genet 1985;22(6): 492–5.

81. Svejgaard A, Svejgaard E, Nielsen LS, et al. Some speculations on the associations between HL-A and disease based on studies of psoriasis patients and their families. Transplant Proc 1973;5(4):1797–8.

82. Szanto E, Linse U. Arthropathy associated with palmoplantar pustulosis. Clin Rheumatol 1991;10(2): 130–5.

83. Keat A, Maini R, Nkwazi G, et al. Role of *Chlamydia trachomatis* and HLA-B27 in sexually acquired reactive arthritis. Br Med J 1978;1(6113):605–7.

84. Ryan TJ, Baker H. The prognosis of generalized pustular psoriasis. Br J Dermatol 1971;85(5):407–11.

85. Tolman MM, Moschella SL. Pustular psoriasis (Zumbusch). Arch Dermatol 1960;81:400–4.

86. von Zumbusch LR. Psoriasis und pustulöses Exanthem. Arch Dermatol Res 1909;99(1):335–46 [in German].

87. Umezawa Y, Ozawa A, Kawasima T, et al. Therapeutic guidelines for the treatment of generalized pustular psoriasis (GPP) based on a proposed classification of disease severity. Arch Dermatol Res 2003;295(Suppl 1):S43–54.

88. Kingery FA, Chinn HD, Saunders TS. Generalized pustular psoriasis. Arch Dermatol 1961;84:912–9.

89. al-Fouzan AS, Nanda A. A survey of childhood psoriasis in Kuwait. Pediatr Dermatol 1994;11(2):116–9.

90. Beylot C, Bioulac P, Grupper C. Generalized pustular psoriasis in infants and children: report of 27 cases. In: Farber EM, Cox AJ, Jacobs PH, editors. Psoriasis. New York: Yorke Medical Books; 1977. p. 171–9.

91. Braverman IM, Cohen I, O'Keefe E. Metabolic and ultrastructural studies in a patient with pustular psoriasis (von Zumbusch). Arch Dermatol 1972; 105(2):189–96.

92. Dawson TA. Tongue lesions in generalized pustular psoriasis. Br J Dermatol 1974;91(4):419–24.

93. Zelickson BD, Muller SA. Generalized pustular psoriasis. A review of 63 cases. Arch Dermatol 1991; 127(9):1339–45.

94. O'Keefe E, Braverman IM, Cohen I. Annulus migrans. Identical lesions in pustular psoriasis, Reiter's syndrome, and geographic tongue. Arch Dermatol 1973;107(2):240–4.

95. Shelley WB. Generalized pustular psoriasis induced by potassium iodide. A postulated role for dihydrofolic reductase. JAMA 1967;201(13): 1009–14.

96. Wagner G, Luckasen JR, Goltz RW. Mucous membrane involvement in generalized pustular psoriasis: report of three cases and review of the literature. Arch Dermatol 1976;112(7):1010–4.

97. Gordon M, Pearlstein HH, Burgoon CF Jr. Pustular psoriasis (Zumbusch). Dermatologica 1969;138(2): 65–74.

98. Warren DJ, Winney RJ, Beveridge GW. Oligaemia, renal failure, and jaundice associated with acute pustular psoriasis. Br Med J 1974;2(5916):406–8.

99. Abou-Samra T, Constantin JM, Amarger S, et al. Generalized pustular psoriasis complicated by acute respiratory distress syndrome. Br J Dermatol 2004;150(2):353–6.

100. Doval IG, Peteiro C, Toribio J. Acute respiratory distress syndrome and generalized pustular psoriasis: another case report. Arch Dermatol 1998; 134(1):103.

101. Griffiths M, Porter W, Fergusson-Wood L, et al. Generalized pustular psoriasis complicated by acute respiratory distress syndrome. Br J Dermatol 2006;155(2):496–7.

102. Sadeh JS, Rudikoff D, Gordon ML, et al. Pustular and erythrodermic psoriasis complicated by acute respiratory distress syndrome. Arch Dermatol 1997;133(6):747.

103. Khan SA, Peterkin GA, Mitchell PC. Juvenile generalized pustular psoriasis. A report of five cases and a review of the literature. Arch Dermatol 1972; 105(1):67–72.

104. Mahe E, Bodemer C, Pruszkowski A, et al. Cyclosporine in childhood psoriasis. Arch Dermatol 2001;137(11):1532.

105. Kalla G, Goyal AM. Juvenile generalized pustular psoriasis. Pediatr Dermatol 1996;13(1):45–6.

106. Kumar B, Dhar S, Handa S, et al. Methotrexate in childhood psoriasis. Pediatr Dermatol 1994;11(3): 271–3.

107. Ryan TJ, Baker H. Systemic corticosteroids and folic acid antagonists in the treatment of generalized pustular psoriasis. Evaluation and prognosis based on the study of 104 cases. Br J Dermatol 1969;81(2):134–45.

108. Pereira T, Vieira A, Fernandes J, et al. Anti-TNF-a therapy in childhood pustular psoriasis. Dermatology 2006;213(4):350–2.

109. Mengesha YM, Bennett ML. Pustular skin disorders: diagnosis and treatment. Am J Clin Dermatol 2002;3(6):389–400.

110. Ozawa A, Ohkido M, Haruki Y, et al. Treatments of generalized pustular psoriasis: a multicenter study in Japan. J Dermatol 1999;26(3):141–9.

111. Robinson A, Van Voorhees AS, Hsu S, et al. Treatment of pustular psoriasis: from the Medical Board of the National Psoriasis Foundation. J Am Acad Dermatol 2012;67(2):279–88.

112. Moy RL, Kingston TP, Lowe NJ. Isotretinoin vs etretinate therapy in generalized pustular and chronic psoriasis. Arch Dermatol 1985;121(10): 1297–301.

113. Collins P, Rogers S. The efficacy of methotrexate in psoriasis–a review of 40 cases. Clin Exp Dermatol 1992;17(4):257–60.

114. Poulalhon N, Begon E, Lebbe C, et al. A follow-up study in 28 patients treated with infliximab for severe recalcitrant psoriasis: evidence for efficacy and high incidence of biological autoimmunity. Br J Dermatol 2007;156(2):329–36.

115. Callen JP, Jackson JH. Adalimumab effectively controlled recalcitrant generalized pustular psoriasis in an adolescent. J Dermatolog Treat 2005; 16(5–6):350–2.

116. Kamarashev J, Lor P, Forster A, et al. Generalised pustular psoriasis induced by cyclosporin a withdrawal responding to the tumour necrosis factor alpha inhibitor etanercept. Dermatology 2002; 205(2):213–6.

117. Dauden E, Santiago-et-Sanchez-Mateos D, Sotomayor-Lopez E, et al. Ustekinumab: effective in a patient with severe recalcitrant generalized pustular psoriasis. Br J Dermatol 2010;163(6):1346–7.

118. Viguier M, Guigue P, Pages C, et al. Successful treatment of generalized pustular psoriasis with the interleukin-1-receptor antagonist Anakinra: lack of correlation with IL1RN mutations. Ann Intern Med 2010;153(1):66–7.

119. Hubler WR Jr. Familial juvenile generalized pustular psoriasis. Arch Dermatol 1984;120(9):1174–8.

120. Oosterling RJ, Nobrega RE, Du Boeuff JA, et al. Impetigo herpetiformis or generalized pustular psoriasis? Arch Dermatol 1978;114(10):1527–9.

121. Bajaj AK, Swarup V, Gupta OP, et al. Impetigo herpetiformis. Dermatologica 1977;155(5):292–5.

122. Beveridge GW, Harkness RA, Livingstone JR. Impetigo herpetiformis in two successive pregnancies. Br J Dermatol 1966;78(2):106–12.

123. Murphy FR, Stolman LP. Generalized pustular psoriasis. Arch Dermatol 1979;115(10):1215–6.

124. Orton DI, George SA. Subcorneal pustular dermatosis responsive to narrowband (TL-01) UVB phototherapy. Br J Dermatol 1997;137(1):149–50.

125. Pierard GE, Pierard-Franchimont C, de la Brassinne M. Impetigo herpetiformis and pustular psoriasis during pregnancy. Am J Dermatopathol 1983;5(3):215–20.

126. Sauer GC, Geha BJ. Impetigo herpetiformis. Report of a case treated with corticosteroid–review of the literature. Arch Dermatol 1961;83: 119–26.

127. Kapoor R, Kapoor JR. Cyclosporine resolves generalized pustular psoriasis of pregnancy. Arch Dermatol 2006;142(10):1373–5.

128. Shaw CJ, Wu P, Sriemevan A. First trimester impetigo herpetiformis in multiparous female successfully treated with oral cyclosporine. BMJ Case Rep 2011 May 12. http://dx.doi.org/10.1136/bcr. 02.2011.3915.

129. Vun YY, Jones B, Al-Mudhaffer M, et al. Generalized pustular psoriasis of pregnancy treated with narrowband UVB and topical steroids. J Am Acad Dermatol 2006;54(2):S28–30.

130. Sheth N, Greenblatt DT, Acland K, et al. Generalized pustular psoriasis of pregnancy treated with infliximab. Clin Exp Dermatol 2009;34(4):521–2.

131. Breier-Maly J, Ortel B, Breier F, et al. Generalized pustular psoriasis of pregnancy (impetigo herpetiformis). Dermatology 1999;198(1):61–4.

132. Bukhari IA. Impetigo herpetiformis in a primigravida: successful treatment with etretinate. J Drugs Dermatol 2004;3(4):449–51.

133. Gimenez Garcia R, Gimenez Garcia MC, Llorente de la Fuente A. Impetigo herpetiformis: response to steroids and etretinate. Int J Dermatol 1989; 28(8):551–2.

134. Winzer M, Wolff HH. Impetigo herpetiformis. Hautarzt 1988;39(2):110–3.

135. Lohrisch I, Heilmann S, Haustein UF. Impetigo herpetiformis and PUVA-treatment (author's transl). Dermatol Monatsschr 1979;165(9):648–52.

136. Liao PB, Rubinson R, Howard R, et al. Annular pustular psoriasis–most common form of pustular psoriasis in children: report of three cases and review of the literature. Pediatr Dermatol 2002;19(1): 19–25.

137. Staughton R. Infantile generalized pustular psoriasis responding to dapsone. Proc R Soc Med 1977;70(4):286–7.

138. Adler DJ, Rower JM, Hashimoto K. Annular pustular psoriasis. Arch Dermatol 1981;117(5):313–4.

139. Vocks E, Worret WI, Ring J. Erythema annulare centrifugum-type psoriasis: a particular variant of acute-eruptive psoriasis. J Eur Acad Dermatol Venereol 2003;17(4):446–8.

140. Singh N, Thappa DM. Circinate pustular psoriasis localized to glans penis mimicking 'circinate balanitis' and responsive to dapsone. Indian J Dermatol Venereol Leprol 2008;74(4):388.

141. Park YM, Kang H, Cho BK. Annular pustular psoriasis localized to the dorsa of the feet. Acta Derm Venereol 1999;79(2):161–2.

142. Rosinska D, Wolska H, Jablonska S, et al. Etretinate in severe psoriasis of children. Pediatr Dermatol 1988;5(4):266–72.

143. Shelnitz LS, Esterly NB, Honig PJ. Etretinate therapy for generalized pustular psoriasis in children. Arch Dermatol 1987;123(2):230.

144. Sneddon IB, Wilkinson DS. Subcorneal pustular dermatosis. Br J Dermatol 1956;68(12):385–94.

145. Chimenti S, Ackerman AB. Is subcorneal pustular dermatosis of Sneddon and Wilkinson an entity sui generis? Am J Dermatopathol 1981;3(4): 363–76.

146. Pinkus H. Is subcorneal pustular dermatosis of Sneddon and Wilkinson and entity sui generis? Am J Dermatopathol 1981;3(4):379–80.

147. Sneddon I, Wilkinson DS. Subcorneal pustular dermatosis differs from subcorneal pustulosis. Am J Dermatopathol 1981;3(4):377.

148. Wolff K. Subcorneal pustular dermatosis is not pustular psoriasis. Am J Dermatopathol 1981;3(4): 381–2.

149. Sanchez NP, Perry HO, Muller SA, et al. Subcorneal pustular dermatosis and pustular psoriasis. A clinicopathologic correlation. Arch Dermatol 1983; 119(9):715–21.

150. Apted J. Subcorneal pustular dermatosis is seen in early infancy. Pediatr Dermatol 1976;1:1–3.

151. Beck AL Jr, Kipping HL, Crissey JT. Subcorneal pustular dermatosis: report of a case. Arch Dermatol 1961;83(4):627.

152. Johnson SA, Cripps DJ. Subcorneal pustular dermatosis in children. Arch Dermatol 1974;109(1):73.

153. Kocak M, Birol A, Erkek E, et al. Juvenile subcorneal pustular dermatosis: a case report. Pediatr Dermatol 2003;20(1):57–9.

154. Sneddon IB, Wilkinson DS. Subcorneal pustular dermatosis. Br J Dermatol 1979;100(1):61–8.

155. Marsden JR, Millard LG. Pyoderma gangrenosum, subcorneal pustular dermatosis and IgA paraproteinaemia. Br J Dermatol 1986;114(1):125–9.

156. Scerri L, Zaki I, Allen BR. Pyoderma gangrenosum and subcorneal pustular dermatosis, without monoclonal gammopathy. Br J Dermatol 1994; 130(3):398–9.

157. Delaporte E, Colombel JF, Nguyen-Mailfer C, et al. Subcorneal pustular dermatosis in a patient with Crohn's disease. Acta Derm Venereol 1992;72(4): 301–2.

158. Cream JJ, Grimes SM, Roberts PD. Subcorneal pustulosis and IgA myelomatosis. Br Med J 1977; 1(6060):550.

159. Todd DJ, Bingham EA, Walsh M, et al. Subcorneal pustular dermatosis and IgA paraproteinaemia: response to both etretinate and PUVA. Br J Dermatol 1991;125(4):387–9.

160. Ellis FA. Subcorneal pustular dermatosis. AMA Arch Derm 1958;78(5):580–8.

161. Weedon D. In: Weedon's skin pathology, vol. 1, 3rd edition. Edinburgh: Churchill Livingstone; 2010.

162. Reed J, Wilkinson J. Subcorneal pustular dermatosis. Clin Dermatol 2000;18(3):301–13.

163. Hashimoto T, Yasumoto S, Nagata Y, et al. Clinical, histopathological and immunological distinction in two cases of IgA pemphigus. Clin Exp Dermatol 2002;27(8):636–40.

164. Harvath L, Yancey KB, Katz SI. Selective inhibition of human neutrophil chemotaxis to N-formyl-methionyl-leucyl-phenylalanine by sulfones. J Immunol 1986; 137(4):1305–11.

165. Walkden V, Roberts A, Wilkinson J. Two cases of subcorneal pustular dermatosis. Response to use of intermittent clobetasol propionate cream. Eur J Dermatol 1994;4(1):44–6.

166. Folkers E, Tafelkruyer J. Subcorneal pustular dermatosis (Sneddon-Wilkinson disease)–therapeutic problems. Br J Dermatol 1978;98(6):681–4.

167. Iandoli R, Monfrecola G. Treatment of subcorneal pustulosis by etretinate. Dermatologica 1987; 175(5):235–8.

168. Cameron H, Dawe RS. Subcorneal pustular dermatosis (Sneddon-Wilkinson disease) treated with narrowband (TL-01) UVB phototherapy. Br J Dermatol 1997;137(1):150–1.

169. Park YK, Park HY, Bang DS, et al. Subcorneal pustular dermatosis treated with phototherapy. Int J Dermatol 1986;25(2):124–6.

170. Bauwens M, De Coninck A, Roseeuw D. Subcorneal pustular dermatosis treated with PUVA therapy. A case report and review of the literature. Dermatology 1999;198(2):203–5.

171. Bonifati C, Trento E, Cordiali Fei P, et al. Early but not lasting improvement of recalcitrant subcorneal pustular dermatosis (Sneddon-Wilkinson disease) after infliximab therapy: relationships with variations in cytokine levels in suction blister fluids. Clin Exp Dermatol 2005;30(6):662–5.

172. Voigtlander C, Luftl M, Schuler G, et al. Infliximab (anti-tumor necrosis factor alpha antibody): a novel, highly effective treatment of recalcitrant subcorneal pustular dermatosis (Sneddon-Wilkinson disease). Arch Dermatol 2001;137(12): 1571–4.

173. Hallopeau FH. Sur une asphyxie locale des extrémités avec polydactylie suppurative chronique et poussées éphémères de dermatite pustuleuse disséminée et symétrique. Bull Soc Fr Dermatol Syphiligr 1890;1:39–45 [in French].

174. Yerushalmi J, Grunwald MH, Hallel-Halevy D, et al. Chronic pustular eruption of the thumbs. Diagnosis: acrodermatitis continua of Hallopeau (ACH). Arch Dermatol 2000;136(7):925–30.

175. Moschella SL. Review of so-called aseptic neutrophilic dermatoses. Australas J Dermatol 1983; 24(2):55–62.

176. Kirkup ME, Lovell CR. Acquired syndactyly secondary to acrodermatitis continua of Hallopeau. Br J Dermatol 2005;152(5):1083–4.

177. Waller JM, Wu JJ, Murase JE, et al. Chronically painful right thumb with pustules and onycholysis. Diagnosis: acrodermatitis continua of Hallopeau. Clin Exp Dermatol 2007;32(5):619–20.

178. Akiyama T, Seishima M, Watanabe H, et al. The relationships of onset and exacerbation of pustulosis palmaris et plantaris to smoking and focal infections. J Dermatol 1995;22(12):930–4.

179. Kubeyinje EP, Belagavi CS. Risk factors for palmoplantar pustulosis in a developing country. East Afr Med J 1997;74(1):54–5.

180. Michaelsson G, Gustafsson K, Hagforsen E. The psoriasis variant palmoplantar pustulosis can be improved after cessation of smoking. J Am Acad Dermatol 2006;54(4):737–8.

181. Rosen K, Mobacken H, Swanbeck G. PUVA, etretinate, and PUVA-etretinate therapy for pustulosis palmoplantaris. A placebo-controlled comparative trial. Arch Dermatol 1987;123(7):885–9.

182. Eriksson MO, Hagforsen E, Lundin IP, et al. Palmoplantar pustulosis: a clinical and immunohistological study. Br J Dermatol 1998;138(3):390–8.

183. Burge S, Ryan T. Acute palmoplantar pustulosis. Br J Dermatol 1985;113(1):77–83.

184. Burden AD, Kemmett D. The spectrum of nail involvement in palmoplantar pustulosis. Br J Dermatol 1996;134(6):1079–82.

185. Piraccini B, Tosti A, Iorizzo M, et al. Pustular psoriasis of the nails: treatment and long-term follow-up of 46 patients. Br J Dermatol 2002;144(5):1000–5.

186. Chamot A, Vion B, Gerster J. Acute pseudoseptic arthritis and palmoplantar pustulosis. Clin Rheumatol 1986;5(1):118–23.

187. Yamamoto T, Kimura K, Katayama I, et al. Successful treatment of severe arthralgia associated with palmoplantar pustulosis with low-dose oral cyclosporine A. J Dermatol 1995;22(7):512.

188. Rosen K, Lindstedt G, Mobacken H, et al. Thyroid function in patients with pustulosis palmoplantaris. J Am Acad Dermatol 1988;19(6):1009–16.

189. Rosen K, Mobacken H, Nilsson LA. Increased prevalence of antithyroid antibodies and thyroid diseases in pustulosis palmoplantaris. Acta Derm Venereol 1981;61(3):237–40.

190. Lundin A, Hakansson L, Michaelsson G, et al. Neutrophil locomotion and serum chemotactic and chemokinetic activities in pustulosis palmoplantaris compared with psoriasis. Arch Dermatol Res 1987;279(6):385–91.

191. Asumalahti K, Ameen M, Suomela S, et al. Genetic analysis of PSORS1 distinguishes guttate psoriasis and palmoplantar pustulosis. J Invest Dermatol 2003;120(4):627–32.

192. Kragballe K, Larsen FG. A hydrocolloid occlusive dressing plus triamcinolone acetonide cream is superior to clobetasol cream in palmo-plantar pustulosis. Acta Derm Venereol 1991;71(6):540–2.

193. Murray D, Corbett MF, Warin AP. A controlled trial of photochemotherapy for persistent palmoplantar pustulosis. Br J Dermatol 1980;102(6):659–63.

194. Ettler K, Richards B. Acitretin therapy for palmoplantar pustulosis combined with UVA and topical 8-MOP. Int J Dermatol 2001;40(8):541–2.

195. Lassus A, Geiger JM. Acitretin and etretinate in the treatment of palmoplantar pustulosis: a double-blind comparative trial. Br J Dermatol 1988;119(6):755–9.

196. Erkko P, Granlund H, Remitz A, et al. Double-blind placebo-controlled study of long-term low-dose cyclosporin in the treatment of palmoplantar pustulosis. Br J Dermatol 1998;139(6):997–1004.

197. Reitamo S, Erkko P, Remitz A, et al. Cyclosporine in the treatment of palmoplantar pustulosis. A randomized, double-blind, placebo-controlled study. Arch Dermatol 1993;129(10):1273–9.

198. Thomsen K, Osterbye P. Pustulosis palmaris et plantaris. Br J Dermatol 1973;89(3):293–6.

199. Ward JM, Corbett MF, Hanna MJ. A double-blind trial of clomocycline in the treatment of persistent palmoplantar pustulosis. Br J Dermatol 1976;95(3):317–22.

200. Thomsen K. Pustulosis palmaris et plantaris treated with methotrexate. Acta Derm Venereol 1971;51(5):397–400.

201. Bissonnette R, Poulin Y, Bolduc C, et al. Etanercept in the treatment of palmoplantar pustulosis. J Drugs Dermatol 2008;7(10):940.

202. Ghate JV, Alspaugh CD. Adalimumab in the management of palmoplantar psoriasis. J Drugs Dermatol 2009;8(12):1136–9.

203. Yawalkar N, Hunger RE. Successful treatment of recalcitrant palmoplantar pustular psoriasis with sequential use of infliximab and adalimumab. Dermatology 2009;218(1):79–83.

204. Mössner R, Thaci D, Mohr J, et al. Manifestation of palmoplantar pustulosis during or after infliximab therapy for plaque-type psoriasis: report on five cases. Arch Dermatol Res 2008;300(3):101–5.

205. Shmidt E, Wetter DA, Ferguson SB, et al. Psoriasis and palmoplantar pustulosis associated with tumor necrosis factor-alpha inhibitors: the Mayo Clinic experience, 1998 to 2010. J Am Acad Dermatol 2012;67(5):e179–85.

206. Morris A, Rogers M, Fischer G, et al. Childhood psoriasis: a clinical review of 1262 cases. Pediatr Dermatol 2001;18(3):188–98.

207. Jarratt M, Ramsdell W. Infantile acropustulosis. Arch Dermatol 1979;115(7):834–6.

208. Kahn G, Rywlin AM. Acropustulosis of infancy. Arch Dermatol 1979;115(7):831.

209. Wilsmann-Theis D, Hagemann T, Dederer H, et al. Successful treatment of acrodermatitis continua suppurativa with topical tacrolimus 0.1% ointment. Br J Dermatol 2004;150(6):1194–7.

210. Bordignon M, Zattra E, Albertin C, et al. Successful treatment of a 9-year-old boy affected by acrodermatitis continua of Hallopeau with targeted ultraviolet B narrow-band phototherapy. Photodermatol Photoimmunol Photomed 2010;26(1):41–3.

211. Lipsker D, Perrigouard C, Foubert A, et al. Anakinra for difficult-to-treat neutrophilic panniculitis: IL-1 blockade as a promising treatment option for neutrophil-mediated inflammatory skin disease. Dermatology 2010;220(3):264–7.

212. Mueller RB, Ogilvie A, Schwarz S, et al. Adalimumab treatment of a patient with psoriasis suppurativa Hallopeau associated osteoarthropathy. Clin Exp Rheumatol 2009;27(5):887.

213. Puig L, Barco D, Vilarrasa E, et al. Treatment of acrodermatitis continua of Hallopeau with TNF-blocking agents: case report and review. Dermatology 2010;220(2):154–8.

214. Ryan C, Collins P, Kirby B, et al. Treatment of acrodermatitis continua of Hallopeau with adalimumab. Br J Dermatol 2009;160(1):203–5.

215. Sopkovich JA, Anetakis Poulos G, Wong HK. Acrodermatitis continua of Hallopeau successfully treated with adalimumab. J Clin Aesthet Dermatol 2012;5(2):60–2.

216. Mang R, Ruzicka T, Stege H. Successful treatment of acrodermatitis continua of Hallopeau by the tumour necrosis factor-alpha inhibitor infliximab (Remicade). Br J Dermatol 2004;150(2):379–80.

217. Rubio C, Martin MA, Arranz Sanchez DM, et al. Excellent and prolonged response to infliximab in a case of recalcitrant acrodermatitis continua of Hallopeau. J Eur Acad Dermatol Venereol 2009; 23(6):707–8.

218. Bonish B, Rashid RM, Swan J. Etanercept responsive acrodermatitis continua of Hallopeau: is a pattern developing? J Drugs Dermatol 2006;5(9): 903–4.

219. Kazinski K, Joyce KM, Hodson D. The successful use of etanercept in combination therapy for treatment of acrodermatitis continua of Hallopeau. J Drugs Dermatol 2005;4(3):360–4.

220. Nikkels AF, Pierard GE. Etanercept and recalcitrant acrodermatitis continua of Hallopeau. J Drugs Dermatol 2006;5(8):705–6.

221. Thielen AM, Barde C, Marazza G, et al. Long-term control with etanercept (Enbrel) of a severe acrodermatitis continua of Hallopeau refractory to infliximab (Remicade). Dermatology 2008;217(2): 137–9.

222. Weisshaar E, Diepgen TL. Successful etanercept therapy in therapy refractory acrodermatitis continua suppurativa Hallopeau. J Dtsch Dermatol Ges 2007;5(6):489–92.

What Do Autoinflammatory Syndromes Teach About Common Cutaneous Diseases Such as Pyoderma Gangrenosum? A Commentary

Daniel Butler, BS[a], Kanade Shinkai, MD, PhD[b],*

KEYWORDS

- Autoinflammation • Pyoderma gangrenosum • Neutrophilic dermatoses
- Pyogenic arthritis syndrome • Deficiency of interleukin 1 receptor agonist
- Familial Mediterranean fever • Cryopyrin-associated periodic syndrome

KEY POINTS

- Pyoderma gangrenosum (PG) is a neutrophilic dermatosis whose pathogenesis is poorly understood. Current PG treatments target a broad spectrum of immunologic mediators, including neutrophils, lymphocytes, and cytokines, with variable success.
- Many autoinflammatory disorders feature cutaneous eruptions, including several presentations of neutrophilic dermatoses.
- Emerging literature highlights the pathophysiologic similarities between autoinflammation and PG; common immunologic pathways shared between these 2 entities may result in alterations in neutrophil recruitment and/or homeostasis, leading to neutrophilic dermatoses.
- Although rare, autoinflammatory disorders may in turn inform the understanding of more common cutaneous disorders, including the neutrophilic dermatoses.

INTRODUCTION

Pyoderma gangrenosum (PG) is a neutrophilic dermatosis marked by ulcerating skin lesions and a chronic or remitting disease course. Despite the recognition of this clinical entity almost 100 years ago by Brocq, the pathogenesis of PG remains poorly understood. Although recent research has begun to elucidate the pathogenesis and components involved in many neutrophilic dermatoses including PG, very little evidence exists that supports a rational therapeutic approach to this clinical entity.[1,2] To date, the conceptual framework of PG treatment has highlighted the equal importance of treating the inflammatory etiology of PG balanced with optimized wound care.[3] Often, multiple immunosuppressive agents are required to achieve remission or control over the progression of PG skin lesions; these agents target a broad array of inflammatory pathways likely involved in PG pathogenesis, including lymphocyte-directed therapy, neutrophil-directed therapy, and cytokine blockade. The broad nature of the available therapies, even in algorithmic format, reveals that there are still significant gaps in the current understanding of the disease.

[a] University of Arizona School of Medicine, 1510 N Campbell Avenue, PO Box 245017, Tucson, AZ 85724, USA;
[b] Department of Dermatology, University of California, San Francisco School of Medicine, 1701 Divisadero Street, 3rd Floor, San Francisco, CA 94115, USA
* Corresponding author.
E-mail address: shinkaik@derm.ucsf.edu

Dermatol Clin 31 (2013) 427–435
http://dx.doi.org/10.1016/j.det.2013.04.004
0733-8635/13/$ – see front matter © 2013 Elsevier Inc. All rights reserved.

Autoinflammatory diseases commonly present with cutaneous manifestations, and many disorders of autoinflammation specifically present with neutrophilic dermatoses; new information on the molecular and cellular pathways underlying autoinflammation thus provides great insights into the understanding of neutrophilic dermatoses, especially PG. This article aims to offer a fresh perspective on the pathogenesis of PG with a focus on emerging and convergent concepts in the pathophysiology of neutrophilic dermatoses and autoinflammation. Specifically, this article offers a series of observations on the natural history of PG, highlighting similarities between PG, other neutrophilic dermatoses, and autoinflammatory disorders, to elucidate key pathways and common connections between the disorders. These observations emphasize the relevance of studying rare autoinflammatory syndromes, as they in turn inform the understanding of more common skin disorders such as PG.

OBSERVATION 1—NEUTROPHILIC DERMATOSES, INCLUDING PG, OCCUR IN ASSOCIATION WITH A BROAD SPECTRUM OF SYSTEMIC DISORDERS

It is well established that many neutrophilic dermatoses, including PG, occur in association with a broad spectrum of systemic conditions, such as malignancy, neutropenia, rheumatologic disease, infection, autoinflammatory syndromes, and immunodeficiency, in addition to being triggered by medications and pathergy. A key question is how such disparate processes result in, or associate with the common phenotype of PG. A unifying hypothesis is that these diseases converge on inflammatory pathways leading to alterations in the recruitment of neutrophils or changes in neutrophil homeostasis; however, a definitive common pathway remains elusive (**Fig. 1A**). Recent research has highlighted numerous pathways that likely play a role in the inflammation of PG, which will be reviewed here. Ultimately, identifying and targeting common inflammatory pathways would maximize the clinical approach to this disorder.

OBSERVATION 2—NEUTROPHILIC DERMATOSES OCCUR IN THE SETTING OF INHERITED DISEASES OF AUTOINFLAMMATION

A significant advancement in the understanding of neutrophilic dermatoses has emerged from the observation that many autoinflammatory syndromes feature neutrophilic dermatoses and that these present across a broad spectrum of clinical and histopathologic phenotypes. Autoinflammatory diseases are defined as a distinct group of disorders that stem from dysregulation of the innate immune system, leading to chronic episodic systemic inflammation with end-organ damage, excessive cytokine production, and typically lacking features of autoimmunity such as autoreactive lymphocytes or autoantibodies. Disorders of autoinflammation commonly present with cutaneous manifestations.[2,4,5] In fact, several monogenic inherited diseases of and likely acquired autoinflammatory syndromes include neutrophilic infiltration patterns in skin, including erysipelas-like dermatoses in familial Mediterranean fever (FMF), neutrophilic urticaria in cryopyrin-associated periodic syndromes (CAPS), and pustular dermatosis in the deficiency of interleukin (IL) 1-receptor antagonist (DIRA) syndrome, among others. The recent elucidation of the genetic and cellular basis of autoinflammation, although rare, thus reveals molecular pathways potentially relevant to more common neutrophilic dermatoses.

Importantly, a notable inherited autoinflammatory syndrome features PG as 1 of its hallmark symptoms. The rare syndrome of pyogenic arthritis, pyoderma gangrenosum, and acne (PAPA) is associated with genetic mutations in the PSTPIP1 protein, resulting in excessive IL-1 signaling. PG lesions are an almost universal manifestation in patients with this syndrome, suggesting a key role for the IL-1 cytokine pathway in the pathogenesis of PG in at least a subset of patients. The recognition of IL-1 signaling pathways in PAPA syndrome has also greatly informed the treatment of this condition. IL-1 blockade has been shown to be an effective therapy for both bone and skin lesions in the syndrome of PAPA; Brenner and colleagues[6] reported successful treatment of PG in the setting of PAPA syndrome with the IL-1 blocking medication, anakinra. Additionally, treatment for this distinct class of diseases is largely directed at cytokine pathways such as tumor necrosis factor (TNF)-alpha and lymphocyte-directed therapy, including corticosteroids, methotrexate, and cyclosporine, suggesting additional putative mechanisms contributing to the pathogenesis of the disease.[6–8]

Use of an IL-1 receptor antagonist for the treatment of PG in PAPA syndrome exemplifies how recognizing the elevation of IL-1 stemming from PAPA mutations led to significant improvements in treating patients with this disease. IL-1 likely plays a central role in a number of diseases of autoinflammation. Emerging genetic information has illuminated that many of the genes underlying autoinflammatory disorders function within a common IL-1 signaling pathway; mutations in these genes

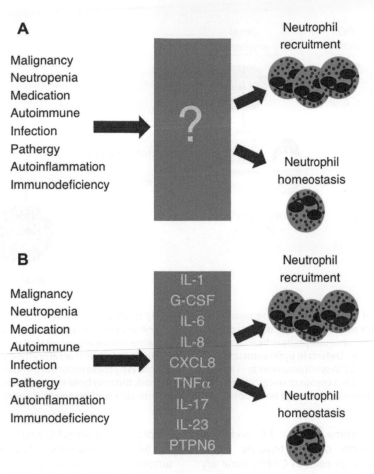

Fig. 1. (*A*) Observation: PG is associated with a broad spectrum of systemic disease processes. Do these diseases share common inflammatory pathways leading to neutrophil recruitment and/or neutrophil homeostasis that result in the making of a neutrophilic dermatosis? (*B*) Observation: the broad spectrum of systemic diseases associated with PG may shares common inflammatory pathways that lead to alterations in neutrophil recruitment and neutrophil homeostasis that result in the phenotype of PG on the skin. Certain disease processes may act through specific inflammatory mediators (eg, neutropenia may trigger IL-1 and G-CSF pathways) that result in neutrophilic infiltration into skin. Treatment of neutrophilic dermatoses seen in association with different underlying systemic processes may thus require therapeutic targeting of distinct inflammatory pathways.

converge on a common cellular phenotype of excessive IL-1 production. Specifically, cryopyrin, pyrin, PSTPIP1, and IL-1RA are the genes involved in CAPS, FMF, PAPA, and DIRA, respectively, all of which regulate IL-1 production (**Fig. 2**).[9–12] Stimulation of the cryopyrin inflammasome results in IL-1 production via the activation of caspase-1 or IL-1 converting enzyme, a protease that cleaves and activates an inactive pro-form of IL-1.[13–15] Mutations in cryopyrin, as seen in CAPS, enhance activity of the cryopyrin inflammasome and result in excess production of IL-1. The inflammasome is in turn regulated by pyrin, a protein associated with gene mutations leading to FMF, with subsequent constitutive activation of the inflammasome complex. Additionally, pyrin uniquely interacts with a key adaptor protein, PSTPIP1, whose mutations in

PAPA syndrome induce activation of pyrin, resulting in increased downstream IL-1 production.[16,17] Mutations in mechanisms designated to dampen IL-1 activity at the cell surface level, as seen in DIRA, result in constitutive activation of the IL-1 receptor. Thus the convergence of these mutations within a common IL-1 pathway and the observation that all of these disorders feature neutrophilic dermatoses as a cutaneous manifestation highlight the importance of the IL-1 signaling pathways in the pathogenesis of neutrophilic dermatoses seen in association with autoinflammation.

In spite of this unifying mechanism, what continues to elude researchers and clinicians is why different defects along the common molecular pathway lead to distinct cutaneous manifestations (see **Fig. 2**). For example, mutations in PSTPIP1

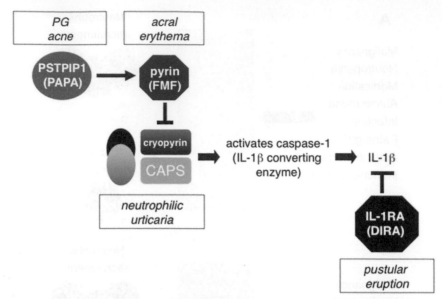

Fig. 2. Activation of the cryopyrin inflammasome results in IL-1β production through the activation of caspase 1. Mutations along this pathway result in distinct presentations of neutrophilic dermatoses on the skin. Defects in cryopyrin in CAPS results in neutrophilic urticaria, whereas PG and acne lesions are associated with PSTPIP1 mutations seen in PAPA syndrome. Defects in pyrin associated with FMF are associated with acral erythema, and the deficiency of IL-1R antagonist in DIRA syndrome results in a pustular eruption. Why these mutations in the IL-1 pathway differentially lead to distinct cutaneous manifestations is not understood, but may hold key information in the molecular determination of distinct patterns of neutrophilic infiltration into skin leading to neutrophilic dermatoses.

seen in PAPA syndrome result in PG and acne, whereas downstream defects typically induce neutrophilic urticaria as seen in CAPS, acral erythema in FMF, or the pustular eruption in DIRA. The differences in these cutaneous findings highlight a fundamental question that remains to be understood; the answer to this fundamental question may hold critical information to subtle differences in immunologic determinants that give rise to distinct presentations of neutrophilic dermatoses as a whole, for example, the molecular or cellular distinctions differentiating Sweet from pustular psoriasis from PG. How newly recognized autoinflammatory disorders featuring neutrophilic dermatoses, such as the deficiency of the IL-36 receptor antagonist (DITRA) or chronic atypical neutrophilic dermatosis with lipodystrophy and elevated temperature (CANDLE) syndromes, intersect with this important IL-1 signaling pathway remains to be seen, and likely will add intriguing new information to the understanding of this complex set of disorders.

OBSERVATION 3—PG IS ALSO ASSOCIATED WITH ACQUIRED AUTOINFLAMMATORY SKIN DISORDERS

Another emerging concept in the understanding of PG is that it occurs in association with likely acquired autoinflammatory disorders, such as

syndromes featuring PG and hidradenitis suppurativa (HS).[18–21] The notion that there exist acquired autoinflammatory disorders is not new, and notable examples include Still disease and Schnitzler syndrome, both associated with excessive IL-1 production with documented treatment response to IL-1 blockade.[22,23] HS is likely in itself an acquired autoinflammatory syndrome, as it features many of the hallmarks of autoinflammatory disorders: systemic inflammation with skin and joint inflammation, excessive cytokine production, fevers, elevated markers of systemic inflammation, and a neutrophilic dermatosis. The association between PG and HS has now been reported in the literature with clinical cases that detail various patterns of presentation. Hsiao and colleagues[20] reported an HS/PG overlap syndrome and noted both concordance and discordance in the patterns of HS and PG, in which PG lesions were seen both within and distinct from areas of HS. Some of the patients partially responded to IL-1R antagonist, specifically anakinra, and 2 patients went on to have complete remission with TNF blockade using infliximab (KS, personal observation). Another example of this association was recently reported by Braun-Falco and colleagues,[21] who described a likely related syndrome consisting of PG, acne, and HS, referred to as PASH. It is intriguing to note that the patient described by this latter group of investigators was found to have a microsatellite repeat motif within the PSTPIP1 gene, the gene associated with PAPA syndrome; the clinical relevance of this molecular finding has not yet been elucidated. The clinical response to IL-1 blockade and the potential aberration in the PSTPIP1 gene noted in these likely related disorders suggest a key role for the IL-1 pathway in this acquired form of autoinflammation.

Taken together, the many examples of inherited and acquired autoinflammatory syndromes suggest a vital role that IL-1 dysregulation may play in the pathogenesis of neutrophilic dermatoses and raise many key questions about the molecular pathways involved in neutrophilic dermatoses. Although rare, these cases of autoinflammation are important to study, because they clearly highlight molecular pathways that may have essential roles in PG pathogenesis.

OBSERVATION 4—PG RESPONDS TO A BROAD SPECTRUM OF CYTOKINE BLOCKADE

It is important to observe that PG responds to blockade of a broad spectrum of cytokine pathways. To date, there is a wealth of literature on the efficacy of TNF-αblockade for the treatment of PG, and new literature supports the beneficial effects of IL-23 blockade. Based on the observation that IL-23 is elevated in a case of PG, there are now several case reports over the past 2 years on the role of ustekinumab (which targets the p40 subunit of IL-23) as a therapeutic option.[24-26] There have been 3 reports of successful use of ustekinumab for PG, including 1 case of peri-stomal PG. Although successful in all cases, there was delayed onset of efficacy. In 2 of the cases, patients did not see evidence of healing until week 4, and in another case, there was no evidence of healing until week 8.[25,26] Although questions remain regarding the IL-23 blockade approach, its reported success highlights a potentially important pathway and therapeutic target for PG.

Additional cytokine pathways, including IL-1β and IL-6, may represent important alternative therapeutic targets for the treatment of common PG. Although it is promising to broaden the treatment options for PG, it also highlights a perplexing aspect of PG pathogenesis: why do some cases of PG respond to certain cytokine blockade, whereas other cases of PG respond to distinct cytokine blockade? Whether this represents divergent pathways in the underlying etiology, and whether these cytokine pathways represent bona fide autoinflammation, remain unknown. Although this expanding palette of treatment options brings hope for clinicians and patients dealing with PG, identification of strategies to clearly define which cytokine pathway is most relevant for any given patient's disease is paramount.

OBSERVATION 5—NEUTROPHILIC DERMATOSES OCCUR IN THE SETTING OF NEUTROPENIA

This paradoxic observation is common in neutrophilic dermatoses such as Sweet syndrome and also in some cases of PG. Neutropenia may be associated with neutrophilic dermatoses in the setting of myelodysplasia, hematologic malignancies, bone marrow transplant patients, and even in medication-induced neutrophilic dermatoses. Although this connection is not fully understood, it is intriguing to speculate whether neutropenia triggers (or subverts) mechanisms of neutrophil recruitment or neutrophil homeostasis that may give rise to neutrophilic dermatoses.

One critical homeostatic pathway involved in bone marrow replacement that may have a key role in the pathogenesis of neutrophilic dermatoses is granulocyte colony-stimulating factor (G-CSF). To date, several reports in the literature have implicated a role for both endogenous and exogenous G-CSF in association with neutrophilic dermatoses.[27-29] Perhaps the most eloquent details of the development of neutrophilic dermatoses in the setting of neutropenia was reported by Uhara and colleagues,[27] who described a patient after induction chemotherapy for Acute Myeloid Leukemia with a striking correlation between the development of neutrophilic dermatoses and endogenous serum G-CSF levels. With the onset of leukopenia, the rise of endogenous G-CSF was associated with the appearance of skin manifestations, initially with folliculitis, and later with nodules consistent with Sweet syndrome. The resolution of these skin lesions also corresponded to falling G-CSF levels.[27] This report suggests that homeostatic mechanisms triggered by neutropenia, such as inflammatory cytokines resulting in bone marrow recruitment and perhaps even fever, may, in certain circumstances, result in neutrophilic dermatoses. Why these neutrophils home to skin and other organs—as many cases of extracutaneous neutrophilic infiltrations have also been described including Sweet syndrome and PG—is not clearly understood. Whether this represents a phenomenon of locus minoris resistentiae, pathergy, or stochastic determination remains unknown.

Perhaps the clearest examples of the association between G-CSF and neutrophilic dermatoses are the common cases of exogenous G-CSF triggering skin conditions such as PG and Sweet syndrome.[28] Impaired clearance of iatrogenic G-CSF may represent 1 proposed mechanism of why this phenomenon occurs. Whereas first-generation G-CSF, filgrastim, a relatively small molecule (18.8 kDa) with a half-life of 3.4 hours, is cleared via renal and neutrophil receptor-mediated mechanisms, newer pegylated forms, such as pegfilgrastim (38.8 kDa), are too large for renal clearance and rely solely on neutrophil receptor-mediated clearance. The resulting half-life of pegylated forms is much longer: 33 hours or 10 times longer than that of filgrastim.[28] With the longer half-life secondary to altered clearance patterns, the question arises if newer pegylated forms of G-CSF increase the risk of neutrophilic dermatoses in the setting of prolonged neutropenia due to elevated G-CSF levels.

Elevated serum or tissue levels of G-CSF may have significant impact on patterns of neutrophil recruitment and neutrophil homeostasis. In vivo, G-CSF derives from vascular endothelium, fibroblasts, and macrophages when triggered by activated T cells and interleukins. Once elaborated, its most important effects are on the bone marrow, where it stimulates proliferation and differentiation of CD34+ stem cell precursors, and also in the periphery, where it activates neutrophils, promotes phagocytosis and superoxide generation, and suppresses apoptosis. The effects of the molecule thus likely play a crucial role in peripheral granulocyte replacement in the setting of leukopenia and also in neutrophil recruitment in infection and inflammation, but what happens when this important homeostatic mechanism is enhanced by G-CSF toxicity?

One hypothesis is that high levels of either endogenous or exogenous G-CSF can result in neutrophilic dermatoses due to its promotion of a series of physiologic aberrations, including escalated neutrophil recruitment and abnormal neutrophil function. High G-CSF levels cause endothelium to migrate and proliferate, as well as induce cytokines such as IL-1β and TNFαthat can trigger subsequent inflammatory pathways that may recruit neutrophils or promote aberrant neutrophil responses. In bone marrow, high G-CSF levels result in the release of immature granulocyte precursors. Neutrophil functioning itself is altered in that the cells have different chemotactic and adherence patterns through changes in surface expression triggered by high levels of G-CSF. Additionally, neutrophil apoptosis is delayed, and phagocytosis is enhanced.[30,31]

Thus the setting of neutropenia offers multiple risk factors to the development of neutrophilic dermatoses:

Neutropenia triggers normal homeostatic mechanisms for neutrophil replacement

G-CSF concentrations rise and potentially alter neutrophil recruitment and functioning

When medical intervention is required, exogenous G-CSF is given to patients

The effects of exogenous G-CSF (especially pegylated forms) may be potentiated through the impairment of normal clearance mechanisms in the setting of neutropenia

The pathways highlighted by this paradoxic clinical scenario may play a common role in the pathogenesis of neutrophilic dermatoses. It is also important to note that in cases of medication-induced neutropenia resulting in Sweet syndrome, G-CSF and additional pathways, including IL-6, IL-1, and IL-3 were identified as having a putative role in the development of neutrophilic dermatosis.[32–34]

OBSERVATION 6—T CELLS LIKELY PLAY A KEY ROLE IN ORCHESTRATING NEUTROPHILIC DERMATOSES

New literature has highlighted the role of certain T cell subsets as mediators in the formation of neutrophilic dermatoses. One study looked at the roles of CXCL8+, CCR6+, CD4+ T cells associated with neutrophilic infiltrates in acute generalized exanthematous pustulosis (AGEP), pustular psoriasis, and Behcet disease.[35] Although a causal association between the T cells and the neutrophilic infiltrate could not be ascertained by these histopathologic studies, it was noted that this T helper subset did not express typical Th1 or Th2 cytokine profiles. It is intriguing to speculate whether this T helper subset may represent Th17 cells; a recentlyrecognized T helper subset implicated in a number of neutrophilic dermatoses, including pustular psoriasis.[36] Highlighting an important role for certain T helper subsets in the orchestration of neutrophilic dermatoses is intuitively appealing, as it is well-known that lymphocyte-directed treatments such as cyclosporine and mycophenolate mofetil are effective for the treatment of this class of skin disorders.

OBSERVATION 7—OTHER SIGNALING PATHWAYS INVOLVED IN NEUTROPHIL RECRUITMENT OR HOMEOSTASIS MAY PLAY A KEY ROLE IN NEUTROPHILIC DERMATOSES

Several reports have suggested a role for defective signaling pathways involved in neutrophil recruitment or homeostasis in the pathogenesis of neutrophilic dermatoses. Nord and colleagues[37] recently described a patient with leukocyte adhesion deficiency, an immunodeficiency stemming from defects in CD18, a key neutrophil homing receptor, who developed a large PG lesion. Another recent report suggests the role of tyrosine phosphatase nonreceptor type 6, PTPN6, another key signaling molecule likely implicated in neutrophil recruitment and homeostasis, in the pathogenesis of neutrophilic dermatoses. A mouse model with impaired PTPN6 function gives rise to marked neutrophilic infiltration into the skin, blood, lungs, and spleen stemming from signaling defects leading to a failure of neutrophil apoptosis.[38] The role of this gene was examined in a human population looking at 23 patients with PG and Sweet syndrome. Whereas only 1 patient with a familial autoinflammatory disorder had a heterozygous mutation of PTPN6, 50% of the subjects had abnormalities in transcriptional regulation or gene splice variants in this gene in comparison to healthy controls. Nesterovitch and colleagues[38] concluded that transcriptional regulation of PTPN6 plays a key role in the pathogenesis of neutrophilic dermatoses, but how this occurs remains unknown.

OBSERVATION 8—A BROAD SPECTRUM OF THERAPEUTIC TARGETS EXISTS AS THE MAINSTAY OF PG TREATMENT

Reviewing the PG treatment literature highlights the role of many immunologic components (cytokines, neutrophils, and lymphocytes) as potentially relevant therapeutic targets. The treatment course of PG is notoriously challenging, and different patients require either distinct treatment strategies (neutrophil-directed vs lymphocyte-directed vs cytokine-directed) or a combined treatment regimen targeting multiple inflammatory pathways. Additional review of the pathogenesis literature as described highlights common inflammatory pathways, including those of autoinflammation, that converge on known cellular functions leading to alterations in neutrophil recruitment and/or neutrophil homeostasis: IL-1, IL-6, TNFα, IL-23, CXCL8, PTPN6 (see **Fig. 1B**). It is intriguing to consider the possibility that there exist different subsets of PG disease, for example, subsets of neutrophilic dermatoses in which particular inflammatory pathways play a more significant role. Furthermore, this may explain the original query of why such seemingly disparate systemic processes (ie, hematologic malignancy, neutropenia, medications, connective tissue disease) give rise to the common phenotype of PG on the skin. For example, in neutropenia, a failing bone marrow must elaborate G-CSF and IL-1 to recruit more neutrophils. In connective tissue disease, IL-1 may be elevated, and T cell subsets and their chemokines such as CXCL8 may play a

key role in orchestrating neutrophilic recruitment into sites of inflammation. In infections and possibly also pathergy, acute-phase reactants and other early inflammatory pathways elaborate IL-1, IL-6, and IL-8, which augment early neutrophil recruitment. In autoinflammation, highly selective pathways such as IL-1β may be the cause of symptoms. Taken together, each systemic process may trigger common mechanisms and inflammatory mediators involved in the qualitative or quantitative aspects of neutrophil biology that give rise to neutrophilic dermatoses. In the future, treatment may be directed at understanding specific pathways that are most relevant to any given patient, and treatment algorithms will be clarified or determined by which inflammatory pathways prevail.

SUMMARY

Neutrophilic dermatoses are a complex class of cutaneous disorders for which the pathogenesis and evidence for treatment remain to be elucidated. Although the literature implicates many distinct inflammatory pathways involved in the development of neutrophilic dermatoses such as PG, recent data highlight the role of certain common pathways that may prevail and also explain the well-established association of PG with a broad spectrum of systemic disorders. Although likely not exclusively an autoinflammatory disorder, PG shares many features with diseases of autoinflammation, including the chronic remitting course, dysregulation of the innate immune system including neutrophils, and a role for excessive cytokine production. Many key questions remain unanswered, but the elucidation of autoinflammatory syndromes may yield critical insights into the molecular and cellular pathways that give rise to neutrophilic dermatoses, as well as answers to the factors that give rise to distinct cutaneous presentations of neutrophilic dermatoses. Thus the study of autoinflammatory syndromes, although rare, is a worthwhile endeavor to inform the understanding and treatment of more common skin diseases such as PG.

REFERENCES

1. Ahronowitz I, Harp J, Shinkai K. Etiology and management of pyoderma gangrenosum: a comprehensive review. Am J Clin Dermatol 2012;13(3): 191–211.
2. Brydges S, Kastner DL. The systemic autoinflammatory diseases: inborn errors of the innate immune system. Curr Top Microbiol Immunol 2006; 305:127–60.

3. Bennett ML, Jackson JM, Jorizzo JL, et al. Pyoderma gangrenosum. A comparison of typical and atypical forms with an emphasis on time to remission. Case review of 86 patients from 2 institutions. Medicine (Baltimore) 2000;79(1):37–46.

4. Farasat S, Aksentijevich I, Toro JR. Autoinflammatory diseases: clinical and genetic advances. Arch Dermatol 2008;144(3):392–402.

5. Simon A, van der Meer JW. Pathogenesis of familial periodic fever syndromes or hereditary autoinflammatory syndromes. Am J Physiol Regul Integr Comp Physiol 2007;292(1):R86–98.

6. Brenner M, Ruzicka T, Plewig G, et al. Targeted treatment of pyoderma gangrenosum in PAPA (pyogenic arthritis, pyoderma gangrenosum and acne) syndrome with the recombinant human interleukin-1 receptor antagonist anakinra. Br J Dermatol 2009; 161(5):1199–201.

7. Tofteland ND, Shaver TS. Clinical efficacy of etanercept for treatment of PAPA syndrome. J Clin Rheumatol 2010;16(5):244–5.

8. Demidowich AP, Freeman AF, Kuhns DB, et al. Brief report: genotype, phenotype, and clinical course in five patients with PAPA syndrome (pyogenic sterile arthritis, pyoderma gangrenosum, and acne). Arthritis Rheum 2012;64(6):2022–7.

9. Aksentijevich I, Masters SL, Ferguson PJ, et al. An autoinflammatory disease with deficiency of the interleukin-1-receptor antagonist. N Engl J Med 2009;360(23):2426–37.

10. Shaw MH, Reimer T, Kim YG, et al. NOD-like receptors (NLRs): bona fide intracellular microbial sensors. Curr Opin Immunol 2008;20(4):377–82.

11. Church LD, Cook GP, McDermott MF. Primer: inflammasomes and interleukin 1beta in inflammatory disorders. Nat Clin Pract Rheumatol 2008; 4(1):34–42.

12. Ting JP, Kastner DL, Hoffman HM. CATERPILLERs, pyrin and hereditary immunological disorders. Nat Rev Immunol 2006;6(3):183–95.

13. Contassot E, Beer HD, French LE. Interleukin-1, inflammasomes, autoinflammation and the skin. Swiss Med Wkly 2012;142:w13590.

14. Shinkai K, Kilcline C, Connolly MK, et al. The pyrin family of fever genes: unmasking genetic determinants of autoinflammatory disease. Arch Dermatol 2005;141(2):242–7.

15. Zeft AS, Spalding SJ. Autoinflammatory syndromes: fever is not always a sign of infection. Cleve Clin J Med 2012;79(8):569–81.

16. Shoham NG, Centola M, Mansfield E, et al. Pyrin binds the PSTPIP1/CD2BP1 protein, defining familial Mediterranean fever and PAPA syndrome as disorders in the same pathway. Proc Natl Acad Sci U S A 2003;100(23):13501–6.

17. Yu JW, Fernandes-Alnemri T, Datta P, et al. Pyrin activates the ASC pyroptosome in response to engagement by autoinflammatory PSTPIP1 mutants. Mol Cell 2007;28(2):214–27.

18. Shenefelt PD. Pyoderma gangrenosum associated with cystic acne and hidradenitis suppurativa controlled by adding minocycline and sulfasalazine to the treatment regimen. Cutis 1996;57(5):315–9.

19. Ah-Weng A, Langtry JA, Velangi S, et al. Pyoderma gangrenosum associated with hidradenitis suppurativa. Clin Exp Dermatol 2005;30(6):669–71.

20. Hsiao JL, Antaya RJ, Berger T, et al. Hidradenitis suppurativa and concomitant pyoderma gangrenosum: a case series and literature review. Arch Dermatol 2010;146(11):1265–70.

21. Braun-Falco M, Kovnerystyy O, Lohse P, et al. Pyoderma gangrenosum, acne, and suppurative hidradenitis (PASH)–a new autoinflammatory syndrome distinct from PAPA syndrome. J Am Acad Dermatol 2012;66(3):409–15.

22. Fleischmann R. Anakinra in the treatment of rheumatic disease. Expert Rev Clin Immunol 2006;2(3): 331–40.

23. Krause K, Weller K, Stefaniak R, et al. Efficacy and safety of the interleukin-1 antagonist rilonacept in Schnitzler syndrome: an open-label study. Allergy 2012;67(7):943–50.

24. Guenova E, Teske A, Fehrenbacher B, et al. Interleukin 23 expression in pyoderma gangrenosum and targeted therapy with ustekinumab. Arch Dermatol 2011;147(10):1203–5.

25. Goldminz AM, Botto NC, Gottlieb AB. Severely recalcitrant pyoderma gangrenosum successfully treated with ustekinumab. J Am Acad Dermatol 2012;67(5):e237–8.

26. Fahmy M, Ramamoorthy S, Hata T, et al. Ustekinumab for peristomal pyoderma gangrenosum. Am J Gastroenterol 2012;107(5):794–5.

27. Uhara H, Saida T, Nakazawa H, et al. Neutrophilic dermatoses with acute myeloid leukemia associated with an increase of serum colony-stimulating factor. J Am Acad Dermatol 2008;59(2 Suppl 1):S10–2.

28. Draper BK, Robbins JB, Stricklin GP. Bullous Sweet's syndrome in congenital neutropenia: association with pegfilgrastim. J Am Acad Dermatol 2005; 52(5):901–5.

29. Kawakami T, Ohashi S, Kawa Y, et al. Elevated serum granulocyte colony-stimulating factor levels in patients with active phase of sweet syndrome and patients with active behcet disease: implication in neutrophil apoptosis dysfunction. Arch Dermatol 2004;140(5):570–4.

30. Spiekermann K, Roesler J, Emmendoerffer A, et al. Functional features of neutrophils induced by G-CSF and GM-CSF treatment: differential effects and clinical implications. Leukemia 1997;11(4):466–78.

31. von den Driesch P. Sweet's syndrome (acute febrile neutrophilic dermatosis). J Am Acad Dermatol 1994; 31(4):535–56 [quiz: 557–60].

32. Hasegawa M, Sato S, Nakada M, et al. Sweet's syndrome associated with granulocyte colony-stimulating factor. Eur J Dermatol 1998;8(7):503–5.

33. Bidyasar S, Montoya M, Suleman K, et al. Sweet syndrome associated with granulocyte colony-stimulating factor. J Clin Oncol 2008;26(26):4355–6.

34. Reuss-Borst MA, Pawelec G, Saal JG, et al. Sweet's syndrome associated with myelodysplasia: possible role of cytokines in the pathogenesis of the disease. Br J Haematol 1993;84(2):356–8.

35. Keller M, Spanou Z, Schaerli P, et al. T cell-regulated neutrophilic inflammation in autoinflammatory diseases. J Immunol 2005;175(11):7678–86.

36. Fischer-Stabauer M, Boehner A, Eyerich S, et al. Differential in situ expression of IL-17 in skin diseases. Eur J Dermatol 2012;22(6):781–4.

37. Nord KM, Pappert AS, Grossman ME. Pyoderma gangrenosum-like lesions in leukocyte adhesion deficiency I treated with intravenous immunoglobulin. Pediatr Dermatol 2011;28(2): 156–61.

38. Nesterovitch AB, Gyorfy Z, Hoffman MD, et al. Alteration in the gene encoding protein tyrosine phosphatase nonreceptor type 6 (PTPN6/SHP1) may contribute to neutrophilic dermatoses. Am J Pathol 2011;178(4):1434–41.

Role of Interleukin 1 in Atopic Dermatitis

William Abramovits, MD[a,b,c,d],
Joaquin J. Rivas Bejarano, MD[e,f,*],
Wendell C. Valdecantos, MD[e]

KEYWORDS

- Atopic dermatitis • Interleukin 1 • Inflammasome • T cells • Eczema • Mononuclear cells
- Neutrophils • Cytokines

KEY POINTS

- Interleukin 1 (Il-1) ligands
- Signal transduction patterns of Il-1 receptors
- Inflammasome-mediated inflammation
- IL-1 activation by inflammasome
- Naturally occurring antagonists
- IL-1/IL-1 receptor antagonist balance
- Role of IL-1 in atopic dermatitis

OVERVIEW OF INTERLEUKIN 1

Interleukin-1 (IL-1) is a potent inflammatory cytokine that plays a central role in the innate immune response.[1] Discovered in the 1970s, it was initially named lymphocyte-activating factor, catabolin, and endogenous pyrogen because of its proinflammatory effects.[2] IL-1 mediates the acute phase of inflammation by inducing local and systemic responses, such as pain sensitivity, fever, vasodilation, and hypotension. It also promotes the expression of adhesion molecules on endothelial cells, which allows the infiltration of inflammatory and immunocompetent cells into the tissues.[3]

IL-1 is secreted mainly by monocytes, tissue macrophages, and dendritic cells, but is also expressed by B lymphocytes, natural killer (NK) cells, and epithelial cells.[4] In the epidermis, IL-1 is produced by keratinocytes under the stimulation of proinflammatory cytokines, with the stratum corneum serving as a major reservoir of active IL-1. The release of IL-1 from the epidermis after activation is a primary event that promotes inflammatory skin conditions through the induction of various cytokines, proinflammatory mediators, and adhesion molecules.[5,6]

IL-1: An Extensive Family of Ligands

IL-1 belongs to a family of ligands and receptors.[7] The classic members IL-1α and IL-1β mediate their biological responses via activation of the IL-1 receptor type I, which is expressed by almost all cell types. The IL-1 receptor antagonist (IL-1Ra), the third member of the IL-1 family, has antiinflammatory activity because of its ability to bind to IL-1

Disclosures: Drs Joaquin Rivas and Wendell Valdecantos are employees of AbbVie.

[a] Department of Medicine, Baylor University Hospital and Texas A&M Medical School, 3500 Gaston Avenue, Dallas, TX 75246, USA; [b] Department of Dermatology, University of Texas Southwestern Medical School, 5323 Harry Hines Boulevard, Dallas, TX 75235, USA; [c] Department of Family Practice, University of Texas Southwestern Medical School, 5323 Harry Hines Boulevard, Dallas, TX 75235, USA; [d] Dermatology Treatment & Research Center, 5310 Harvest Hill Road, Dallas, TX 75230, USA; [e] Global Medical Affairs, Immunology, AbbVie, 1 North Waukegan Road North, Chicago, IL 60064, USA; [f] Biology Department, LoneStar College, 2700 WW Thorne Drive, WN Building #210, Houston, TX 77073, USA
* Corresponding author. 3510 London Lane, Missouri City, TX 77459.
E-mail address: Bejarano.0214@yahoo.com

Dermatol Clin 31 (2013) 437–444
http://dx.doi.org/10.1016/j.det.2013.04.008

receptor type I, thus preventing the binding of the proinflammatory molecules IL-1α and IL-1β.[4]

With the ongoing discovery of the mechanisms and pathways of inflammation, receptor response, and cytokine expression, the IL-1 family has expanded to the current 11 members shown in **Table 1**. The IL-1R family has also expanded to 9 distinct genes and includes coreceptors, decoy receptors, binding proteins, and inhibitory receptors.[8]

For some investigators, the properties of IL-1 still remain the model for mediating inflammation, describing IL-1 as capable of initiating its action by binding to the ligand-binding chain (IL-1RI), following a series of events that includes recruitment of the coreceptor chain (accessory protein or IL-1RAcP). As a consequence, a complex is formed of IL-1RI plus IL-1 plus the coreceptor, initiating the signal by recruitment of the adaptor protein MyD88 to the Toll-IL-1 receptor (TIR) domain. This concept established the share of functions by different cytokines that attach to the same type of receptors, which is followed by the phosphorylation of several kinases, the nuclear factor (NF) kappa light chain enhancer of activated B cells (NF-κB) translocates to the nucleus, and the expression of a large range of inflammatory genes takes place.

Signal transduction in IL-1–stimulated cells has been reviewed in detail by Weber and colleagues[9] with similar statements and conclusions. IL-33, a cytokine with high level of involvement in atopic dermatitis (AD) immunopathogenesis, has been included in the IL-1 family of ligands. IL-33 binds to ST2, a member of the TIR superfamily that does not activate NF-κB and has been suggested as an important effector molecule of T-helper type 2 (Th2) cell responses; it also recruits the IL-1RAcP. T-helper type 2 (Th2)–like properties characterize IL-33. The 6 proinflammatory members of the IL-1 family each recruit the IL-1RAcP coreceptor with the TIR domain and MyD88 docks to each, making their pathogenic action a common mechanism. IL-1Ra, IL-1α, and IL-1β have a similar affinity to IL-1RI. The IL-1 ligands, their coreceptors, and main properties are presented in **Table 1**.[1,10,11]

From this perspective, the expression of IL-1 receptor stimulation has complex implications: ligands mediate their biological responses via activation of specific receptors and share the target for the immunoglobuline (Ig)-like receptor binder, where all ligands can stimulate the IL-1 receptor. This characteristic is unique for the IL-1 family of receptors because of the presence of the TIR domain in the cytoplasmic segment of each member in this class.

Particular attention should be given to IL-37 and IL-33, because of their capacity to interact with the IL-1 receptor and to translocate directly to the nucleus. These unique ligands of the IL-1 family, on interaction with the IL-1 receptor, function as proinflammatory (IL-33) and as antiinflammatory (IL-37) cytokines, which is a special property of the ligands, working as a guarantee of the inflammatory response; for example, expression of the N-terminal amino acids of IL-1α stimulates IL-8 production in the presence of complete blockade of the IL-1RI on the cell surface. Because of this property, the ligands mentioned earlier were named by Dinarello and colleagues[8] as dual-function cytokines.

With the exception of IL-1Ra, each member of the IL-1 family is first synthesized as a precursor without a clear signal peptide for processing and

Table 1
The IL-1 receptor family of ligands

Name	Receptor	Coreceptor	Property
IL-1α	IL-1R1	IL-1RacP	Proinflammatory
IL-1β	IL-1R1	IL-1RacP	Proinflammatory
IL-1Ra	IL-1R1	NA	Antagonist IL-1α and β
IL-18	IL-18Rα	IL-18Rβ	Proinflammatory
IL-36Ra	IL-1Rp2	NA	Antagonist IL-36α, β, γ
IL-36α	IL-1Rp2	IL-1RAcP	Proinflammatory
IL-37	IL-18Rα	Unknown	Antiinflammatory
IL-36β	IL-1Rp2	IL-1RAcP	Proinflammatory
IKL-36γ	IL-1Rp2	Unknown	Proinflammatory
IL-38	Unknown	IL-1RAcP	Unknown
IL-33	ST2	IL-1RAcP	Th2 Response, Proinflammatory

Abbreviations: IL-1RI, type 1 interleukin 1 ligand–binding chain; IL-1RAcP, interleukin 1 receptor accessory protein coreceptor chain; IL-1Rp, interleukin 1 receptor protein; IL-1Ra, interleukin 1 receptor antagonist.

secretion, and none are found in the Golgi apparatus. IL-1α and IL-33 are similar in that their precursor forms can bind to their respective receptor and trigger signal transduction; both have a dual function: in addition to binding to their respective cell surface receptors, the intracellular precursor forms translocate to the nucleus and influence transcription, and their nuclear function is transcription of proinflammatory genes. IL-37 is a unique ligand in the IL-1 family because it functions as an antiinflammatory cytokine; activation of this cytokine generates a net decrease in inflammation.[11–14] **Fig. 1** shows a summary of Il-1 receptor signaling and includes all activation details for each member of the IL-1 receptor family, as proposed by Dinarello and colleagues[8] in 2009 with some additions based on the latest discoveries.[7]

Characterization of Il-1

IL-1α is a unique member of the cytokine family synthesized as a precursor protein Pro-IL-1α, with the mature form resulting from the removal of N-terminal amino acids. Both Pro-IL-1α and mature IL-1α are biologically active.[8] IL-1α expression can promote local inflammation by functioning both as secreted and membrane-bound proteins.[15]

Other publications assign proinflammatory properties of IL-1α in connection to the development of atherosclerotic vascular disease.[16]

IL-1β is the best-studied cytokine of the IL-1 family; it plays a central role in defensive mechanisms against pathogens. However, its expression can be triggered by a variety of host-derived or environmental cellular stressors, including skin

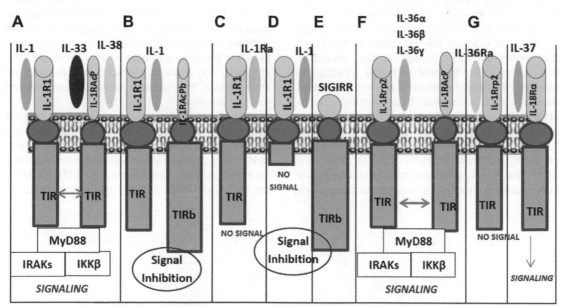

Fig. 1. Signaling patterns for the IL-1 ligands. (A) IL-1/IL-1RI/IL-1RAcP/IL-33 binding. Formation of the receptor heterodimeric complex. The TIR domain of each receptor chain recruits MyD88, followed by phosphorylation of IL-1R–associated kinases (IRAKs) and inhibitor of NFB kinase (IKK), resulting in a signal to the nucleus. (B) Formation of the hemodymeric complex (brain and spinal cord) between the variant IL-1RAcPb and IL-1 or IL-1 and IL-1RI. This complex fails to recruit MyD88, and there is inhibition of the IL-1 signal. The failure to recruit MyD88 may be because of an altered TIR domain (TIRb). (C) IL-1Ra binds to IL-1RI, but there is no signal because there is failure to form a complex with IL-1RAcP. (D) IL-1 binds to the IL-1RII but, lacking a cytoplasmic segment, there is no signal. (E) Because of an altered TIR domain (indicated as TIRb), SIGIRR inhibits IL-1 and TLR signaling. SIGIRR can form a complex with IL-33 (not shown) and inhibit IL-33 signaling. (F) IL-1Rrp2 binds IL-36, IL-36, or IL-36 and forms a complex with IL-1RAcP. The TIR domain of each receptor chain approximates and recruits MyD88. (G) IL-36Ra binds to IL-1Rrp2 but fails to form a complex with IL-1RAcP. Thus, IL-36Ra prevents the binding of IL-36, IL-36, or IL-36 to IL-1Rrp2, and IL-36Ra is the natural receptor antagonist IL-36. IKK, inhibitor of NFB kinase; IL-1-Ra, interleukin 1 receptor antagonist; IL-1RAcP, interleukin 1 receptor accessory protein coreceptor chain; IL-1RI, type 1 interleukin 1 ligand-binding chain; IL-1Rp, interleukin 1 receptor protein; MyD88, intracellular adaptor protein; SIGIRR, single IL-1–related receptor; TIR, Toll-IL-1 receptor domain; TIRb, altered TIR domain; TLR, Toll-like receptors. (*Data from* Dinarello CA. Interleukin-1 in the pathogenesis and treatment of inflammatory diseases. Blood 2011;117(14):3720–32; and Dinarello CA. Immunologic and inflammatory functions of the interleukin-1 family. Annu Rev Immunol 2009;27:519–50.)

irritants. It had been mentioned as mediator of inflammatory responses by supporting T-cell survival, upregulating the IL-2 receptor on lymphocytes, enhancing antibody production of B cells, and promoting B-cell proliferation and T-helper 17 cell differentiation. Recent studies have suggested that IL-1β does not only induce urticarial rashes in autoinflammatory diseases but is also important in the expression of other allergy-related diseases such as bronchial asthma, contact hypersensitivity, and AD.[1]

IL-1 and Inflammasome-mediated Inflammation

The expression of IL-1β from cells requires NF-κB–mediated transcriptional upregulation of pro–IL-1β and caspase-1–driven conversion of pro–IL-1β into its active form. Caspase-1 activity is controlled by a cytosolic multiprotein complex or activation scaffold, also known as the inflammasome.[1]

The complex detects pathogens and danger signals and induces the activation of the proinflammatory cytokines, which, in turn, attract inflammatory cells to deal with the infection or stressor. In autoinflammatory as well as allergic diseases such as contact hypersensitivity, bronchial asthma, and AD, dysfunctional inflammasome processing has been shown to account for IL-1β–induced inflammation. It is an IL-1 activating platform; cryopyrin (NLRP3, NLRP1), IPAF, and AIM2, are the key pathways to produce its activation, and have a role as key molecules in regulating

the inflammatory cytokine processing platform. **Fig. 2** shows a model proposed by Goldbach-Mansky[17] of the mechanisms mentioned earlier. Cryopyrin, apoptosis speck protein (ASC), cardinal, and 2 procaspase-1 molecules assemble to form the cryopyrin inflammasome that activates caspase-1. Active caspase-1 enzymatically cleaves inactive IL-1β into its active form.

The activation mechanisms of the inflammasome have been studied to determine what subfamilies of NOD receptors produce cytokine activation and release on presentation of different activators. At present, there are 4 accepted mechanisms for which the inflammasome is activated: NLRP3 (activated by several mechanisms, including extracellular ATP from the foreign invaders, crystal molecules engulfed by the phagocytes, secreting lysosomes detected by the inflammasome or activated reactive oxygen species [ROS]. The final product is membrane pore formation), NLRP1 (found in experimental murine models, by an undefined mechanism, assuming to have similar pathways than NLRP3), IPAF (activated by gram-negative bacteria with type III or IV secreting substances), and AIM2 (a cytosolic double-stranded DNA sensor that induces caspase-1–dependent IL-1β maturation).[18]

For the nucleotide-binding domain–like receptor protein 3 inflammasome (NLRP3), the most accepted and studied inflammasome, the pathway starts with cell activation via pattern recognition receptors such as Toll-like receptors (TLRs), leading to NF-kB–induced upregulation of pro–IL-1b

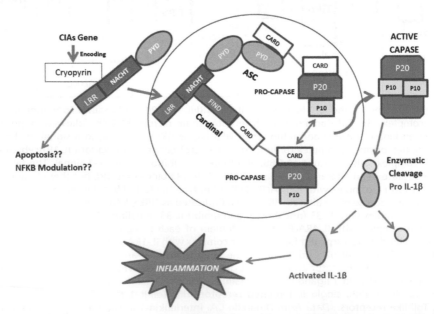

Fig. 2. Mechanism of inflammasome activation of IL-1. (*Adapted from* Goldbach-Mansky R. Blocking IL-1 in rheumatic diseases. Ann N Y Acad Sci 2009;1182:111–23; with permission.)

expression. Specific pathogen-associated molecular patterns (PAMPs) and danger-associated molecular patterns (DAMPs) can activate NLRP3, which, via recruitment of ASC and procaspase-1, results in assembly of the inflammasome. Procaspase-1 is cleaved into active caspase-1, which in turn promotes the processing of pro–IL-1β into the biologically active IL-1β. The major currently accepted models for NLRP3 inflammasome activation are presented in **Fig. 3**. The postulated mechanisms are not exclusive: the NLRP3 agonist, ATP, triggers P2X7-dependent pore formation by the pannexin-1 hemichannel,

allowing extracellular NLRP3 agonists to enter the cytosol and directly engage NLRP3. Crystalline or particulate NLRP3 agonists are engulfed, and their physical characteristics lead to lysosomal rupture. The NLRP3 inflammasome senses lysosomal content in the cytoplasm; for example, via cathepsin-B–dependent processing of a direct NLRP3 ligand. All DAMPs and PAMPs, including ATP and particulate/crystalline activators, trigger the generation of ROS. An ROS-dependent pathway triggers NLRP3 inflammasome complex formation. Caspase-1 clustering induces autoactivation and caspase-1–dependent maturation and

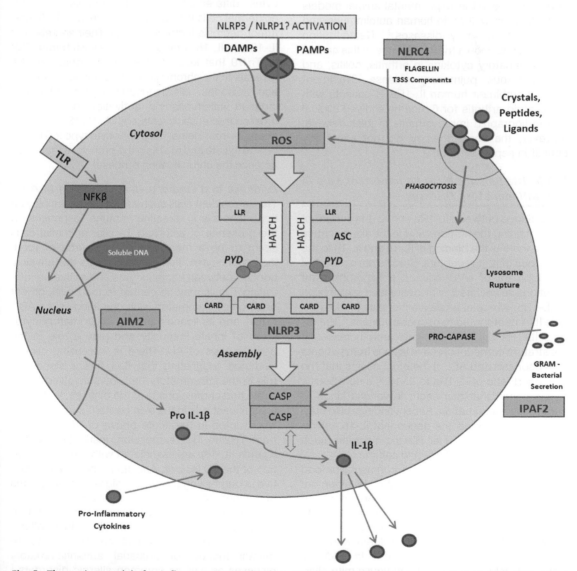

Fig. 3. The major models for inflammasome activation. CARD, N-terminal caspase recruitment; LRR, C-terminal leucine-rich repeats; NACHT, nucleotide-binding area oligomerization domain; NLR, Nodlike receptors; PPR, pattern recognition receptors; PYD, pyrin domains; ROS, reactive oxygen species. (*Data from* Schroder K, et al. The inflammasomes. Cell 2010;140:821–32.)

secretion of proinflammatory cytokines, such as IL-1b and IL-18.

Naturally Occurring Antagonists

IL-1Ra is the only known naturally occurring receptor antagonist. It competitively binds the IL-1 receptor to antagonize IL-1 activity without any agonist function.[5] There are 2 isoforms of IL-Ra: a secretory form (sIL-1Ra) and an intracellular form (icIL-1Ra). The sIL-1Ra is mainly secreted by activated monocytes, macrophages, and neutrophils, whereas the icIL-1Ra remains in the cytoplasm of keratinocytes and other epithelial cells, monocytes, and fibroblasts.[5,19] Endogenous IL-1Ra is expressed in experimental animal models of disease as well as in human autoimmune and chronic inflammatory diseases.[20] Neutralization of IL-1Ra has shown the importance of this natural antiinflammatory cytokine in arthritis, colitis, and granulomatous pulmonary disease. Treatment with recombinant human IL-1Ra in patients with rheumatoid arthritis for 6 months showed clinical and radiographic improvements in joint disease; however, the same therapy did not show any benefit in sepsis syndrome.[19]

IL-1/IL-1Ra Balance Plays an Important Role in Skin Inflammatory Diseases

The balance between IL-1Ra and IL-1 is important in maintaining the homeostasis in the skin because IL-1Ra inhibits the binding of IL-1α and IL-1β to the two types of IL-1 receptors. Studies have reported development of UVB-induced polymorphic light eruptions associated with decreased expression of IL-1Ra, whereas a relative increase in bioavailable IL-1 contributed to psoriasis vulgaris.[4] The ratio of IL-1Ra to IL-1α was significantly increased in the stratum corneum of active lesions from patients with psoriasis and AD.[5] It therefore seems that the increased ratio of IL-1Ra to IL-1α is a nonspecific phenomenon that can occur in various kinds of cutaneous inflammation. Recent findings also suggest that inflammasome-dependent IL-1β activation plays a role in other allergic disorders such as contact hypersensitivity and asthma.[1]

In AD, T-cell responses to environmental or food allergens are associated with the development and aggravation of the disease. An enhanced endogenous secretion of IL-1α leading to increased IL-2 activity in blood mononuclear cells following allergen exposure in children with food sensitive AD has been reported.[19] In addition, both ultraviolet B irradiation and house mite allergens have been shown to induce inflammasome-dependent IL-1b secretion from keratinocytes.[1] Staphylococcus aureus or herpes simplex virus infections are also correlated with disease exacerbation in AD. Hemolysis and bacterial lipoproteins from microbes can activate the NLRP3 inflammasome, leading to disease exacerbation in AD.[1]

Acute and Chronic Phases of immunoglobulin E and T-cell–mediated AD

In the acute phase of AD, Langerhans cells are activated on binding of allergens by means of specific immunoglobulin (Ig) E and FcϵRI. They produce monocyte chemotactic protein 1 (MCP-1) and IL-16. Allergen-derived peptides are presented to T cells by Langerhans cells that induce a Th2 profile. After migration into the skin, the recruited monocytes differentiate into inflammatory dendritic epidermal cells (IDEC) and produce IL-1, IL-6, and tumor necrosis factor α (TNF-α). Their secretion of IL-12 and IL-18 contributes to the switch from Th2 to Th1/0 that leads to the chronic phase of the disease. In the chronic phase and during exacerbation episodes, allergen-induced and pathogen-induced inflammasome activation become the most characteristic events, with IL-12/18 producing changes from Helper T Lymphocyte type 2 (TH2) to TH1 to initiate and maintain the pathways that characterize the chronification process.

Evidence that supports the role of IL-1 in AD
Tissue-resident cells such as keratinocytes play an important role in directing immune responses. In the presence of activated T cells, epithelial cells seem to be a more significant source of IL-1β than monocytes. IL-1 secretion and the physical contact between keratinocytes and activated infiltrating T cells may be central to the development of chronic inflammatory skin conditions such AD.[6]

IL-1 and its ligands are key inflammatory cytokines of innate immunity and play a role in the pathogenesis of AD. There is increasing clinical evidence suggesting that IL-1 has a significant role in the inflammatory pathways involved in the acute and chronic phase of the disease. IL-1 plays a significant role in the skin barrier function, which is disrupted in the acute phase of AD. Changes from TH2 to TH1 expression, instigated by IL-1 ligands (IL-18), are associated with the chronification of the AD lesions. Anti–IL-1 blockade is effective in depressing the clinical signs and symptoms of a variety of inflammatory disorders.

IL-1-neutralizing drugs have been shown to completely suppress or markedly reduce inflammatory responses in clinical studies and experimental models of urticarial autoinflammatory diseases as well as common allergic disorders.[1] In the United States, some IL-1–neutralizing drugs have been approved for use in specific inflammatory diseases, including anakinra (Kineret), a combinant human IL-1 receptor antagonist that binds to IL-1 receptor type 1 and that was approved by the US Food and Drug Administration (FDA) for the treatment of rheumatoid arthritis in 2001; rilonacept (Arcalyst), a soluble IL-1 receptor immunoglobulin recombinant human IL-1 receptor–immunoglobulin fusion protein that exerts its mechanism of action by binding to IL-1α and IL-1β and was approved by the FDA for the treatment of Cryopirin-associated periodic syndrome (CAPS) in February 2008; canakinumab (Ilaris), a humanized anti–IL-1β antibody that binds to IIL-1β and was approved by the FDA for the treatment of CAPS in July 2009. Other treatments include colchicine, TNF blockade, thalidomide, azathioprine, nonsteroidal antiinflammatory drugs, and corticosteroids.[17]

Important findings support the role of the inflammasome and IL-1β in autoinflammatory as well as allergic diseases such as AD. Dysfunctional inflammasome processing has been shown to account for IL-1β–induced inflammation, supporting the crucial role for IL-1β and inflammasomes in a variety of allergy-related disorders including AD.[1]

Watanabe and colleagues[21] conducted an in vivo/in vitro study to determine whether the inflammasome contributes to contact hypersensitivity (CS) or to eczema. The results show the involvement of IL-1β-processing inflammasome CS. The proinflammatory stimulus was caused by NALP3 inflammasome-dependent IL-1β production in the skin. In CS or in eczema, delayed-type hypersensitivities, the immune response depends on the concomitant activation of the innate and adaptive immune systems, including IL-1β/IL-18 activation in the skin.

There is an increase of IL-2 activity in mononuclear cells from patients with food-sensitive AD following allergen exposure. Soluble IL-2 receptor (sIL-2R) is an indirect marker of T-cell activation by IL-2; raised concentrations have been described in adults with AD. In vitro studies suggest that IL-2 secretion by TH cells is antigen driven and also dependent on IL-1 expression by cells of the macrophage/monocyte series. Some data suggest that IL-1 upregulates the expression of high-affinity receptors for IL-2 on TH1 cells. In addition, there is an enhanced endogenous secretion of IL-1α and increased stimulation of IL-2 receptors in children with AD.[19,22]

Transgenic mice expressing IL-18 from the keratin 5 promoter show many features of AD: acanthosis, a mixed inflammatory cell infiltrate, increased cytokine and chemokine expression, an infiltrate composed of eosinophils, neutrophils, and mast cells, increase in serum IgE levels, and increased B cells in the draining lymph node.

These findings suggest that IL-18 (an IL-1R ligand) is a causative cytokine for the typical clinical and histopathologic features of the chronic phase of AD.[23]

Rania and colleagues[24] recently published the results of a study including 20 atopic patients and 20 apparently healthy individuals serving as controls. Skin biopsies from all participants were examined for detection of IL-1β and 33. Both cytokines were significantly highly expressed in atopics, which could explain a role of both of them in the pathogenesis of atopy and in the trafficking of leucocytes during the inflammation caused by AD. The IL-33 receptor, consisting of ST2 and IL-1 receptor accessory protein, was widely expressed as well, particularly by Th2 cells and mast cells. IL-33 is host protective against helminthic infection by promoting Th2-type immune responses. IL-33 can also promote the pathogenesis of asthma by expanding Th2 cells and mediates joint inflammation, AD, and anaphylaxis by mast cell activation.

IL-33 seems to drive Th2 responses, suggesting roles in allergic and atopic diseases, as well as in fibrosis. IL-33 exerts its effects by activating the suppression of tumorigenicity 2 (ST2)/IL-1aR receptor on different types of cells, including mast cells and Th2 cells. The ST2 receptor is either expressed on the cell surface or shed from these cells (soluble ST2, sST2), thereby functioning as a decoy receptor. After binding to its receptor, IL-33 activates NF-kβ, suggesting that it regulates the outcome of diseases such as AD.[25]

In a study by Nutan and colleagues,[26] 45 subjects with AD were treated with betamethasone ointment and their IL-1β levels were measured before and following treatment. The IL-1β levels were increased in proportion to the severity of disease activity; following improvement they decreased in a statistically significant manner.

REFERENCES

1. Krause K, Metz M, Makris M, et al. The role of interleukin-1 in allergy-related disorders. Curr Opin Allergy Clin Immunol 2012;12(5):477–84.
2. O'Neill LA. The interleukin-1 receptor/Toll-like receptor superfamily: 10 years of progress. Immunol Rev 2008;226:10–8.
3. Contassot E, Beer HD, French LE. Interleukin-1, inflammasomes, autoinflammation and the skin. Swiss Med Wkly 2012;142:w13590.
4. Jensen LE. Targeting the IL-1 family members in skin inflammation. Curr Opin Investig Drugs 2010;11(11):1211–20.
5. Terui T, Hirao T, Sato Y, et al. An increased ratio of interleukin-1 receptor antagonist to interleukin-1

alpha in inflammatory skin diseases. Exp Dermatol 1998;7(6):327–34.

6. Renne J, Schäfer V, Werfel T, et al. Interleukin-1 from epithelial cells fosters T cell-dependent skin inflammation. Br J Dermatol 2010;162(6):1198–205.

7. Dinarello CA. Interleukin-1 in the pathogenesis and treatment of inflammatory diseases. Blood 2011; 117(14):3720–32.

8. Dinarello CA. Immunological and inflammatory functions of the interleukin-1 family. Annu Rev Immunol 2009;27:519–50.

9. Weber A, Wasiliew P, Kracht M. Interleukin-1 (IL-1) pathway. Sci Signal 2010;3:cm1.

10. Huising MO, Stet RJ, Savelkoul HF, et al. The Molecular evolution of the IL-1 family of cytokines. Dev Comp Immunol 2004;28(5):395–413.

11. Carriere V, Roussel L, Ortega N, et al. IL-33, the IL-1-like cytokine ligand for ST2 receptor, is a chromatin-associated nuclear factor in vivo. Proc Natl Acad Sci U S A 2007;104(1):282–7.

12. Werman A, Werman-Venkert R, White R, et al. The precursor form of IL-1alpha is an intracrine proinflammatory activator of transcription. Proc Natl Acad Sci U S A 2004;101(8):2434–9.

13. Sharma S, Kulak N, Nold MF, et al. The IL-1 family member 7b translocates to the nucleus and down-regulates proinflammatory cytokines. J Immunol 2008;180(8):5477–82.

14. Nold MF, Nold-Petry CA, Zepp JA, et al. IL-37 is a fundamental inhibitor of innate immunity. Nat Immunol 2010;11(11):1014–22.

15. Di Paolo NC, Shayakhmetov DM. Interleukin-1 receptor 2 keeps the lid on interleukin-1α. Immunity 2013;38(2):203–5.

16. Banerjee M, Saxena M. Interleukin-1 (IL-1) family of cytokines: role in type 2 diabetes. Clin Chim Acta 2012;413(15–16):1163–70.

17. Goldbach-Mansky R. Blocking IL-1 in rheumatic diseases. Ann N Y Acad Sci 2009;1182:111–23.

18. Schroder K, Tschopp J. The inflammasomes. Cell 2010;140:821–32.

19. Agata H, Kondo N, Fukutomi O, et al. Interleukin-2 production of lymphocytes in food sensitive atopic dermatitis. Arch Dis Child 1992;67(3):280–4.

20. Arend WP, Malyak M, Guthridge CJ, et al. Interleukin-1 receptor antagonist: role in biology. Annu Rev Immunol 1998;16:27–55.

21. Watanabe H, Gaide O, Petrilli V, et al. Activation of the IL-1 beta processing inflammasome is involved in contact hypersensibility. J Invest Dermatol 2007; 127:1956–63.

22. Greally P, Hussain NJ, Price JF, et al. IL-1 alpha and soluble IL-2 receptors in atopic dermatitis. Arch Dis Child 1992;67:1413.

23. Blumberg H, Hugen D, Tomeblood E, et al. Opposing activities of two novel members of the IL-1 ligand family regulate skin inflammation. J Exp Med 2007; 204(11):2603–26.

24. Rania M, Hay A, Hoha F, et al. The role of IL-1 beta and IL-33 in atopic dermatitis. Our Dermatol Online 2013;4(1):11–4.

25. Ferda C, et al. IL-33: a novel danger signal system in atopic dermatitis. J Invest Dermatol 2012;132(5): 1326–9.

26. Nutan F, Kanwar AJ, Parsad D. The effect of topically applied corticosteroids on interleukin 1beta levels in patients with atopic dermatitis. J Eur Acad Dermatol Venereol 2012;26(8):1020–2.

Psoriasis as Autoinflammatory Disease

Joaquin J. Rivas Bejarano, MD[a,b],*,
Wendell C. Valdecantos, MD[a]

KEYWORDS

- Psoriasis • Autoinflammatory disease • Genetics • Immunopathogenesis • TH cells • TNF-α
- Cytokines • Inflammasome

KEY POINTS

- Psoriasis immunopathogenesis.
- Inflammatory cycle.
- Psoriasis causes and genetic and clinical features.
- Autoinflammatory versus autoimmune.
- Role of Th1-Th2 activation and balance on psoriasis.
- T-cell activation.
- Pathogenic mechanisms of self-immunity.
- Immune links of psoriasis to autoinflammation.
- Inflammasome-mediated inflammation.

INTRODUCTION

This article presents a summary of the evidence that can be used to establish a link between the recently introduced autoinflammatory diseases (AIDs) and psoriasis, a member of the papulosquamous disorders, the primary lesions of which are characterized by scaly plaques. These entities have some common characteristics among their phenotypic features, genetic components, and the mechanism of tissue damage exerted through intricate immunopathologic pathways and players.

The main concepts regarding the disease state of psoriasis are discussed and these lead to the establishment of a link that can change the perspective on the clinical and pathophysiologic nature of psoriasis as a chronic, recurrent disease with important genetically defined features, and an associated or concomitant systemic inflammatory state that involves a multifactorial cellular and molecular network, transforming the old perception of psoriasis as a localized autoimmune skin disease, to the new perspective of psoriasis as a systemic inflammatory disease with autoinflammatory features and severe associated comorbid conditions.

The extension of the skin lesion to a systemic inflammatory stage, as shown in several studies and publications, manifests in different body systems, creating the need for a more comprehensive approach to the affected patients.

From the point of view of several investigators, the concurrent inflammation seen in the different types of psoriasis compromises innate and adaptive immune system components and has a well-defined network of chemokines and messengers that can be compared with the cellular and chemical networks found in the patient with AID, requiring the identification of the possible links between them and the subsequent potential consideration of psoriasis as an AID.

Several years of intense studies of the pathogenic components, immune mediators, and involved

Disclosures: Drs Joaquin Rivas and Wendell Valdecantos are employees of AbbVie.
[a] Immunology, Global Medical Affairs, AbbVie, 1 North Waukegan Road, North Chicago, IL 60064, USA;
[b] Biology Department, LoneStar College, 2700 WW Thorne Drive, WN Building #210, Houston, TX 77073, USA
* Corresponding author. 3510 London Lane, Missouri City, TX 77459.
E-mail address: bejarano.0214@yahoo.com

Dermatol Clin 31 (2013) 445–460
http://dx.doi.org/10.1016/j.det.2013.04.009
0733-8635/13/$ – see front matter © 2013 Elsevier Inc. All rights reserved.

pathways of psoriasis enhanced knowledge about the disease state and its clinical associated conditions. The concept of activated T cells has gained a key role, suggesting autoimmunity as a basic mechanism of the disease. In later publications and discoveries, after evaluating the different psoriasis phenotypes, analysis of the variable course of the disease with periodic outbreaks, as well as results from immunotyping studies, justified an extension of the autoimmunity concept. Current evidence establishes that innate immunity and autoinflammation play significant roles.

AIDS: A NEW CATEGORY

The AIDs, a concept recently introduced in the medical literature, are a category of illnesses characterized by seemingly unprovoked episodes of inflammation, without high-titer autoantibodies or antigen-specific T cells, in which, as in the autoimmune diseases, the capability of self-recognition is disturbed, initiating an attack on the body's own tissues. The distorted and abnormal response generates a cellular network with the implicated chemokine chain reaction that, in turn, generates an inflammatory response. The mechanisms for which the inflammation is generated and the abnormal action of the innate immune system are currently not completely understood. In 2008, Yao and colleagues[1] proposed the new classification, with the identification of the genes underlying hereditary components associated with gene mutations for the periodic fever syndromes. Soon after the new nosology was proposed, Masters and colleagues[2] published an article in which 6 categories of AIDs were defined: interleukin (IL)-1β activation disorders (inflammasomopathies), nuclear factor (NF)-κB activation syndromes, protein misfolding disorders, complement regulatory diseases, disturbances in cytokine signaling, and macrophage activation syndromes. More conditions, mostly included because of their clinical manifestations, have recently been added to the classification, with a special consideration of their complexity and their heritable linkage.[3–5] Details of the newest classification are discussed elsewhere in this issue by Abramovits. The diseases are characterized by spontaneous activation of cells of innate immunity in the absence of ligands. Autoantibodies are usually not found.[6]

AUTOIMMUNE VERSUS AUTOINFLAMMATORY

Differentiated by the absence or presence of specific antibodies, the activation of different immune systems, and their genetic features, the disorders share common characteristics in that both result from the immune system targeting and aggressively injuring self-tissues, with a resulting increased inflammation as an expression of the tissue damage mechanisms. These common grounds could create confusion in diagnosis. This conceptualization was defined by The National Institute of Arthritis and Musculoskeletal and Skin Diseases (NIAMS), a part of the US Department of Health and Human Services, National Institutes of Health (NIH), in March 2010[7] (discussed later). Their publication established several different types of AID.

The mechanism for which the local or systemic damage is produced in autoinflammatory syndromes is complex, involving cellular and cytokine networks, and probably involves a systemic disruption of the molecular basis of mediating and controlling inflammation. These disorders were defined, until recently, by phenotypic features, including recurrent attacks of fever, abdominal pain, arthritis, or cutaneous signs, which occasionally overlap inducing doubts and consequently an inaccurate diagnosis. To date, the improved knowledge of the pathophysiology, the mechanisms of the disease, and the molecular effects of the mediators has allowed an expansion of their classification.

Autoimmune disorders are a consequence of an inappropriate immune response of the body against substances and tissues whose presence is recognized as normal in the body. The immunologic hallmark is the formation of specific antibodies against the target organ or tissue; the immune system mistakes some part of the body as a pathogen and attacks its own cells. This response may be restricted to certain organs (eg, in autoimmune thyroiditis) or involve a particular tissue in different places (eg, Goodpasture disease, which may affect the basement membrane in both the lung and the kidney).

It is important not to confuse autoinflammatory syndromes with autoimmune diseases, which are caused by the body's adaptive immune system developing antibodies to antigens that then attack healthy body tissues.[7] Autoimmunity and autoinflammation share some common characteristics: both lead to self-directed inflammation, but with different mechanisms. Although autoimmunity involves adaptive immune activation, autoinflammation involves innate immune activation. Autoinflammation is genetically related to perturbations of innate immune function, including proinflammatory cytokine signaling abnormalities, or bacterial sensing, or local tissue abnormalities. The clinical and pathophysiologic expressions of autoinflammation are determined by cells of the innate immune system, including neutrophils and macrophages or nonimmune cells.

Recent discoveries on the contribution of the innate immunity mechanisms in inflammatory disorders have led to a new examination of the current nosology of this large group of diseases. Some investigators suggest a classification with 2 poles. The first is defined by the predominance of autoinflammation, whereas, in the second, 1 autoimmunity predominates.[8]

MECHANISMS OF SELF-IMMUNITY

The challenge of the immune system is to produce a response to invasive foreign antigens without breaking down the natural immunologic tolerance, reacting to self-components of the recognized structures of the human body. The cellular structures that identify the exposed epitopes and warrant the proper response and mechanisms to inactivate or eliminate self-reactive cells and non-self structures are the preexistent genetically encoded receptors. The discriminating actions and the capability of producing an immune response with the included mechanisms of self-tolerance is the responsibility of the cellular receptors located at the B and T cells. A well-known array of factors, genetically and environmentally associated, could induce altered autoimmunity by breaking down

the self-tolerance, preventing the response to self-epitopes.

However, to provide some benefits, a grade of immune tolerance is needed. The concept is exemplified by the following examples: the recognition of neoplastic cells by CD8+ T cells (a contribution that reduces the possibility of cancerous developments at a tissue level), the rapid immune response in the early stages of an infection when the availability of foreign antigens limits the response, or during the inflammatory process involved in the production of healing and repairs following tissue injuries. Stefanova and colleagues[9] (2002) showed that self–major histocompatibility complex (MHC) recognition maintains the responsiveness of CD4+ T cells when foreign antigens are absent.

To explain the origin and mechanisms of immunologic tolerance, several theories have been proposed. The most important hypotheses considered to explain these concepts are represented in **Fig. 1**.[10,11]

Loss of Tolerance

A challenge to this process was reported by investigators around the world, with evidence that shows that the antibody responses are produced by B lymphocytes during spontaneous human autoimmunity. Loss of tolerance by T cells has

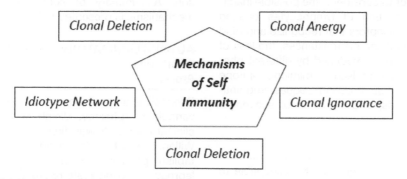

Accepted theories to explain the mechanisms of Immunological Tolerance: **Clonal Deletion theory:** Burnet et al. Self-reactive lymphoid cells are destroyed during the development of the immune system in an individual. **Clonal Anergy theory:** Nossal et al, self-reactive T- or B-cells become inactivated in the normal individual and cannot amplify the immune response. **Idiotype Network theory:** Jerne et al, a network of antibodies capable of neutralizing self-reactive antibodies exists naturally within the body. **Clonal Ignorance theory:** auto-reactive T cells that are not represented in the thymus will mature and migrate to the periphery, where they will not encounter the appropriate antigen because it is at inaccessible tissues. Consequently, auto-reactive B cells, that escape deletion, cannot find the antigen or the specific helper T-cell. **Suppressor population or Regulatory T cell theory:** regulatory T-lymphocytes (commonly CD4+FoxP3+ cells, among others) function to prevent, downregulates, or limit auto aggressive immune responses in the immune system.

Fig. 1. The accepted mechanisms of self immunity.

been hard to show, and where there is evidence for an abnormal T-cell response it is usually not of the antigen recognized by autoantibodies. Some instances supporting this statement are that (1) there are autoantibodies to immunoglobulin (Ig) G heavy chain constant region of the immunoglobulin molecule domains (Fc) but apparently no corresponding T-cell response in rheumatoid arthritis (RA); (2) there are autoantibodies to DNA that cannot evoke a T-cell response, and limited evidence for T-cell responses implicates nucleoprotein antigens in systemic lupus erythematous (SLE); (3) there are autoantibodies to tissue transglutaminase but the T-cell response is to the foreign protein gliadin in celiac disease. The discrepancy created the presumption of human autoimmune disease, in most cases (with probable exceptions including type I diabetes) based on a loss of B-cell tolerance, which makes use of normal T-cell responses to foreign antigens in a variety of aberrant ways.[12] The failure of these mechanisms probably leads to autoimmunity.

Role of Th1/Th2 Balance in Self-immunity

Several investigators consider the balance between Th1/Th2 an important player; it may induce particular responses to determined self-antigens producing the expression of cytokines and inflammatory mediators with clinical manifestations of specific diseases.

Another factor to consider is the possible inactivation or destruction of lymphocytes bearing B-cell or T-cell receptors that recognize and bind self-epitopes; in these circumstances, the loss of self-tolerance can be mediated by different phenomena, such as molecular mimicry, epitope spreading, loss of suppression, sequestered antigens, neoantigens, and induction of scavenger receptors.

Involved Genetic Factors

Certain individuals are genetically susceptible to developing autoimmune diseases. This susceptibility is associated with multiple genes in conjunction with other risk factors. Genetically predisposed individuals do not always develop autoimmune disease; an environmental condition is needed to induce the expression of the genetically preestablished condition.

Three main sets of genes are suspected in many autoimmune diseases. These genes are related to: immunoglobulin, T-cell receptors, and the MHCs. The first two, which are involved in the recognition of antigens, are inherently variable and susceptible to recombination. These variations enable the immune system to respond to a wide variety of invaders, but may also give rise to lymphocytes capable of self-reactivity.

There is also strong evidence to suggest that certain MHC class II allotypes correlated with human leukocyte antigen (HLA) DR2 are strongly positively correlated with SLE.[13] HLA DR3 is strongly correlated with Sjögren syndrome, myasthenia gravis, SLE, and diabetes mellitus (DM) type 1; HLA DR4 is correlated with the genesis of RA, type 1 DM, and pemphigus vulgaris.

A few publications establish the correlation between the MHC class I molecules and the generation of autoimmunity, the association between HLA B27 and ankylosing spondylitis being the most consistent finding reported. The polymorphisms within class II MHC promoters and autoimmune disease may have some type of correlation.

Most recent data associate protein tyrosine phosphatase, nonreceptor type 22 (PTPN22) with multiple autoimmune diseases including type I DM, RA, SLE, Hashimoto thyroiditis, Graves disease, Addison disease, myasthenia gravis, vitiligo, systemic sclerosis, juvenile idiopathic arthritis, and psoriatic arthritis (PsA).

Pathogenesis of Autoimmune Disease

Several operative mechanisms have been reported to be involved in the pathogenesis of autoimmune diseases, besides the previously mentioned genetic predisposition and environmental modulation. A summary of some of the important mechanisms is presented in **Fig. 2**.[14–16]

AUTOINFLAMMATORY FEATURES OF PSORIASIS
Psoriasis

Psoriasis is a papulosquamous skin disease with variable morphology, distribution, severity, and clinical course. It was first described by Robert Willan,[17] a British dermatologist who helped establish psoriasis as a separate entity from leprosy.[18,19] Widely referred to as psoriasis vulgaris, after the most common clinical type, the condition affects an estimated 2% of the general population[18] and predominantly is a disease of white people. A bimodal age of onset has been reported for psoriasis, with the mean age of onset for the first presentation ranging from 15 to 20 years of age, with a second peak occurring at 55 to 60 years.[19]

Cause

The cause of psoriasis is complex, with evidence that both multiple genes and environmental factors are involved. Population studies report that the incidence of psoriasis is greater in first-degree

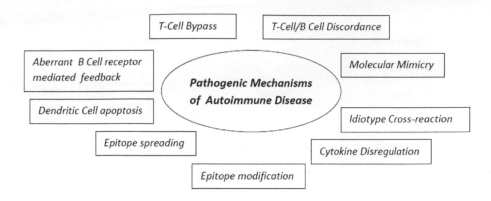

Fig. 2. Autoimmune diseases. Pathogenic mechanisms.

and second-degree relatives of patients than in the general population.[18] About 30% of patients have an affected first-degree relative, whereas the risk of having the disease is 2 to 3 times greater in monozygotic than in dizygotic twins.[19] Early onset (before age 40 years) psoriasis has been reported to have a stronger genetic basis, because a greater proportion of patients had a family history of psoriasis, more severe disease, and stronger HLA associations (HLA-Cw6, HLA-DR7, HLA-B13, and HLA-Bw57).[20,21] Major susceptibility loci for psoriasis have been established at chromosome 6p21.3 (PSOR1), whereas other associations have been reported on chromosomes 17q (PSORS2), 4q (PSORS3), 1cenq21 (PSORS4), 3q21 (PSORS5), 19p (PSORS6), 1p (PSORS7), and 4q31 (PSOR9).[20,21] Environmental factors also play an important role in the pathogenesis of psoriasis, including

infection, skin trauma, drugs, and stress.[22] Beta-hemolytic streptococcus infection of the pharynx and tonsils often precedes the first manifestation of the disease. Infections may also trigger a rare generalized pustular form, called von Zumbusch psoriasis.[21] Mechanical trauma to the skin can trigger the development of psoriatic lesions at the site of the trauma in individuals predisposed to developing the disease, an isomorphic reaction known as the Koebner phenomenon. A positive Koebner predicts subsequent disease activity.[23] The use of medications, such as beta-blockers, cloroquine, tetracyclines, interferons, nonsteroidal antiinflammatory drugs (NSAIDs), and lithium, has also been associated with the onset of psoriasis.[23] Furthermore, lifestyle factors, including alcoholism, smoking, stress, and obesity, have been reported to negatively affect the disease.[24] Fig. 3 shows an integrated perspective of these factors.

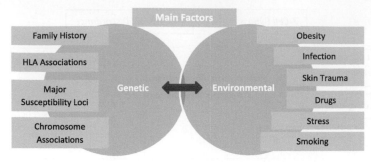

Fig. 3. Causes of psoriasis.

Clinical features

Psoriasis generally manifests as chronic inflammation of the skin characterized by disfiguring, scaling, and erythematous plaques accompanied by pain and pruritus. The disease waxes and wanes during a patient's lifetime, and is often modified by treatment, with few spontaneous remissions.[22] Plaque psoriasis (also called psoriasis vulgaris) is the most common form, affecting 80% to 90% of patients. Plaque psoriasis typically presents as raised areas of inflamed skin covered with a silvery white scale. The scale can easily be removed from a psoriatic plaque, and may reveal focal bleeding points (the Auspitz sign). Lesions often begin as small papules that expand and coalesce to form extensive psoriatic plaques. Lesions are typically distributed symmetrically on the scalp, elbows, knees, and lumbosacral area.[21] Skin involvement may range from only a few plaques to numerous lesions covering almost the entire body surface. Other classifications of psoriasis include inverse psoriasis, erythrodermic psoriasis, pustular psoriasis, and guttate psoriasis (**Table 1**). The clinical findings in individual patients frequently overlap in more than one type of psoriasis.

Approximately half of patients with psoriasis have distinctive nail changes related to the disease. These changes include pitting, onycholysis (nail plate separation), oil spots (orange-yellow subungual discoloration), and dystrophy. Fingernails are more commonly affected than toenails. Psoriatic nail disease occurs more frequently in patients with PsA.[19,21]

Impact of psoriasis

Although psoriasis is rarely life-threatening, the disease negatively affects quality of life and represents a psychosocial and financial burden for patients and the health care system. Psoriasis decreases the quality of life at least as much as diabetes, ischemic heart disease, or chronic obstructive pulmonary disease.[19] Patients also suffer from disfigurement and from social stigmatization, leading to higher rates of depression, anxiety, sexual dysfunction, poor self-esteem, and suicidal thoughts than are found in the general population, even in less severe disease. Moreover, patients with a diagnosis of psoriasis usually require lifelong care with the associated expenses caused by the chronicity of the disease. In the United States, the annual per capita health care and out-of-pocket (OOP) costs for individuals with psoriasis have been reported to be significantly greater than those for individuals without the condition. United States national annual estimates of health care, OOP, and total direct medical expenses for psoriasis were $3.67 billion, $1.49 billion, and $5.17 billion, respectively.[25]

Diagnosis

The diagnosis is made clinically, based on the characteristic appearance of the lesions. A skin biopsy may be necessary to exclude other conditions. Disease severity is loosely based on the amount of body surface area (BSA) involved, with mild being less than 3% BSA involved; moderate, 3% to 10% BSA involved; and severe, greater than 10% BSA involved, although any percentage of involvement on critical areas such as the face or hands may convey a severe rating. The Psoriasis Area and Severity Index (PASI), a measure of overall disease severity and coverage that assesses BSA, erythema, induration, and scaling, is often used in clinical trials but rarely in the clinic.

Histopathologic features: immunopathogenesis

In psoriasis, keratinocyte migration from the basal layer of the epidermis to the skin surface takes only 3 days, in contrast with normal skin development, which takes approximately 4 weeks. Keratinocyte hyperproliferation and abnormal apoptosis result in parakeratosis, characterized by the accumulation of partially differentiated keratinocytes that retain their nuclei and that form the basis of the scaly plaque formation in psoriasis. As such,

Table 1
Clinical types of psoriasis

Type	Description	Skin Areas Involved
Plaque psoriasis	Well-defined, sharply demarcated, erythematous plaques that vary in size from 1 cm to several centimeters	Scalp, trunk, buttocks, and limbs, extensor surfaces such as the elbows and knees
Inverse psoriasis (flexural)	Erythematous plaques with minimal scaling because of the moist nature of involved areas Can be confused with candida, intertrigo, and dermatophyte infections	Skin fold areas, including the axillary, genital, perineal, intergluteal, and inframammary areas
Erythrodermic psoriasis	Generalized erythema with varying degrees of scaling Can be a life-threatening condition because of hypothermia, hypoalbuminemia, and high-output cardiac failure	Affects almost the entire body surface area
Pustular psoriasis	Raised bumps that are filled with noninfectious pus (pustules) Rare Represents active, unstable disease	May be generalized (von Zumbusch disease) or localized to the palms and soles (palmoplantar pustulosis)
Guttate psoriasis (eruptive)	Droplike (1–10 mm) salmon pink papules, usually with a fine scale Occurs in less than 2% of patients with psoriasis Often preceded by history of upper respiratory infection with group A beta-hemolytic streptococci Usually self-limiting	Primarily on the trunk and the proximal extremities

the illness was initially considered to be a condition primarily of abnormal keratinocyte proliferation and maturation with secondary inflammation. With the identification of cytokines like tumor necrosis factor alpha (TNF-α) and various interleukins in psoriatic plaques, researchers switched focus to identifying and localizing many different types of cytokines within normal and diseased skin.[26]

In 1991, the initial version of the cytokine network theory of psoriasis was proposed to explain its immunopathogenesis.[27] Cytokines are small, biologically active proteins that regulate the growth, function, and differentiation of cells and coordinate the immune response and inflammation. The theory suggested that the dendritic cells (DCs) secreting TNF-α in the dermis played a central role in the initiation and maintenance of the disease.[27] Available data at that time showed that TNF-α could induce relevant adhesion molecules, growth factors, and chemokines.

Clinical research provided further evidence that highly specific reagents targeting TNF-α were observed to improve skin and, in some circumstances, joint disease activity.[28,29] However, TNF-α has pleiotropic biological effects and redundancy with other cytokines. Thus, a single cytokine such as TNF-α cannot fully account for the inflammatory process in psoriasis considering the diversity and complexity of the cytokine network.

Current evidence suggests that psoriasis is a complex immune-mediated inflammatory disease driven primarily by T cells, particularly Th1 and Th17 cells. This shift in paradigm toward T cells was in part caused by the therapeutic success observed in psoriasis with medications that inhibit T-cell functions, such as cyclosporine A, a substance that diminishes T-cell proliferation and cytokine production.[23,26]

T-cell activation (Th1 and Th17)

T cells are generally accepted to be the key players in initiating and maintaining pathologic changes in psoriasis. For reasons not yet completely understood, DCs in the skin become activated to recognize and capture a cutaneous antigen, then migrate to the lymph nodes where they stimulate T cells by presenting them with the antigen. This process triggers the proliferation of antigen-recognizing T cells and memory effector cells.[30] However, the antigen responsible for T-cell activation in the skin has to still be conclusively identified. After antigen stimulation, T cells enter the circulatory system and interact with adhesion molecules in endothelial cells of blood vessels. Adhesion molecules, particularly P-selectin and E-selectin, are expressed in higher concentrations in psoriasis.[23] This interaction with adhesion molecules allows the migration of T cells, as well as macrophages, DCs, natural killer (NK) cells, and neutrophils through the blood vessel wall into the skin and around dermal blood vessels. The lymphocytic infiltrate and resident T cells play important roles in preceding and driving the epidermal changes.[30]

Psoriasis has traditionally been classified as a T-cell helper 1 (Th1) disease because of a predominance of Th1 pathway cytokines, such as TNF-α, interferon gamma (IFN-γ), IL-2, and IL-12 in psoriatic plaques.[19] Increased levels of Th1 cytokines in serum have also been reported, and the circulating levels of TNF-α, IFN-γ, IL-2, and IL-18 seem to be correlated with the severity of psoriasis.[30]

IFN-γ is secreted by Th1 cells, DCs, and NK cells, and seems to play a key role in the early stages of the clinical presentation. IFN-γ accelerates the migration of immune cells into the skin and activates monocytes, macrophages, DCs, and endothelial cells. It also stimulates epidermal cell proliferation and inhibits the apoptosis of keratinocytes, causing the hyperproliferation of keratinocytes observed in psoriatic plaques.[30] IL-12 secreted by DC plays a major role in the development of Th1 cell-mediated immune responses. Together with IL-2 from T cells, these cytokines regulate the transcription of IFN-γ and TNF-α. IL-2 is likewise responsible for the differentiation, proliferation, and maturation of T cells into memory effector cells. IL-18, a cytokine important in cellular adhesion, also contributes to secretion of IFN-γ.[30]

TNF-α is an important cytokine of the Th1 pathway. It has pronounced proinflammatory effects and is produced by DCs, T cells, macrophages, and keratinocytes in psoriasis. TNF-α stimulates the proliferation of T cells, other cytokines, and adhesion molecules. In particular, TNF-α induces the expression of IL-6 and C-reactive protein (CRP) in psoriasis. IL-6 induces T-cell activation, stimulates the proliferation of keratinocytes, and mediates the acute-phase response.[30] TNF-α also increases expression of IL-18, a

cytokine that provides a strong chemotactic signal for the recruitment of neutrophils. In conjunction with IFN-γ, TNF-α promotes inflammatory cell infiltration of the skin by increasing the expression of intercellular adhesion molecule 1 (ICAM-1). Improvement of cutaneous symptoms with biologic therapies that specifically neutralize TNF-α in patients with psoriasis provide additional evidence of the central role of TNF-α in the immunopathology of the disease.

More recently, studies reported the critical contribution of Th17 pathway–associated cytokines, particularly IL-23 and IL-17, in the pathogenesis of psoriasis.[31,32] In this new paradigm, the activated DCs in the dermis produce IL-23 and IL-12, which stimulate resident Th17, Th22, and Th1 cells. IL-23 secreted by DCs activates Th17 cells to produce IL-17A and IL-17F, which drive keratinocyte responses. The stimulated epidermis can produce abundant cytokines and inflammatory mediators, including IL-8, chemokine CXC ligand (CXCL), monocyte chemotactic protein (MCP)-1, chemokine CC ligand (CCL) 2, CXCL1, CXCL2, CXCL3, and CCL20. The chemokines attract neutrophils, DCs, and chemokine CC receptor (CCR) and Th17 cells. Also produced are CXCL9, CXCL10, and CXCL11, which further recruit circulating CXCR3 and Th1 cells into the dermis and epidermis. Such chemokine induction and leukocyte recruitment can occur within hours of tissue injury in the skin.[31] Details of this new perspective are presented in **Fig. 4**.

Clinical studies investigating individual cytokine antagonists for the treatment of psoriasis provide additional support for a central role of IL-23 and IL-17, along with TNF-α, in driving the disease process. Biologic therapies that inhibit TNF-α and IL-12/23p40 have already been approved in recent years for extensive psoriasis, whereas agents such as anti–IL-23p19 and anti–IL-17 are currently showing promise in clinical trials.

IL-22, produced by Th22 cells, mediates the crosstalk between the immune system and keratinocytes, stimulating epidermal hyperplasia and hypogranulosis. It also induces production of cytokines, chemokines, and acute-phase proteins from various inflammatory cells and regulates the differentiation and migration of keratinocytes. IL-22 production is upregulated in psoriatic skin, with increased levels in the peripheral blood, and seems to correlate with the severity of the disease.[30]

Other cells involved in psoriasis

Additional inflammatory cells and mediators also play important roles in the immunopathology of psoriasis. Vascular endothelial growth factor

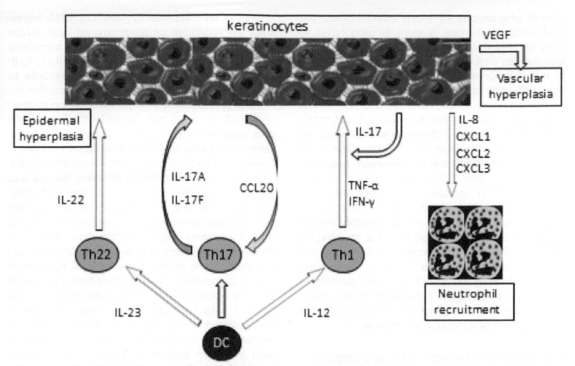

Fig. 4. The Th17 pathway in the inflammatory cycle of psoriasis. DC, dentritic cells; N, neutrophils; VEGF, vascular endothelial growth factor.

(VEGF) induces vascular dilation and hyperplasia, whereas activation of the keratinocytes also induces IL-17C, further perpetuating the inflammatory cycle.[31] Macrophages produce TNF-α and contribute to angiogenesis by releasing proteases, growth factors, and other cytokines.[30] Mast cells secrete large amounts of TNF-α, IFN-γ, IL-8, and other mediators such as VEGF, to recruit neutrophils and lymphocytes during innate and T-cell–mediated inflammation.[30] Neutrophils seem to recruit and activate T lymphocytes, modulate T-cell–mediated hypersensitivity responses, and influence the proliferation and differentiation of keratinocytes.[30] Elastase, a primary protease released at inflammatory sites by activated neutrophils, seems to mediate inflammation and tissue damage by inducing the activation of other inflammatory cells and the degradation of matrix proteins and clotting factors. Elastase has also been reported to induce keratinocyte proliferation by epidermal growth factor receptor activation and may modify cytokine and receptor functions.[30]

Signs and symptoms of psoriasis as a consequence of inflammation

The clinical features of psoriasis are direct consequences of the pathophysiologic events resulting from the dysregulated immune response. The

hyperplasia and altered differentiation of epidermal keratinocytes manifest as thick, scaly plaques, providing the classic feature of psoriasis. The keratinocyte response is primarily driven by Th1 and Th17 pathway cytokines, such as IFN-γ, IL-22, and TNF-α. These cytokines are amplified by the further secretion of proinflammatory cytokines by activated macrophages and DCs, as well as by the keratinocytes themselves. Although IFN-γ has been reported to have a direct inhibitory effect on keratinocytes, it seems that its proinflammatory effects of increasing leukocyte migration and activation outweigh this inhibition.[23]

The erythema characteristic of psoriatic lesions is caused by the increased, dilated, and tortuous capillaries that extend between the epidermal columns into the dermis. Vascular proliferation results in superficial dermal microvascular plexus in lesions and is triggered by local expression of angiogenic factors, such as TNF-α, transforming growth factor alpha (TGF-α), IL-8, thymidine phosphorylase, endothelial cell–stimulating angiogenesis factor, angiopoietin, and VEGF.[30]

In addition to skin plaques, psoriasis can present with extracutaneous conditions including arthritis, atherosclerosis, inflammatory bowel disease, obesity, atherosclerosis, type 2 DM, and depression. It seems that, regardless of the various clinical phenotypes of these comorbidities, the dysfunctional immune system is recognized to have an important role in the expression of these diseases as well. Th1 and Th17 cells are essential in the pathogenesis and progression of atherosclerosis, with atherosclerosis sharing a myriad of common cytokines, chemokines, and innate mechanisms with psoriasis, including those mediated by TNF-α.[33,34] Activated macrophages are linked to the development of Crohn disease in the gastrointestinal tract,[35] whereas migratory macrophages and TNF-α are linked to obesity-induced insulin resistance.[36] Adipocytes have been reported to produce proinflammatory cytokines under the influence of inflammatory mediators such as TNF-α, suggesting that an interplay may exist between adipocytes and the inflammation that drives psoriasis.[37] TNF-α levels were also significantly increased in acutely depressed patients, supporting the hypothesis that an activation of the TNF-α system may contribute to the development of a depressive disorder.[38]

THE IMMUNE COMPONENTS OF PSORIASIS LINKED TO AUTOINFLAMMATION

As a common factor, neutrophil migration is observed in autoinflammatory cryopyrin-associated periodic syndrome (CAPS) as well as reported on common inflammatory keratoses like psoriasis. The molecular pathogenesis is associated in both conditions with an abnormal regulation of the innate immune response and Th17 cell differentiation via IL-1 signaling.[39]

In AID, the innate or primitive immune system causes inflammation for unknown reasons, also having hereditary components usually associated with a gene mutation. The previously mentioned considerations also apply to psoriasis, and considerable evidence supports its genetic links.

In psoriasis, the movement of immune cells from basal to superficial layers of the skin produces a stimulation of the superficial keratinocytes inducing their proliferation. Because of the characteristics of the disease, in terms of genetic links, immunopathogenic mechanisms and clinically associated comorbid conditions, psoriasis does not seem to be a true autoimmune disease.[18] The typical characteristics of autoimmune diseases are not the same as the immune response of psoriasis, in which the cycle of chronic inflammation does not seem to be caused by outside antigens (although DNA does have an immunostimulatory effect). Dendritic and T cells move from the dermis to the epidermis, secreting TNF-α, IL-1β, and IL-6, which cause inflammation, and IL-22, which causes keratinocytes to proliferate.[18]

DNA is an inflammatory stimulus. DNA stimulates the receptors on plasmacytoid DCs, which produce IFN-γ, another inflammatory stimulator that also produces cytokines, such as IL-1, IL-6, and TNF-α, causing more inflammatory cells to arrive and producing further inflammation.[18]

As described earlier, the psoriatic lesion is characterized by a chronic, persistent inflammation and stimulus to the superficial layer of the epidermis. This inflammation is mediated by a link between innate and adaptive immune systems by the DCs. They are increased in psoriatic lesions and induce the proliferation of T cells and Th1 cells. Some of these cells are producers of TNF-α, which induces chemotaxis for immune cells producing and stimulating more inflammation. TNF-α is involved in the early stages of inflammation and maintaining the status; these effects have been well documented.[18] T cells move from the dermis into the epidermis, attracted to the epidermis by alpha-1 beta-1 integrin, a signaling molecule on the collagen in the epidermis. Psoriatic T cells secrete IFN-γ and IL-17, which is also associated with IL-22, an inducer of keratinocyte proliferation.[18,40] Defects in regulatory T cells and in the regulatory cytokine IL-10 are also involved in the chronic inflammatory process.[18,40]

Special attention has been paid to pustular psoriasis, a clinical variety of psoriasis that is now being considered as a separate entity and included in the latest classification of AIDs. There are several publications available in which some of correlated clinical variations of the pustular disease, such as generalized pustular psoriasis (GPP), palmoplantar pustulosis, and acrodermatitis continua, have been described by some investigators.[17,41,42] These entities had shown different genotypic markers.[42,43] The GPP genotype shows that a homogenous mutation of a gene encoding an IL-36 receptor antagonist leads to deficiency of the IL-36 receptor, thereby causing GPP.[44,45] GPP shows several features in common with autoinflammatory disorders, including an intermittent course of disease, fever, neutrophilia, and signs of systemic inflammation. IL-36 is a member of the IL-1 family of ligands, meaning that the expression of IL-36 stimulation can lead to an interaction and expression of the IL-1 receptors with the consequent protein expression, with clinical features of the AIDs. Exacerbation of the psoriatic clinical manifestations as a consequence of corticosteroid withdrawal or overtreatment with ultraviolet light showed the clinical evolution or transformation of the psoriatic plaque into the more severe pustular forms of the disease, becoming generalized with a more advanced and aggressive inflammatory stage. The hyperinflammatory reaction, unique for this form of the disease, is the reflection of a latent autoinflammatory component present in all psoriatic patients.

Pathologic reports in multiple publications showed that all the tissue changes in psoriasis are the consequence of a dysregulated immune response. The adaptive autoimmune dysregulation by activated Th1 cells causes autoimmunity.[46] As explained earlier, the increased numbers of activated T cells, DCs, and neutrophils in lesional skin interact with keratinocytes, causing the increased production of cytokines and chemokines, along with their altered functions.[46]

Another factor to consider is the presence of HLA-Cw*0602 positivity in psoriatic patients. These self-proteins possess the capacity to activate peripheral blood T cells (eg, CD8+ T cells), showing that self-peptides are presented to the immune system by HLA-Cw6. Several epitopes that immunologically reveal molecular mimicry with keratinocyte-derived proteins have been found in these patients, indicating that keratinocyte proteins serve as targets for streptococcal-induced autoimmune responses, causing guttate psoriasis.

The Involvement of Th17 Cells; Another Link to Autoinflammation

The observations discussed earlier give the impression of a purely Th1-mediated immunopathology; however, there is a role for Th17 cells to be considered. The activation and recruitment of Th17 cells is pivotal, and Th17 and Th17-associated cytokines play a significant role in initiating and maintaining psoriatic changes.[46–48] Cytokines overproduced in lesional skin comprise TNF-α, IFN type 1 and 2, IL-1, IL-8, IL-12, IL-22, IL-23, and IL-17A.[49,50] In this scenario, IL-22, IL-23, and IL-17A produced by activated Th17 subpopulations sustain a persistent inflammatory milieu. These cytokines (in concert with others, eg, IL-8 and TNF-α) stimulate keratinocytes to proliferate and secrete proinflammatory cytokines and antimicrobial peptides (AMPs).[51]

In addition, macrophage activation, a phenomenon initially studied to explain psoriatic inflammation and other inflammatory events, including cardiovascular events in atheromatous plaque and plaque rupture events, as well as other systemic inflammatory diseases, implicates the adaptive system in the disease process of psoriasis.[52–54]

Considering the factors mentioned earlier, the inflammatory process in psoriasis can be considered to be caused by the uncontrolled activation of a trio of activated immune cells, namely Th1, Th17, and Th22 cells.

The Genetic Components of Psoriasis: an Important Link to Autoinflammation

Genetic risk factors significantly contribute to the susceptibility of psoriasis, genetic factors being considered more important than environmental factors.[2] A major genetic risk factor is HLA-Cw*0602 (designated PSORS1), which has been reported to be present in 65% of psoriatic patients.[55,56] This MHC class 1 molecule is also present in approximately 20% of the normal population who do not develop the disease. HLA-Cw6 has been considered as a marker of early onset psoriasis[11] and is strongly associated with guttate psoriasis.[43]

Effects of Inflammasome-mediated Inflammation

Inflammasomes are a typical component of autoinflammation and have also been reported to have a role in psoriatic inflammation.[57] An important signal activating inflammasome-mediated inflammation is cytosolic DNA.[58] The cytosolic DNA acts as a signal capable of activating inflammasomes via the DNA sensor AIM2. This form of cytosolic DNA is abundant in psoriatic keratinocytes.[59] Cytosolic DNA triggers the release of IL-1β via AIM2, increased amounts of which are also located within psoriatic keratinocytes. As a result, IL-1β is activated in psoriatic skin, thereby initiating an innate (autoinflammatory) cascade. The leading enzyme in the activation process is caspase-5, which is increased in psoriatic keratinocytes but not in keratinocytes from other skin diseases.[57]

As mentioned earlier, these findings place psoriasis, especially the pustular subtypes (eg, GPP), among the autoinflammation pathways. McGonagle and colleagues[60] and McGonagle and McDermott[61] studied psoriatic nail disease and juxta-articular enthesitis, emphasizing the close association of nail psoriasis with distal PsA, suggesting events of autoinflammatory immune activation.

Some patients affected by psoriasis reported the association of the flaring episodes with local trauma and stress; factors that suggest the generation of autoinflammatory tissue factors. Associated local infections that generate the interaction of antigen-presenting cells with bacterial compounds can be responsible for dysregulated autoinflammatory immune activation.[62]

The Systemic Inflammatory Stage of Psoriasis

Analysis from epidemiologic data reported a higher risk of comorbidity on patients with PsA compared with patients with psoriasis alone.[62]

The prevalence of hypertension, metabolic syndrome, hyperlipidemia, obesity, type 2 DM, and at least 1 cardiovascular event was significantly increased in those patients. It seems that in patients with psoriasis, inflammation of the joints, in addition to the inflammatory skin disease, aggravates the risk of metabolic syndrome signs and its complications. There is also evidence that the severity, as well as the duration, of disease plays a role. Severe psoriasis of long duration has been accepted as an independent risk factor for atherosclerosis, myocardial infarction, and stroke. Different theories have been studied, all of them trying to find the factors that stimulate and maintain the chronic, severe, systemic inflammatory stage that predispose to the associated comorbidities. A large number of publications implicate TNF-α, IFN-γ, IL-1, fat cells, and other proinflammatory cytokines such as IL-6 and CRPs as important players in the process (**Fig. 5**).[63–65]

CONCLUSIVE REMARKS

Psoriasis is a heterogeneous disorder; the diverse immunopathogenesis and the intricate role of inflammatory cells, proinflammatory chemokines, and genetic and environmental factors that drive the clinical presentations of the disease limits the possibility of classifying psoriasis as a purely autoimmune disorder.

The intervention of activated T cells and the concurrent innate immune activation causes are instrumental in causing polygenic autoinflammatory and autoimmune diseases. Some findings suggest that the heterogeneity of clinical phenotypes may be regulated by both innate and adaptive immune pathways.

The presence of a combination of environmental, immunogenic, and genetic factors produces the diverse spectrum of psoriatic disorders. Many investigators consider that evidence for autoimmunity in the general sense is limited. Support for their opinion includes the absence of shared genetic risk factors for autoimmune diseases such as PTPN22 polymorphisms, absence of B-cell activation and disease-specific antibodies, and a lack of defined autoantigens, except for the specific conditions mentioned in this article. The genetic components of psoriasis and its clinical variations are different from the genetic components of typical autoimmune diseases.

The neutrophils, widely considered an important component of autoinflammatory pathogenesis, have been found in early psoriatic lesions. Their

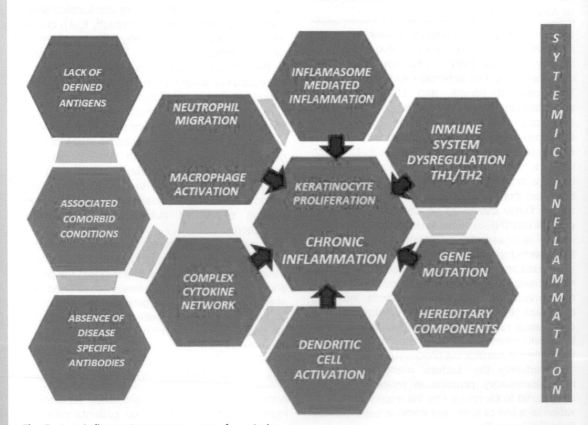

Fig. 5. Autoinflammatory components of psoriasis.

function is modulated by T lymphocytes and by monocytes. Many psoriasis-associated proinflammatory molecules, including angiopoietin-1, cathelicidins, CCR6, CD15, CD40, CD40L, CD69, CXCL10, Fas ligand, folic acid pathways, and associated molecules (homocysteine, NF-kappaB, vascular cell adhesion molecule 1, and VEGF), GM-CSF, IFN-γ, IL-1β, IL-4, IL-6, IL-8, IL-12, IL-15, IL-17, IL-20, IL-22BP, and IL-23, leukotriene B4, S100A7-9 and S100A12, sphingosine 1 phosphate, TGF-β-1, and TNF-α, are secreted by or are affected by neutrophils. These findings make the neutrophils important mediators and players in the immune response of the psoriatic patient.[66]

The chronic inflammatory stage of the psoriatic patient is characterized by prominent skin infiltration by neutrophils and microabscess formation. Through the progressive inflammatory stage, several cellular phenomena occur, including the adhesion of leukocytes and subsequent transmigration through the activated endothelium with the consequent accumulation of these cells in skin (Wetzel and colleagues[67] proposed that Thy-1, a human adhesion molecule on activated endothelial cells, is the mediator for the adhesion of neutrophils via the interaction with the 2-integrin Mac-1).

Newly discovered evidence integrates distinctive components of autoinflammation into the psoriatic inflammatory process. Inflammasome-mediated inflammation, dual involvement of Th1/Th2 in the different stages of the disease, the associated systemic inflammatory stage that produces associated or concomitant severe associated comorbidities, the established and well-defined genetic predisposition factors, the altered immunologic pathways, and the dysregulated immune response without clear evidence of causative antigens are some of the evidence-based factors actively participating in psoriatic inflammation that alter the classification of psoriasis from the autoimmune family and tend to change the perception to autoinflammation pathways. Some clinical variations of the disease including the pustular forms (guttate psoriasis) and PsA have been included in the new classification of autoinflammatory diseases. Evidence has been published regarding the association of autoinflammatory immune activation and correlation between PsA, nail psoriasis, and juxta-articular enthesitis.

Taken together, these data provide circumstantial evidence leading to a new perspective for psoriasis as an AID. Psoriasis is an inflammatory disease showing dysregulated innate immunity and is genetically distinct from autoimmunity, with combined adaptive and innate immune responses. Classic autoimmune diseases, with autoantibody and MHC class II associations, have adaptive immune genetic associations, including cytotoxic T-lymphocyte antigen 4 and PTPN22, which regulates some signaling pathways in T and B cells, characteristics not present in psoriasis.

GLOSSARY OF TERMS

Autoimmunity is the failure of an organism in recognizing its own constituent parts as self, which allows an immune response against its own cells and tissues. Any disease that results from such an aberrant immune response is termed an autoimmune disease. It is often attributed to a lack of germ development of a target body with the consequent immune response acting against its own cells and tissues. The immune system has the constant task of differentiating between the body's self and targets that are nonself. The main objective of its function is to remove nonself antigens, and a complex process of inflammation is involved in the mechanism of elimination.

An autoantigen is an antigen that, despite being a normal tissue constituent, is the target of a humoral (antibody) or cell-mediated immune response.

With AIDs, the term autoinflammatory syndrome has been attributed to the group of disorders characterized by unexplained recurrent attacks of inflammation without any evidence that this process is related to rejection of autoantigen. AIDs are caused by genetic mutations in molecules that are involved in regulating the innate immune response, an intricate defense system that evolved to quickly recognize and act against infectious agents and other danger signals produced by the human body. As per the International Society of Systemic Autoinflammatory Diseases (ISSAID), AIDs are defined as illnesses caused by primary dysfunction of the innate immune system. The new concept includes a large number of diseases, initially focusing on hereditary recurrent fevers, to include familial Mediterranean fever, mevalonate kinase deficiency, TNF receptor–associated periodic syndrome, CAPS, and NAPS12/NLRP12-associated periodic syndromes.

An antigen can be defined as any substance capable, under appropriate conditions, of inducing a specific immune response and of reacting with the products of that response; that is, with specific antibody or specifically sensitized T lymphocytes, or both. They may be soluble substances, such as toxins and foreign proteins, or particulate, such as bacteria and tissue cells; however, only the portion of the protein or polysaccharide molecule known as the antigenic determinant combines with antibody or a specific receptor on a lymphocyte.

The immune system is a complex network of specialized cells and organs that work together to defend the body against attacks by foreign invaders. The innate immune system is the more primitive part of the immune system. It uses types of white blood cells (granulocytes and monocytes) to destroy harmful substances. In this system, immune cells have receptors that have evolved to target specific proteins and other antigens that are commonly found on pathogens. The adaptive immune system is characterized by the response of cells to proteins and other antigens that they may never have encountered before, and that are presented to them by other cells. There is an interaction between both systems; the innate system often passes antigens on to the adaptive system.

Inflammation is a localized protective response elicited by injury or destruction of tissues, which serves to destroy, dilute, or separate the injurious agent and the injured tissue. It is characterized in the acute form by the classic signs of pain, heat, redness, swelling, and loss of function. It involves a multipart series of events, including arteriolar, capillary, and venular vasodilation, with increased permeability and blood flow; exudation of fluids, including plasma proteins; and migration of white blood cells into the inflammatory focus.

Idiotypes are antigenic epitopes found in the antigen-binding portion (Fab) of the immunoglobulin molecule.

Inflammasomes are cytosolic multiprotein complexes that recognize pathogen-associated molecular patterns. Recognition of pathogen-associated molecular patterns is followed by production of the proinflammatory cytokines IL-1b and IL-18.

Epitope, also known as antigenic determinant, is the part of an antigen that is recognized by the immune system, specifically by antibodies, B cells, or T cells. The part of an antibody that recognizes the epitope is called a paratope. Although epitopes are usually nonself proteins, sequences derived from the host that can be recognized are also epitopes.

PTPN23 is the approved symbol from the Human Genome Organisation Gene Nomenclature Committee (HGNC) database for tyrosine protein phosphatase nonreceptor type 23, which is an enzyme that in humans is encoded by the PTPN23 gene.

Th cells are a subgroup of lymphocytes, a type of white blood cell, that play an important role in the immune system, particularly in the adaptive immune system. They help the activity of other immune cells by releasing T-cell cytokines. They are essential in B-cell antibody class switching, in the activation and growth of cytotoxic T cells, and in maximizing bactericidal activity of phagocytes such as macrophages. Mature Th cells express the surface protein CD4 and are referred to as CD4+ T cells. CD4+ T cells are generally treated as having a predefined role as helper T cells within the immune system. For example, when an antigen-presenting cell expresses an antigen on MHC class II, a CD4+ cell aids those cells through a combination of cell-to-cell interactions (eg, CD40 and CD40L) and through cytokines. Nevertheless, there are rare exceptions; for example, subgroups of regulatory T cells, NK T cells, and cytotoxic T cells express CD4 (although cytotoxic examples have been observed in extremely low numbers in specific disease states, they are usually considered nonexistent). All of these CD4+ T-cell groups are not considered T helper cells.

Tolerance is defined as the process by which the immune system does not attack an antigen. This process can be natural or self-tolerance, in which the body does not post an immune response to self-antigens, or induced, created by manipulating the immune system. It occurs in 3 forms: central, peripheral, and acquired, based on whether or not the mechanisms listed earlier operate in the central lymphoid organs (thymus and bone marrow) or the peripheral lymphoid organs (lymph node, spleen, and so forth), where self-reactive B cells may be destroyed. The mechanism of central tolerance is simply an induced and triggered apoptotic death, mediated by surface expression of IgM of developing B cells within the bone marrow; similarly, the binding of peptide-MHC complex by T-cell receptors of single positive (CD4+CD8−) thymocytes, causing them to undergo apoptotic death. The process eliminates potential autoreactive B and T cells before entering the general circulation and peripheral tissues, before producing systemic damage. For peripheral tolerance, many mechanisms have been suggested, all implicated in the control or elimination of autoreactive cells from the B or T lymphocytes after they move from the lymphoid tissue at the thymus or the bone marrow. For example, anergy (inhibition of the required steps on signaling by binding of T-cell receptors to pMHC I and II) and suppression (induction of tolerance to self-epitopes by regulatory cells, including, as shown in multiple studies, by the effect of activated specific T cells [CD4+ and CD8+] that induce inhibitory effects on antibody production). These theories are not mutually exclusive.

REFERENCES

1. Yao Q, Furst D. Autoinflammatory diseases: an update of clinical and genetic aspects. Rheumatology 2008;47(7):946–95.
2. Masters S, Simon A, Aksentijevich I, et al. Horror autoinflammaticus: the molecular pathophysiology of autoinflammatory diseases. NIH Public Access. Author Manuscript. Annu Rev Immunol 2009;27: 621–68.
3. Houten SM, Kuis W, Duran M, et al. Mutations in MVK, encoding mevalonate kinase, cause hyperimmunoglobulinaemia D and periodic fever syndrome. Nat Genet 1999;22:175–7.
4. Galon J, Aksentijevich I, McDermott MF, et al. TNFRSF1A mutations and autoinflammatory syndromes. Curr Opin Immunol 2000;12:479–86.
5. Amagay M, Kouji M. Overview of autoimmunity and autoinflammation. Inflamm Reagen Jan 2011;31(1): 50–1.
6. Lamprecht P, Gross WL. Autoinflammatory syndromes. Internist (Berl) 2009;50(6):676–84. http://dx.doi.org/10.1007/s00108-009-2302-5 [in German].
7. The NOMID Alliance: The NOMID Alliance is a 501 (c) (3) non-profit public charity dedicated to promoting awareness, proper diagnosis and treatment, and improved care for people with CAPS (Cryopyrin-Associated Periodic Syndromes) and other autoinflammatory diseases. Awareness publication of the NIAMS and NIH. Information clearinghouse. Available at: www.niams.nih.gov. Accessed March, 2010.
8. Stankovic K, Grateau G. What's new in autoinflammatory diseases? Rev Med Interne 2008;29(12): 994–9 [in French].
9. Stefanova I, Dorfman JR, Germain RN. Self-recognition promotes the foreign antigen sensitivity of naive T lymphocytes. Nature 2002;420(6914):429–34.
10. Pike B, Boyd A, Nossal G. Clonal anergy: the universally anergic B lymphocyte. Proc Natl Acad Sci U S A 1982;79(6):2013–7.
11. Jerne N. Towards a network theory of the immune system. Ann Immunol (Paris) 1974;125C(1–2):373–89.
12. Edwards JC, Cambridge G, Abrahams VM. Do self-perpetuating B lymphocytes drive human autoimmune disease? Immunology 1999;97:1868–76.
13. Klein J, Sato A. The HLA system. Second of two parts. N Engl J Med 2000;343(11):782–6.
14. Edwards JC, Cambridge G. B-cell targeting in rheumatoid arthritis and other autoimmune diseases. Nat Rev Immunol 2006;6(5):394–403. http://dx.doi.org/10.1038/nri1838.
15. Kubach J, Becker C, Schmitt E, et al. Dendritic cells: sentinels of immunity and tolerance. Int J Hematol 2005;81(3):197–203. http://dx.doi.org/10.1532/IJH97.04165.
16. Srinivasan R, Houghton AN, Wolchoks JD. Induction of autoantibodies against tyrosinase-related proteins following DNA vaccination: unexpected reactivity to a protein paralogue. Cancer Immun 2002;2:8.
17. Willam R. On cutaneous diseases. Philadelphia: Kimber & Conrad; 1809. Early Autoimmune imprints. Second Series No. 19235.
18. Nestle FO, Kaplan DH, Barker J. Psoriasis. N Engl J Med 2009;361(5):496–509.
19. Griffiths CE, Barker JN. Pathogenesis and clinical features of psoriasis. Lancet 2007;370(9583): 263–71.
20. Rahman P, Elder JT. Genetic epidemiology of psoriasis and psoriatic arthritis. Ann Rheum Dis 2005; 64(Suppl 2):ii37–9.
21. Langley RG, Krueger GG, Griffiths CE. Psoriasis: epidemiology, clinical features, and quality of life. Ann Rheum Dis 2005;64(Suppl 2):ii18–23.
22. Menter A, Gottlieb A, Feldman S, et al. Guidelines of care for the management of psoriasis and psoriatic arthritis. J Am Acad Dermatol 2008;58:826–50.
23. Sabat R, Philipp S, Hoflich C, et al. Immunopathogenesis of psoriasis. Exp Dermatol 2007;16(10):779–98.
24. Naldi L, Chatenoud L, Linder D, et al. Cigarette smoking, body mass index, and stressful life events as risk factors for psoriasis: results from an Italian case-control study. J Invest Dermatol 2005;125(1):61–7.
25. Gunnarsson C, Chen J, Rizzo JA, et al. The direct healthcare insurer and out-of-pocket expenditures of psoriasis: evidence from a United States national survey. J Dermatolog Treat 2012;23(4):240–54.
26. Nickoloff BJ, Qin JZ, Nestle FO. Immunopathogenesis of psoriasis. Clin Rev Allergy Immunol 2007; 33(1–2):45–56.
27. Nickoloff BJ. The cytokine network in psoriasis. Arch Dermatol 1991;127:871–84.
28. Gottlieb AB. Psoriasis: emerging therapeutic strategies. Nat Rev Drug Discov 2005;4:19–34.
29. Krueger JG. The immunologic basis for the treatment of psoriasis with new biologic agents. J Am Acad Dermatol 2002;46:1–23.
30. Coimbra S, Figueiredo A, Castro E, et al. The roles of cells and cytokines in the pathogenesis of psoriasis. Int J Dermatol 2012;51(4):389–95.
31. Lowes MA, Russell CB, Martin DA, et al. The IL-23/T17 pathogenic axis in psoriasis is amplified by keratinocyte responses. Trends Immunol 2013;34(4): 174–81. http://dx.doi.org/10.1016/j.it.2012.11.005. pii:S1471–4906(12)00199-8.
32. Mudigonda P, Mudigonda T, Feneran AN, et al. Interleukin-23 and interleukin-17: importance in pathogenesis and therapy of psoriasis. Dermatol Online J 2012;18(10):1.
33. Alexandroff AB, Pauriah M, Lang CC, et al. Atherosclerosis as a systemic feature of psoriasis. Clin Exp Dermatol 2011;36(5):451–2.

34. Armstrong AW, Voyles SV, Armstrong EJ, et al. A tale of two plaques: convergent mechanisms of T-cell-mediated inflammation in psoriasis and atherosclerosis. Exp Dermatol 2011;20(7):544–9.

35. Rogler G. Update in inflammatory bowel disease pathogenesis. Curr Opin Gastroenterol 2004;20:311–7.

36. Arkan MC, Hevener AL, Greten FR, et al. IKK-beta links inflammation to obesity-induced insulin resistance. Nat Med 2005;11:191–8.

37. Reich K. The concept of psoriasis as a systemic inflammation: implications for disease management. J Eur Acad Dermatol Venereol 2012;26(Suppl 2):3–11.

38. Himmerich H, Fulda S, Linseisen J, et al. Depression, comorbidities and the TNF-alpha system. Eur Psychiatry 2008;23(6):421–9.

39. Kambe N, Satoh S, Nakamura Y, et al. Autoinflammatory diseases and the inflammasome: mechanisms of IL-1β activation leading to neutrophil-rich skin disorders. Inflamm Regen 2011;31(1):72–80.

40. Christophers E. Psoriasis: heterogeneity, innate immunity and comorbidities. Expet Rev Dermatol 2012;7(2):195–202.

41. Hebra F. On diseases of the skin including the exanthemata. London: New Sydenham Society; 1868.

42. Von Zumbusch L. Psoriasis und pustulöses exanthem. Arch Dermatol Syph 1910;99:335–46.

43. Asumalahti K, Ameen M, Suomela S, et al. Genetic analysis of PSORS1 distinguishes guttate psoriasis and palmoplantar pustulosis. J Invest Dermatol 2003;120(4):627–32.

44. Marrakchi A, Guigue P, Renshaw BR, et al. Interleukin-36-receptor antagonist deficiency and generalized pustular psoriasis. N Engl J Med 2011;365(7):620–8.

45. Onoufradis A, Simpson MA, Pink AE, et al. Mutations in IL36RN/IL1F5 are associated with severe episodic inflammatory skin disease known as generalized pustular psoriasis. Am J Hum Genet 2011;89(3):432–7.

46. Bowcock AM, Krueger JG. Getting under the skin: the immunogenetics of psoriasis. Nat Rev Immunol 2005;5(9):699–711.

47. Jabbari A, Johnson-Huang LM, Krueger JG. Role of the immune system and immunological circuits in psoriasis. G Ital Dermatol Venereol 2011;146(1):17–30.

48. Gudjonsson JE, Ding J, Johnston A, et al. Assessment of the psoriatic transcriptosome in a large sample: additional regulated genes and comparisons with in vitro models. J Invest Dermatol 2010;130(7):1829–40.

49. Elder JT, Bruce AT, Gudjonsson JE, et al. Molecular dissection of psoriasis: integrating genetics and biology. J Invest Dermatol 2009;130(5):1213–26.

50. Prens E. Linking innate and adaptive immunity in psoriasis. Presented at: Psoriasis: From Gene to Clinic. London, December 1–3, 2011.

51. Schön MP, Ruzicka T. Psoriasis: the plot thickens. Nat Immunol 2001;2(2):91.

52. Zur Stadt U, Beutel K, Kolberg S, et al. Mutation spectrum in children with primary hemophagocytic lymphohistiocytosis: molecular and functional analyses of PRF1, UNC13D, STX11, and RAB27A. Hum Mutat 2006;27:62–8.

53. Janka GE. Familial and acquired hemophagocytic lymphohistiocytosis. Eur J Pediatr 2007;166:95–109.

54. Hansson GK. Inflammation, atherosclerosis, and coronary artery disease. N Engl J Med 2005;352:1685–95.

55. Branderup F, Holm N, Grunnet N, et al. Psoriasis in monozygotic twins: variations in expression in individuals with identical genetic constitution. Acta Derm Venereol 1982;62(3):229–36.

56. Henseler T, Christophers E. Psoriasis of early and late onset: characterization of two types of psoriasis vulgaris. J Am Acad Dermatol 1985;13(3):450–6.

57. Salskov-Iversen ML, Johansen C, Kragballe K, et al. Caspase-5 expression is upregulated in lesional psoriatic skin. J Invest Dermatol 2011;131(3):670–6.

58. Lande R, Gregorio J, Facchinetti V, et al. Plasmacytoid dendritic cells sense self-DNA coupled with antimicrobial peptide. Nature 2007;449(7162):564–9.

59. Dombrowski Y, Peric M, Koglin S, et al. Cytosolic DNA triggers inflammasome activation in keratinocytes in psoriatic lesions. Sci Transl Med 2011;3(82):82ra38.

60. McGonagle D, Ash Z, Dickie L, et al. The early phase of psoriatic arthritis. Ann Rheum Dis 2011;70(Suppl 1):71–6.

61. McGonagle D, McDermott MF. A proposed classification of the immunologic diseases. PLoS Med 2006;3:1242–8.

62. Husted JA, Thavaneswaran A, Chandran V, et al. Cardiovascular and other comorbidities in patients with psoriatic arthritis: a comparison with patients with psoriasis. Arthritis Care Res 2011;63(12):1729–35.

63. Shapiro J, Cohen AD, David M, et al. The association between psoriasis, diabetes mellitus, and atherosclerosis in Israel: a case control study. J Am Acad Dermatol 2007;56(4):629–34.

64. Gelfand JM, Neimann AL, Shiin DB, et al. Risk of myocardial infarction in patients with psoriasis. JAMA 2006;296(14):1735–41.

65. Federman DG, Shelling M, Prodanovich S, et al. Psoriasis: an opportunity to identify cardiovascular risk. Br J Dermatol 2009;160(1):1–7.

66. Aronson PJ. A review of the role of neutrophils in psoriasis and related disorders. Dermatol Online J 2008;14(7):7.

67. Wetzel A, Wetzig T, Haustein UF, et al. Increased neutrophil adherence in psoriasis: role of the human endothelial cell receptor Thy-1 (CD90). J Invest Dermatol 2006;126:441–52.

Autoinflammatory Disorders, Pain, and Neural Regulation of Inflammation

Michael C. Chen, PhD*, Matthew H. Meckfessel, PhD

KEYWORDS

- Autoinflammatory disorders • Neural crosstalk • IL-1β • Inflammasome • Pain • Neuromodulation

KEY POINTS

- Current dermatologic disorders with predominant inflammatory components, such as rosacea and acne, possess hallmark features of autoinflammatory disorders.
- The contribution of interleukin-1 beta (IL-1β) in mediating pain through underlying neural pathways is underappreciated in the context of autoinflammatory disorders, and needs to be further explored.
- Disorders marked by increases in IL-1β in the absence of adaptive immune activation, in conjunction with inexplicable pain and inflammation, may be considered diagnostic criteria for classifying autoinflammatory disorders.
- Further exploration into the causative link between inflammation and the nervous system may lead to new therapeutic modalities for autoinflammatory disorders, such as neuromodulation.

INTRODUCTION

Autoinflammatory disorders are a newly described class of disorders marked predominantly by dysregulation of the innate immune system.[1] This heterogeneous class of disorders is clinically distinct from autoimmune disorders.[1–3] Autoinflammatory disorders are currently recognized as "clinical disorders marked by abnormally increased inflammation, mediated predominantly by the cells and molecules of the innate immune system, with a significant host predisposition."[1] Increased levels of interleukin-1 beta (IL-1β) cause abnormal inflammatory responses and are central to these disorders. Infection has yet to be found during episodic flares and does not seem to be a precipitating factor in the disorders. High-titer antibodies and antigen-specific autoreactive T cells are also absent.

A large number of disorders are now recognized as autoinflammatory and the number continues to grow. Affected systems are diverse and include skin, joints, and the nervous system.[1] The hereditary periodic fever (HPF) syndromes were among the first to be labeled as autoinflammatory.[2] Gout, type 2 diabetes, obesity-induced insulin resistance, Blau syndrome, and others are now classified as autoinflammatory.[1,4] Some autoinflammatory disorders, including pyogenic arthritis-pyoderma gangrenosum-acne (PAPA) syndrome and Blau syndrome, affect the skin.[5,6] Other dermatologic disorders with an inflammatory component, such as rosacea or acne, may potential be autoinflammatory disorders.

Many of the autoinflammatory disorders have a strong pain component that is overlooked. Episodic flares in the HPF syndromes and gout can cause debilitating pain. Cytokines, including

Funding Sources/Support: Galderma Laboratories, L.P., Fort Worth, TX.
Conflict of Interest: None.
Galderma Laboratories, LP, 14501 North Freeway, Fort Worth, TX 76177, USA
* Corresponding author.
E-mail address: michael.chen@galderma.com

Dermatol Clin 31 (2013) 461–470
http://dx.doi.org/10.1016/j.det.2013.04.002

IL-1β, and other inflammatory mediators are known to play important roles in neuronal perception of pain.[7] Thus abnormal innate immune responses may abnormally affect neuronal perception of pain. The nervous system plays an important role in regulating inflammation and inflammatory pain.[8] Neural-inflammation crosstalk may be disrupted in autoinflammatory disorders and contribute to the symptoms. Although crosstalk between inflammation and perception of pain is known to occur, it has not been highlighted in autoinflammatory disorders. Highlighting the inflammatory/neural crosstalk may allow a richer understanding of autoinflammatory disorders and potentially help to broaden the current disorder classification. This article provides an overview of current autoinflammatory disorders and how inexplicable inflammation and pain may factor into classifying new autoinflammatory disorders.

THE INFLAMMASOME

Identification of the inflammasome and its physiologic role helped to elucidate autoinflammatory disorders as being caused by dysregulation of the innate immune system. The inflammasome is a complex of proteins composed of a sensor protein, the adapter protein apoptosis-associated speck-like protein with CARD domain (ASC), and caspase-1.[9] Four sensor proteins have been identified: NLRP1, NLRP3, NLRC4, and AIM2.[10] Binding of stimuli to the sensor protein promotes assembly of the complex and activation of caspase-1. The NLRP1, NLRC4, and AIM2 inflammasomes are activated by specific microbial stimuli, whereas NLRP3 can be activated by a broad range of microbial and sterile stimuli.[4,9] Once activated, the inflammasome processes proIL-1β into its active form. IL-1β is a potent regulator of inflammatory responses. Activation of IL-1β in response to inflammatory stimuli is a 2-step process.[11] The first step involves increased production of proIL-1β. Basal expression of proIL-1β is low and is induced by nuclear factor (NF)-κB.[11] Activation of NF-κB occurs through pathogen-associated molecular patterns (PAMPs) that stimulate phagocytic cells or through primary cytokines.[12] The second step is activation of inflammasomes.

The NLRP3 inflammasome is the most studied inflammasome. Microbial activation can occur through bacteria, fungi, and viruses.[13–15] Unlike other inflammasomes, the NLRP3 inflammasome can be activated in sterile environments by nonmicrobial stimuli; extracellular ATP, monosodium crystals, calcium pyrophosphate dehydrate crystals, cholesterol crystals, and oligomers of islet amyloid polypeptide are all capable of activating

NLRP3 inflammasomes.[16–19] Several of these nonmicrobial activators are also involved in the pathogenesis of other diseases with a strong inflammatory component such as gout and type 2 diabetes. Thus a broad range of stimuli or genetic defects can cause dysregulation of the innate immune system and induce an autoinflammatory response. In the established HPF syndromes and the emerging autoinflammatory disorders, dysregulation of the innate immune system, specifically the inflammasome, is at the epicenter and abnormal inflammasome activity results in increased IL-1β levels.

INFLAMMASOME AUTOACTIVATION DISORDERS

Familial Mediterranean fever (FMF) is an HPF disorder. Patients with FMF experience episodic bouts of fever and serosal inflammation lasting up to 3 days and occurring every 10 days to once a year.[20] During attacks, patients also experience debilitating muscle and joint pain.[21] Defects in the MEFV gene encoding for pyrin have been found to cause FMF.[22] Pyrin is a regulator of capsase-1 activation. The defective pyrin protein causes an overactive inflammasome, which leads to increased levels of IL-1β.[23]

Mutations in the PSTPIP1 (proline-serine-threonine-phosphatase interacting protein 1) gene have been identified as the cause of PAPA syndrome.[24] PAPA syndrome is an autosomal dominant hereditary syndrome that has some clinical similarities to FMF. Sterile arthritis of the knees, elbows, and ankles develops in early childhood in patients with PAPA.[25] Symptoms also include cystic acne and pyoderma gangrenosum, which last into adulthood and may cause debilitating pain.[5] Infection has yet to be found in cultures from skin lesions or joint fluids.[5,24] PSTPIP1 interacts with pyrin to regulate inflammasome activity.[26] Mutations result in hyperphosphorylation of PSTPIP1 disrupting regulation of the NLRP3 inflammasome, which causes increased production of IL-1β.

The cryopyrin-associated periodic syndromes (CAPSs) are a group of 3 syndromes that are also HPF syndromes: familial cold autoinflammatory syndrome (FCAS), Muckle-Wells syndrome (MWS), and neonatal-onset multisystem inflammatory disease (NOMID). FCAS is the least severe and is characterized by cold-induced fever and rashes.[11] MWS is more severe and is accompanied by hearing loss and arthritis. NOMID is the most severe and is characterized by chronic fever, hives, hearing loss, overgrowth of the epiphyses of the long bones, chronic meningitis, cerebral atrophy, and delayed atrophy.[27] All 3 are caused by inherited or de novo mutations in the *NLRP3/CIAS1* gene (previously called cryopyrin).[28,29] The encoded NLRP3 protein is defective in regulation and is constitutively active.[30] Subjects afflicted with any of the CAPSs have increased levels of IL-1β. Biologic therapies for the CAPSs target IL-1β and are effective in managing the disorders.[31,32] Although CAPS is caused by defects in *NLRP3*, the causes of increased levels of IL-1β and the origin of the IL-1β remain unknown. It is also unknown why CAPSs only affect certain organs and not others. Mouse models of CAPS have been developed which will help to address these questions.[33,34]

METABOLITE AUTOINFLAMMATORY DISEASES

Gout is an autoinflammatory disorder marked by severe swelling and pain of the joints. Attacks are recurring and acute, and, if left untreated, can progress into chronic tophaceous gout.[35] Gout is caused by an accumulation of monosodium urate (MSU) crystals. However, MSU crystals are not the sole causative agent in gout.[36] One study investigated what effect MSU crystals or free fatty acids (FFAs) had on human peripheral blood mononuclear cells (PBMCs) and murine macrophages in vitro.[37] Neither produced IL-1β when exposed to MSU crystals or FFAs alone. When PBMCs or murine macrophages were simultaneously exposed to both, large amounts of IL-1β were produced. Thus accumulation of MSU crystals and FFAs activate the NLRP3 inflammasome, resulting in increased levels of IL-1β.[17] This finding is consistent with the clinical manifestation of gout frequently occurring during night. Released IL-1β then binds IL-1 receptors on macrophages, which leads to additional production of proinflammatory cytokines and chemokines.[38]

Mevalonate kinase deficiency (MKD; formerly called hyperimmunoglobulinemia D syndrome [HIDS]) is an HPF syndrome caused by a recessively inherited defect in the mevalonate kinase gene.[39] Mevalonate kinase is the second enzyme in the mevalonate pathway of cholesterol synthesis. Deficiencies result in reduced levels of downstream metabolites. Episodic attacks last longer than those associated with FMF. Symptoms can include abdominal pain, headache, cervical lymphadenopathy, arthritis, and diarrhea.[40] Dysregulation of the inflammasome in HIDS has also been identified.[41] Experiments that inhibited mevalonate kinase by alendronate in human PBMCs treated with lipopolysaccharide (LPS) resulted in a 20-fold increase in *NLRP3* expression and increased levels of secreted IL-1β. When treated

with alendronate or LPS alone, NLRP3 expression was only increased approximately 2.5-fold. Basal levels of *NLRP3* in PBMCs isolated from 2 subjects with MKD were also increased. When these PBMCs were stimulated with just LPS, levels of IL-1β increased. Thus a functioning mevalonate kinase gene and downstream metabolites are necessary for proper inflammasome regulation. Similar to gout, it also seems that multiple stimuli are required to elicit an autoinflammatory response in MKD.

Type 2 diabetes is now recognized as an autoinflammatory disease.[36] High levels of glucose stimulate beta cells to produce IL-1β, indicating a direct role for IL-1β in the disease.[42] Glucose, FFAs, and leptin all induce production of IL-1β from human islets.[43–45] Adipocyte differentiation and insulin resistance are controlled by caspase-1 activation and production of IL-1β.[46] Inhibition of IL-1β improves insulin sensitivity. Taken together, these results highlight the central role of IL-1β in type 2 diabetes and confirm its classification as autoinflammatory.

NF-κB DISEASES

Tumor necrosis factor (TNF) receptor–associated periodic syndrome (TRAPS) was the first disorder to be recognized as autoinflammatory.[47] TRAPS is a dominantly inherited disorder characterized by episodic periods of fever, abdominal pain, migratory erythema, myalgia, and periorbital edema.[48] Molecular cloning identified a missense mutation in the *TNFRSF1A* gene, which encodes for a TNF receptor.[47] Mutations result in increased activity of NF-κB and, ultimately, increased production of IL-1β.

Blau syndrome is an autosomal dominant hereditary disease with a childhood onset.[6] Symptoms include iritis, skin rash, granulomatous arthritis, and periarticular synovial cysts. Blau syndrome is caused by mutations in the *NOD2* gene.[49–51] NOD2 is a cytosolic protein that recognizes muramyl dipeptide (MDP), the minimal active peptidoglycan motif common to bacteria.[52,53] On MDP recognition, NOD2 activates and interacts with RIP2 activating NF-κB. Mutations in NOD2 cause excessive activation and signaling of NF-κB, resulting in increased IL-1β levels.[51]

AUTOINFLAMMATORY DISORDERS DOWNSTREAM OF IL-1β

Deficiency of the IL-1 receptor agonist (DIRA) is a recently described autoinflammatory disorder.[54,55] Symptoms present within 2.5 weeks of birth and include fetal distress, pustular rash, joint swelling, oral mucosal lesions, pain with movement, and cutaneous pustulosis.[54] The pathogenesis of DIRA is caused by deletion or truncation of the *IL1RN* gene.[55,56] Patients with DIRA fail to produce a functioning IL-1 receptor agonist (IL1RA), which plays a crucial role in modulating the effects of IL-1β at the receptor level. Other autoinflammatory disorders can be traced to mutations or changes to stimuli upstream of IL-1β production or activation, but DIRA is unique because the disorder is caused by defects downstream of IL-1β.

AUTOINFLAMMATORY PAIN

There are 3 types of recognized pain: nociceptive, neuropathic, and inflammatory.[57] Nociceptive pain is the result of noxious stimuli activating sensory neurons. Nociceptors respond to temperature, chemical, and mechanical stimuli. Neuropathic pain arises from damage or dysfunction to the nervous system. Normal sensory cells generate action potentials from the end of the nerve at the receptive field. Damaged nerve cells can generate pathologic ectopic discharges from the site of injury, and healthy nerve fibers near damaged nerves can also spontaneously generate pain.[58,59] Ectopic and spontaneous pain are examples of neuropathic pain. Inflammatory pain results from damaged tissue, cancer cells, and other inflamed tissues, which release inflammatory mediators known as an inflammatory soup that modulates nociceptors to perceive pain.[57] Posttranslational modification to nociceptors alters their response, making them more sensitive to pain. Peripheral nociceptors are normally dormant in the absence of stimuli. When activated, they produce an acute response that provides a warning of eminent danger and plays an essential function in an organism's survival.

In particular, IL-1β hypersensitizes nociceptors and proinflammatory cytokines play an important role in hyperalgesia and inflammatory pain.[60–62] Part of this response is alterations of periphery nociceptors that reduce their threshold and increase their sensitivity.[63] The goal of hyperalgesia is to heighten pain awareness to prevent further injury to the afflicted area. Dysregulation of IL-1β can result in increased nociceptor sensitization and eventually neuropathic pain.[64] Attacks and increased levels of IL-1β are episodic in the HPF syndromes; associated pain is acute and does not progress into neuropathic pain. Other autoinflammatory disorders that are not episodic may have associated chronic pain.

The symptoms of gout are extremely painful. Gout initially presents as acute flares, but can progress into a chronic state. Activation of IL-1β produces increased levels of inflammatory mediators and chemokines, which create an influx of neutrophils into the joint. In addition to the direct role that IL-1β has in modulating pain, neutrophils may also have hyperalgesic properties.[65] Chemokines are also important in modulating pain.[66] Thus IL-1β may not only increase pain in gout but also amplify it. Treatment of gout with anakinra, a recombinant IL-1 receptor antagonist, or canakinumab, an anti–IL-1β monoclonal antibody, improves symptoms of acute and chronic tophaceous gout.[67–69] Blocking or inhibiting the effects of IL-1β in treating gout reinforces the central role IL-1β has in autoinflammation as well as pain.

Given the important role that IL-1β plays in pain modulation, subjects with type 2 diabetes frequently experience peripheral neuropathic pain.[70] However, only 3% to 25% of subjects experience peripheral neuropathic pain.[71] Why only a small portion of subjects with type 2 diabetes experience peripheral neuropathic pain is unclear. Clinical trials with anakinra in subjects with type 2 diabetes showed improvements in beta-cell function and inflammation.[72,73] Current pain management therapies for type 2 diabetes do not target IL-1β function. Treatments include lipoic acid, tricyclic antidepressants, gabapentin, pregabalin, duloxetine, and oxycodone.[71] Because of the central role IL-1β plays in pain, IL-1β antagonists and blockers could be potential therapeutic agents for pain relief as well as for helping to manage symptoms in subjects with type 2 diabetes.

The link between autoinflammation and pain is further underscored in animal models. One study screened N-ethyl-N-nitrosourea (ENU)–mutated mice to identify a mouse model for pain.[74] This line showed abnormal nociceptor responses and was hypersensitive to pain. The line also showed symptoms of autoinflammation. These mice showed normal behavior and were otherwise healthy. A mutation in the *PSTPIP2* gene, the same gene implicated in PAPA syndrome, was identified as the causative factor. A successful screen for a pain model in mice yielded a mutation known to cause an autoinflammatory disorder. The identification of this mouse model highlights the importance of pain in autoinflammatory disorder and how the two are interconnected.

POTENTIAL AUTOINFLAMMATORY DISORDERS

All of the disorders discussed thus far have 2 commonalities: unprovoked inflammation and pain. Dysregulation of the innate immune system is the causative agent in these diseases. However, the underlying cause of many disorders has yet to be identified. Are other disorders with seemingly inexplicable inflammation and a pain component autoinflammatory?

INTERSTITIAL CYSTITIS

Interstitial cystitis (IC) is a chronic inflammatory disorder affecting the bladder. IC is characterized by pelvic or perineal pain, urinary urgency and frequency, and nocturia.[75] IC is also marked with a strong pain component and is frequently called painful bladder syndrome. In the absence of a causative factor in IC, management is difficult. Current strategies to manage the symptoms of IC include behavior modification, pentosan polysulfate sodium, amitriptyline, hydroxyzine, and dimethyl sulfoxide.[76] IC is clinically distinct from other bladder and urinary disorders even though symptoms overlap. The cause of IC is not well understood. No diagnostic exists for IC and diagnostic tests are used to rule out other diseases.[77] Markers of inflammation have been identified in subjects with IC. Infiltration of mast cells into the bladder was identified in histologic analysis.[78] Urine samples collected over 24 hours in subjects with IC were increased in antiproliferative factor, epidermal growth factor, insulin growth factor–binding protein 3, and IL-6 compared with healthy subjects.[79] Urine and serum levels of nerve growth factor are also increased in subjects with IC.[80] However, urine markers do not always correlate with biopsy findings.[81] No direct evidence indicates that IC is an autoimmune disease, and there is no evidence of infection.[82,83] Does that indicate that IC is an autoinflammatory disease? Immunohistochemical analysis of tissue from the urothelial layer of the bladder showed the presence of NLRP3.[84] This finding suggests that the inflammasome may play a role in mediating bladder inflammation. The presence of mast cells may also indicate that IC is an autoinflammatory disorder. Mast cells are the source of IL-1β in urticarial rash in CAPS disorders.[85] Given the chronic inflammation, absence of an autoimmune response or infection, infiltrated mast cells, and the presence of NLRP3 in urothelial tissue from the bladder, it is plausible that dysregulation of the NLRP3 inflammasome and increased IL-1β may play a role in the cause of IC. Future studies in patients with IC should address this possibility.

ROSACEA

Rosacea is a chronic disease of the face characterized by flushing, persistent erythema, telangiectasia, papules, and pustules. Rosacea flares are frequently triggered by external stimuli such as ultraviolet (UV) light or temperature changes. The molecular and cellular mechanisms underlying rosacea have yet to be identified. Clinical and histopathologic analyses indicate that rosacea is the result of inflammatory processes.[86] Dysregulation of the innate immune system and an abnormal response to innocuous stimuli have been proposed as underlying causes of rosacea.[87] UV light, a rosacea trigger, is known to induce IL-1β and TNF-α in human skin.[88] UV light also activates inflammasomes in keratinocytes.[89] Biopsies taken from patients with rosacea revealed an increase in mast cells.[90] As discussed earlier, mast cells are a source of IL-1β production. Subjects with rosacea can also experience pain with changes in temperature that are normally perceived as benign.[91] Abnormal signaling by the transient receptor potential (TRP) channels TRPA1 and TRPV1 are thought to play a role in temperature pain. These receptors are located on periphery neurons and may release neurotransmitters that could increase inflammation. An abnormal response to stimuli, infiltration of mast cells, and the presence of pain indicate that rosacea has commonalities with other autoinflammatory disorders.

SUMMARY

Autoinflammatory disorders constitute a large and growing class of disorders (summarized in **Table 1**). Disorders that are seemingly unrelated, such as FMF, type 2 diabetes, and gout, are all similar because of dysregulation of the innate immune system, specifically IL-1β. Although the inflammatory components of these disorders are well recognized, the neural components underlying pain and regulation are not. Crosstalk between the neural networks and inflammatory machinery allows additional levels of regulation to fine tune inflammatory responses. Inflammation modulates pain responses to help protect the organism against further harm, whereas neurotransmitters inhibit inflammatory mediators to ease inflammation. This interplay is highlighted in the mouse model identified from a screen for a pain model that also had autoinflammatory disease. Further emphasizing the link between inflammation and the nervous system is that therapeutic neuromodulation of IC provides symptomatic relief of inflammatory symptoms.[92] Perhaps neuromodulation could also be a therapeutic option for other autoinflammatory disorders. The neural regulation of the inflammatory component in autoinflammatory disorders warrants further investigation. It is conceivable that mutations or deficiencies in the nervous system could elicit unwarranted

Table 1
Autoinflammatory disorders discussed in this review and their causes

Inflammasome Autoactivation Disorders Metabolite Disorders	
FMF	*MEFV*
PAPA	*PSTPIP1*
CAPS	*NLRP3*
NF-kB Disorders	
Blau syndrome	*NOD2*
TRAPS	*TNFRSF1A*
Metabolite Disorders	
Gout	MSU crystals and FFAs
MKD	Melavonate kinase
Type 2 diabetes	Glucose, FFAs, leptin
Potential Autoinflammatory Disorders	
Rosacea	Unknown
IC	Unknown

inflammatory responses. Perhaps neural dysfunction is the causative agent in disorders with an inflammatory component that have not had the underlying mechanisms identified.

Fig. 1 provides an overview of autoinflammatory disorders discussed in this article and their interplay with neural pathways. Other disorders with unexplained inflammation and pain may be

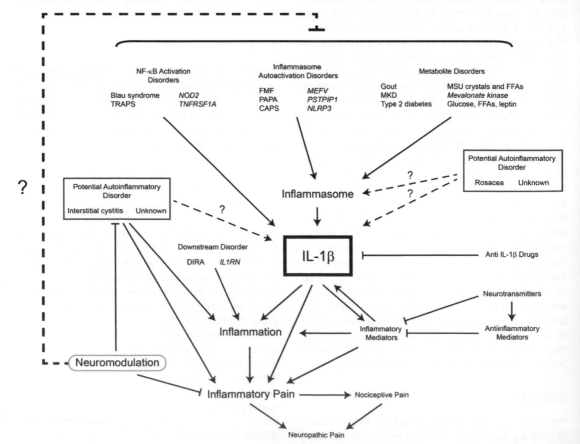

Fig. 1. Overview of known autoinflammatory disorders, potential autoinflammatory disorders, and their interplay with pain. Known and possible therapeutic options are also shown.

autoinflammatory disorders. IC and rosacea each are marked by inflammation and pain. Thus, in the absence of an autoimmune component, these two diseases may be autoinflammatory. Other diseases that fit these criteria may also be classified as autoinflammatory as their causes become better understood, such as psoriasis or Behçet Disease. Taken together, the body of evidence supports a larger role for neural networks in pain and inflammatory regulation in autoinflammatory disorders than is currently appreciated.

REFERENCES

1. Kastner DL, Aksentijevich I, Goldbach-Mansky R. Autoinflammatory disease reloaded: a clinical perspective. Cell 2010;140(6):784–90.
2. Brydges S, Kastner DL. The systemic autoinflammatory diseases: inborn errors of the innate immune system. Curr Top Microbiol Immunol 2006; 305:127–60.
3. Kambe N, Satoh T, Tanizaki H, et al. Enhanced NF-kappaB activation with an inflammasome activator correlates with activity of autoinflammatory disease associated with NLRP3 mutations outside of exon 3: comment on the article by Jeru et al. Arthritis Rheum 2010;62(10):3123–4 [author reply: 3124–5].
4. Menu P, Vince JE. The NLRP3 inflammasome in health and disease: the good, the bad and the ugly. Clin Exp Immunol 2011;166(1):1–15.
5. Smith EJ, Allantaz F, Bennett L, et al. Clinical, molecular, and genetic characteristics of PAPA syndrome: a review. Curr Genomics 2010;11(7): 519–27.
6. Pastores GM, Michels VV, Stickler GB, et al. Autosomal dominant granulomatous arthritis, uveitis, skin rash, and synovial cysts. J Pediatr 1990;117(3): 403–8.
7. Basbaum AI, Bautista DM, Scherrer G, et al. Cellular and molecular mechanisms of pain. Cell 2009;139(2):267–84.
8. Kavoussi B, Ross BE. The neuroimmune basis of anti-inflammatory acupuncture. Integr Cancer Ther 2007;6(3):251–7.
9. Gross O, Thomas CJ, Guarda G, et al. The inflammasome: an integrated view. Immunol Rev 2011; 243(1):136–51.
10. Franchi L, Eigenbrod T, Munoz-Planillo R, et al. The inflammasome: a caspase-1-activation platform that regulates immune responses and disease pathogenesis. Nat Immunol 2009;10(3): 241–7.
11. Ozkurede VU, Franchi L. Immunology in clinic review series; focus on autoinflammatory diseases: role of inflammasomes in autoinflammatory syndromes. Clin Exp Immunol 2012;167(3):382–90.
12. Bauernfeind FG, Horvath G, Stutz A, et al. Cutting edge: NF-kappaB activating pattern recognition and cytokine receptors license NLRP3 inflammasome activation by regulating NLRP3 expression. J Immunol 2009;183(2):787–91.
13. Franchi L, Munoz-Planillo R, Reimer T, et al. Inflammasomes as microbial sensors. Eur J Immunol 2010;40(3):611–5.
14. Joly S, Sutterwala FS. Fungal pathogen recognition by the NLRP3 inflammasome. Virulence 2010;1(4): 276–80.
15. Rathinam VA, Fitzgerald KA. Inflammasomes and anti-viral immunity. J Clin Immunol 2010;30(5): 632–7.
16. Ferrari D, Pizzirani C, Adinolfi E, et al. The P2X7 receptor: a key player in IL-1 processing and release. J Immunol 2006;176(7):3877–83.
17. Martinon F, Petrilli V, Mayor A, et al. Gout-associated uric acid crystals activate the NALP3 inflammasome. Nature 2006;440(7081):237–41.
18. Duewell P, Kono H, Rayner KJ, et al. NLRP3 inflammasomes are required for atherogenesis and activated by cholesterol crystals. Nature 2010; 464(7293):1357–61.
19. Masters SL, Dunne A, Subramanian SL, et al. Activation of the NLRP3 inflammasome by islet amyloid polypeptide provides a mechanism for enhanced IL-1beta in type 2 diabetes. Nat Immunol 2010; 11(10):897–904.
20. Sohar E, Gafni J, Pras M, et al. Familial Mediterranean fever. A survey of 470 cases and review of the literature. Am J Med 1967;43(2):227–53.
21. Feng J, Zhang Z, Li W, et al. Missense mutations in the MEFV gene are associated with fibromyalgia syndrome and correlate with elevated IL-1beta plasma levels. PLoS One 2009;4(12):e8480.
22. Ancient missense mutations in a new member of the RoRet gene family are likely to cause familial Mediterranean fever. The International FMF Consortium. Cell 1997;90(4):797–807.
23. Yildirim K, Uzkeser H, Keles M, et al. Relationship between serum interleukin-1beta levels and acute phase response proteins in patients with familial Mediterranean fever. Biochem Med (Zagreb) 2012;22(1):109–13.
24. Nesterovitch AB, Hoffman MD, Simon M, et al. Mutations in the PSTPIP1 gene and aberrant splicing variants in patients with pyoderma gangrenosum. Clin Exp Dermatol 2011;36(8):889–95.
25. Contassot E, Beer HD, French LE. Interleukin-1, inflammasomes, autoinflammation and the skin. Swiss Med Wkly 2012;142:w13590.
26. Shoham NG, Centola M, Mansfield E, et al. Pyrin binds the PSTPIP1/CD2BP1 protein, defining familial Mediterranean fever and PAPA syndrome as disorders in the same pathway. Proc Natl Acad Sci U S A 2003;100(23):13501–6.

27. Prieur AM. A recently recognised chronic inflammatory disease of early onset characterised by the triad of rash, central nervous system involvement and arthropathy. Clin Exp Rheumatol 2001; 19(1):103–6.

28. Hoffman HM, Mueller JL, Broide DH, et al. Mutation of a new gene encoding a putative pyrin-like protein causes familial cold autoinflammatory syndrome and Muckle-Wells syndrome. Nat Genet 2001;29(3):301–5.

29. Feldmann J, Prieur AM, Quartier P, et al. Chronic infantile neurological cutaneous and articular syndrome is caused by mutations in CIAS1, a gene highly expressed in polymorphonuclear cells and chondrocytes. Am J Hum Genet 2002;71(1): 198–203.

30. Agostini L, Martinon F, Burns K, et al. NALP3 forms an IL-1beta-processing inflammasome with increased activity in Muckle-Wells autoinflammatory disorder. Immunity 2004;20(3):319–25.

31. Hoffman HM, Throne ML, Amar NJ, et al. Efficacy and safety of rilonacept (interleukin-1 Trap) in patients with cryopyrin-associated periodic syndromes: results from two sequential placebo-controlled studies. Arthritis Rheum 2008;58(8):2443–52.

32. Lachmann HJ, Kone-Paut I, Kuemmerle-Deschner JB, et al. Use of canakinumab in the cryopyrin-associated periodic syndrome. N Engl J Med 2009;360(23):2416–25.

33. Brydges SD, Mueller JL, McGeough MD, et al. Inflammasome-mediated disease animal models reveal roles for innate but not adaptive immunity. Immunity 2009;30(6):875–87.

34. Meng G, Zhang F, Fuss I, et al. A mutation in the Nlrp3 gene causing inflammasome hyperactivation potentiates Th17 cell-dominant immune responses. Immunity 2009;30(6):860–74.

35. Dalbeth N, Haskard DO. Mechanisms of inflammation in gout. Rheumatology (Oxford) 2005;44(9): 1090–6.

36. Dinarello CA. Blocking interleukin-1beta in acute and chronic autoinflammatory diseases. J Intern Med 2011;269(1):16–28.

37. Joosten LA, Netea MG, Mylona E, et al. Engagement of fatty acids with Toll-like receptor 2 drives interleukin-1beta production via the ASC/caspase 1 pathway in monosodium urate monohydrate crystal-induced gouty arthritis. Arthritis Rheum 2010;62(11):3237–48.

38. Kingsbury SR, Conaghan PG, McDermott MF. The role of the NLRP3 inflammasome in gout. J Inflamm Res 2011;4:39–49.

39. Simon A, Cuisset L, Vincent MF, et al. Molecular analysis of the mevalonate kinase gene in a cohort of patients with the hyper-igd and periodic fever syndrome: its application as a diagnostic tool. Ann Intern Med 2001;135(5):338–43.

40. Goldfinger S. The inherited autoinflammatory syndrome: a decade of discovery. Trans Am Clin Climatol Assoc 2009;120:413–8.

41. Pontillo A, Paoluzzi E, Crovella S. The inhibition of mevalonate pathway induces upregulation of NALP3 expression: new insight in the pathogenesis of mevalonate kinase deficiency. Eur J Hum Genet 2010;18(7):844–7.

42. Maedler K, Sergeev P, Ris F, et al. Glucose-induced beta cell production of IL-1beta contributes to glucotoxicity in human pancreatic islets. J Clin Invest 2002;110(6):851–60.

43. Boni-Schnetzler M, Thorne J, Parnaud G, et al. Increased interleukin (IL)-1beta messenger ribonucleic acid expression in beta -cells of individuals with type 2 diabetes and regulation of IL-1beta in human islets by glucose and autostimulation. J Clin Endocrinol Metab 2008;93(10):4065–74.

44. Boni-Schnetzler M, Boller S, Debray S, et al. Free fatty acids induce a proinflammatory response in islets via the abundantly expressed interleukin-1 receptor I. Endocrinology 2009;150(12):5218–29.

45. Maedler K, Sergeev P, Ehses JA, et al. Leptin modulates beta cell expression of IL-1 receptor antagonist and release of IL-1beta in human islets. Proc Natl Acad Sci U S A 2004;101(21):8138–43.

46. Stienstra R, Joosten LA, Koenen T, et al. The inflammasome-mediated caspase-1 activation controls adipocyte differentiation and insulin sensitivity. Cell Metab 2010;12(6):593–605.

47. McDermott MF, Aksentijevich I, Galon J, et al. Germline mutations in the extracellular domains of the 55 kDa TNF receptor, TNFR1, define a family of dominantly inherited autoinflammatory syndromes. Cell 1999;97(1):133–44.

48. Turner MD, Chaudhry A, Nedjai B. Tumour necrosis factor receptor trafficking dysfunction opens the TRAPS door to pro-inflammatory cytokine secretion. Biosci Rep 2012;32(2):105–12.

49. Tromp G, Kuivaniemi H, Raphael S, et al. Genetic linkage of familial granulomatous inflammatory arthritis, skin rash, and uveitis to chromosome 16. Am J Hum Genet 1996;59(5):1097–107.

50. Miceli-Richard C, Lesage S, Rybojad M, et al. CARD15 mutations in Blau syndrome. Nat Genet 2001;29(1):19–20.

51. van Duist MM, Albrecht M, Podswiadek M, et al. A new CARD15 mutation in Blau syndrome. Eur J Hum Genet 2005;13(6):742–7.

52. Girardin SE, Boneca IG, Viala J, et al. Nod2 is a general sensor of peptidoglycan through muramyl dipeptide (MDP) detection. J Biol Chem 2003; 278(11):8869–72.

53. Inohara N, Ogura Y, Fontalba A, et al. Host recognition of bacterial muramyl dipeptide mediated through NOD2. Implications for Crohn's disease. J Biol Chem 2003;278(8):5509–12.

54. Aksentijevich I, Masters SL, Ferguson PJ, et al. An autoinflammatory disease with deficiency of the interleukin-1-receptor antagonist. N Engl J Med 2009;360(23):2426–37.

55. Reddy S, Jia S, Geoffrey R, et al. An autoinflammatory disease due to homozygous deletion of the IL1RN locus. N Engl J Med 2009;360(23):2438–44.

56. Jesus AA, Osman M, Silva CA, et al. A novel mutation of IL1RN in the deficiency of interleukin-1 receptor antagonist syndrome: description of two unrelated cases from Brazil. Arthritis Rheum 2011;63(12):4007–17.

57. Scholz J, Woolf CJ. Can we conquer pain? Nat Neurosci 2002;5(Suppl):1062–7.

58. Janig W, Grossmann L, Gorodetskaya N. Mechano- and thermosensitivity of regenerating cutaneous afferent nerve fibers. Exp Brain Res 2009;196(1):101–14.

59. Wu G, Ringkamp M, Hartke TV, et al. Early onset of spontaneous activity in uninjured C-fiber nociceptors after injury to neighboring nerve fibers. J Neurosci 2001;21(8):RC140.

60. Binshtok AM, Wang H, Zimmermann K, et al. Nociceptors are interleukin-1beta sensors. J Neurosci 2008;28(52):14062–73.

61. Watkins LR, Maier SF. Beyond neurons: evidence that immune and glial cells contribute to pathological pain states. Physiol Rev 2002;82(4):981–1011.

62. Milligan ED, Twining C, Chacur M, et al. Spinal glia and proinflammatory cytokines mediate mirror-image neuropathic pain in rats. J Neurosci 2003; 23(3):1026–40.

63. Hucho T, Levine JD. Signaling pathways in sensitization: toward a nociceptor cell biology. Neuron 2007;55(3):365–76.

64. Ren K, Torres R. Role of interleukin-1beta during pain and inflammation. Brain Res Rev 2009;60(1): 57–64.

65. Cunha TM, Verri WA Jr. Neutrophils: are they hyperalgesic or anti-hyperalgesic? J Leukoc Biol 2006; 80(4):727–8 [author reply: 729–30].

66. Kiguchi N, Kobayashi Y, Kishioka S. Chemokines and cytokines in neuroinflammation leading to neuropathic pain. Curr Opin Pharmacol 2012; 12(1):55–61.

67. So A, De Smedt T, Revaz S, et al. A pilot study of IL-1 inhibition by anakinra in acute gout. Arthritis Res Ther 2007;9(2):R28.

68. McGonagle D, Tan AL, Shankaranarayana S, et al. Management of treatment resistant inflammation of acute on chronic tophaceous gout with anakinra. Ann Rheum Dis 2007;66(12):1683–4.

69. So A, De Meulemeester M, Pikhlak A, et al. Canakinumab for the treatment of acute flares in difficult-to-treat gouty arthritis: results of a multicenter, phase II, dose-ranging study. Arthritis Rheum 2010;62(10):3064–76.

70. Boulton AJ, Malik RA, Arezzo JC, et al. Diabetic somatic neuropathies. Diabetes Care 2004;27(6): 1458–86.

71. Tesfaye S, Boulton AJ, Dyck PJ, et al. Diabetic neuropathies: update on definitions, diagnostic criteria, estimation of severity, and treatments. Diabetes Care 2010;33(10):2285–93.

72. Larsen CM, Faulenbach M, Vaag A, et al. Interleukin-1-receptor antagonist in type 2 diabetes mellitus. N Engl J Med 2007;356(15):1517–26.

73. Larsen CM, Faulenbach M, Vaag A, et al. Sustained effects of interleukin-1 receptor antagonist treatment in type 2 diabetes. Diabetes Care 2009; 32(9):1663–8.

74. Chen TC, Wu JJ, Chang WP, et al. Spontaneous inflammatory pain model from a mouse line with N-ethyl-N-nitrosourea mutagenesis. J Biomed Sci 2012;19:55.

75. Marshall K. Interstitial cystitis: understanding the syndrome. Altern Med Rev 2003;8(4):426–37.

76. Lau TC, Bengtson JM. Management strategies for painful bladder syndrome. Rev Obstet Gynecol 2010;3(2):42–8.

77. Moutzouris DA, Falagas ME. Interstitial cystitis: an unsolved enigma. Clin J Am Soc Nephrol 2009; 4(11):1844–57.

78. Sant GR, Kempuraj D, Marchand JE, et al. The mast cell in interstitial cystitis: role in pathophysiology and pathogenesis. Urology 2007;69(Suppl 4): 34–40.

79. Erickson DR, Xie SX, Bhavanandan VP, et al. A comparison of multiple urine markers for interstitial cystitis. J Urol 2002;167(6):2461–9.

80. Liu HT, Kuo HC. Increased urine and serum nerve growth factor levels in interstitial cystitis suggest chronic inflammation is involved in the pathogenesis of disease. PLoS One 2012;7(9): e44687.

81. Erickson DR, Tomaszewski JE, Kunselman AR, et al. Urine markers do not predict biopsy findings or presence of bladder ulcers in interstitial cystitis/painful bladder syndrome. J Urol 2008;179(5): 1850–6.

82. van de Merwe JP. Interstitial cystitis and systemic autoimmune diseases. Nat Clin Pract Urol 2007; 4(9):484–91.

83. Grover S, Srivastava A, Lee R, et al. Role of inflammation in bladder function and interstitial cystitis. Ther Adv Urol 2011;3(1):19–33.

84. Kummer JA, Broekhuizen R, Everett H, et al. Inflammasome components NALP 1 and 3 show distinct but separate expression profiles in human tissues suggesting a site-specific role in the inflammatory response. J Histochem Cytochem 2007;55(5): 443–52.

85. Nakamura Y, Kambe N, Saito M, et al. Mast cells mediate neutrophil recruitment and vascular

leakage through the NLRP3 inflammasome in histamine-independent urticaria. J Exp Med 2009; 206(5):1037–46.

86. Gerber PA, Buhren BA, Steinhoff M, et al. Rosacea: the cytokine and chemokine network. J Investig Dermatol Symp Proc 2011;15(1):40–7.

87. Yamasaki K, Gallo RL. The molecular pathology of rosacea. J Dermatol Sci 2009;55(2):77–81.

88. Brink N, Szamel M, Young AR, et al. Comparative quantification of IL-1beta, IL-10, IL-10r, TNFalpha and IL-7 mRNA levels in UV-irradiated human skin in vivo. Inflamm Res 2000;49(6):290–6.

89. Faustin B, Reed JC. Sunburned skin activates inflammasomes. Trends Cell Biol 2008;18(1):4–8.

90. Schwab VD, Sulk M, Seeliger S, et al. Neurovascular and neuroimmune aspects in the pathophysiology of rosacea. J Investig Dermatol Symp Proc 2011;15(1):53–62.

91. Aubdool AA, Brain SD. Neurovascular aspects of skin neurogenic inflammation. J Investig Dermatol Symp Proc 2011;15(1):33–9.

92. Peters KM. Neuromodulation for the treatment of refractory interstitial cystitis. Rev Urol 2002; 4(Suppl 1):S36–43.

Autoinflammatory Syndromes

John J. Cush, MD

KEYWORDS

- Autoinflammatory • CAPS • Periodic fever • Still disease

KEY POINTS

- Autoinflammatory disorders are enigmatic and diagnostic challenges for clinicians.
- Advances in understanding of genetic perturbations and role of the inflammasome have improved diagnostic and treatment approach to these disorders.
- Many of the autoinflammatory disorders are suggested on the basis of individual age, duration of (febrile) attacks, and cutaneous manifestations.
- Although many of the monogenic autoinflammatory disorders begin in neonates and children, adults may also be affected with new-onset or continued inflammatory disease.

INTRODUCTION

The autoinflammatory syndromes comprise a clinically distinct set of disorders unified by recurrent febrile episodes accompanied by inflammatory cutaneous, mucosal, serosal, and osteoarticular manifestations.[1–3] Although these rare disorders often have a striking onset and inflammatory features, they are without an infectious or autoimmune cause. Instead, many are unified by a genetically driven dysregulated innate immune response with resultant activation of the inflammasome and cytokine excess. Hence, these disorders respond to interleukin (IL)-1 or tumor necrosis factor (TNF)-α and generally not to immunosuppressives. Manifestations include periodic fevers, neutrophilic rashes or urticaria, serositis, hepatosplenomegaly, lymphadenopathy, elevated acute phase reactants, neutrophilia, and a long-term risk of secondary amyloidosis.

The identification of the genetic origins underlying certain disorders has rapidly advanced understanding of the immunopathogenesis of autoinflammatory disorders. Affected individuals often have first- or second-degree relatives with similar features. A monogenic defect has been identified for familial Mediterranean fever (FMF), TNF receptor–associated periodic syndrome (TRAPS), hyperimmunoglobulinemia D with periodic fever syndrome (HIDS), and cryopyrin-associated periodic syndromes (CAPS)—which include a spectrum of disorders: familial cold autoinflammatory syndrome (FCAS), Muckle-Wells syndrome (MWS), and neonatal-onset multisystem inflammatory disease (NOMID). Additional disorders also fall under the autoinflammatory umbrella, because they manifest similar inflammatory features but may or may not have an identifiable genetic cause. Etiologic defects have been discovered for cyclic neutropenia; pyogenic arthritis, pyoderma gangrenosum, and acne (PAPA) syndrome; pyoderma gangrenosum, acne, and suppurative hidradenitis (PASH) syndrome; deficiency of the IL-1 receptor antagonist (IL-1Ra) (DIRA); and deficiency of the IL-36R antagonist (DITRA). Those without a known cause include systemic-onset juvenile idiopathic arthritis (SoJIA);

Disclosures: Clinical investigator for Genentech, Pfizer, UCB, Celgene, Novartis, Amgen, NIH, and CORRONA; advisor and consultant to Janssen, Abbott, UCB, Pfizer, BMS, Amgen, Genentech, Savient, and Celgene. Dr Cush holds no stock or investments in these companies and does not partake in industry "speaker's bureaus" or give industry-guided "promotional lectures."
Funded by: NIH U19 082715.
Baylor Research Institute, Rheumatology Research, 9900 North Central Expressway, Suite 550, Dallas, TX 75231, USA
E-mail address: cushj@msn.com

Dermatol Clin 31 (2013) 471–480
http://dx.doi.org/10.1016/j.det.2013.05.001
0733-8635/13/$ – see front matter © 2013 Elsevier Inc. All rights reserved.

adult-onset Still disease (AOSD); periodic fever, aphthous stomatitis, pharyngitis, and adenopathy (PFAPA) syndrome (or Marshall syndrome); and Schnitzler syndrome.[1-5]

Although these disorders are often rare, some are more frequently seen than others. A federally funded German registry was established in 2009 and in a 9-month period they identified 117 patients (65 male and 52 female; ages 1–21 years) with a diagnosis of FMF (n = 84), SoJIA (n = 22), clinically confirmed AIDS (n = 5), TRAPS (n = 3), CAPS (n = 1), HIDS (n = 1), and PFAPA (n = 1).[6] This review focuses on the distinguishing clinical features, onset, fever/flare duration, etiology, and effective treatments—each of which is crucial to establishing an accurate diagnosis.

ETIOLOGY

Immune responses are either innate or adaptive. The adaptive immune response recognizes self from nonself and generates antigen-specific cellular and cytokine responses, and, with activation-driven autoantibody production, the adaptive responses can establish immunologic memory or immune tolerance. By contrast, the innate immune response acts with immediacy to danger or pathogen signals, termed *pathogen-associated molecule patterns* (*PAMPs*) and endogenous *damage-associated molecular patterns* (*DAMPs*). PAMPs and DAMPs activate intracellular inflammasomes to set forth an inflammatory cascade of effector molecules.[3,4] For example, the NLRP3 inflammasome is a cytosolic scaffold of proteins triggered by PAMPs (microbial pathogens, monosodium urate, and toxins) and DAMPs (ATP, membrane disruption, oxygen radicals, and hypoxia). A disrupted, dysregulated innate immune system yields a proinflammatory state, with the final common pathway being activation of the NLRP3 gene and the inflammasome, with resultant unopposed cytokine excess. Activation of the inflammasome yields increased production of proinflammatory cytokines, such as IL-1, IL-18, TNF-α, IL-6, IL-17, type 1 interferons (IFN-α and IFN-β), and the complement system. The inflammasome is a complex of proteins that activates caspase-1, leading to cleavage of inactive pro-IL-1β to active IL-1β. The critical role of the inflammasome in these disorders has led some to refer to the autoinflammatory disorders as *inflammasomopathies*.[7]

TRAPS

TRAPS is also known as familial Hibernian fever, owing to a higher frequency of this syndrome in those of Irish, Scottish, or Austrian or Northern European dissent. Nevertheless, it has been described in other ethnic groups, including Mediterraneans. TRAPS differs from FMF and HIDS by having febrile attacks that last 1 to 3 weeks and occasionally up to 6 weeks. Characteristic features include fever, arthralgia, myalgia, migratory rash, abdominal pain, pleuritis, conjunctivitis, periorbital edema, oral ulcers, and scrotal swelling. Skin manifestations include migratory macular erythematous rash or patches, ecchymoses, edematous dermal plaques, serpiginous or annular lesions, and periorbital edema.[5,8,9] Limited skin biopsies showed perivascular and interstitial lymphocytic and mononuclear infiltrates without evidence of granulomatous or vasculitic change.

The genetics underlying this disorder was clarified by studies of a large Irish multiplex family who demonstrated an autosomal dominant syndrome characterized by recurrent fever, rash, and abdominal pain. Fevers last more than 5 days and less than 6 weeks. The vast majority (75%–88%) has childhood onset, usually as toddlers at approximately age 3 years and most occurring before age 10 years. Adult onset may occur. Manifestations of TRAPS depend on the mutations for the gene encoding p55 TNF receptor type I (CD120a). There are 46 known missense mutations involving TNF receptor type I, all of which are localized to distal chromosome 12p. The R92Q and P46L mutations are seen in 4% and 1% of the population, respectively, and tend to have low penetrance and less severe disease. The R92Q and T61I polymorphisms may be found with an adult onset and are often associated with rheumatoid arthritis, lupus, or multiple sclerosis. There is effective treatment with etanercept, which has been shown to reduce the frequency and severity of flares.[9] There are reports of efficacy with anakinra and worsening with infliximab.

HYPER IgD SYNDROME

HIDS is a rare disorder that begins early in life, usually before 2 years of age. Most reports have been seen in those of northern European, Dutch, or French ancestry.[1,2,10,11] HIDS has inflammatory symptoms lasting 3 to 7 days with recurrent fever, chills, cervical lymphadenopathy, abdominal pain, hepatosplenomegaly, diarrhea, arthralgia or arthritis, aphthous ulcers, skin rash (usually palmar/plantar), and headaches. Vaccinations may precipitate in inflammatory attacks in some patients. High levels of erythrocyte sedimentation rate (ESR), C-reactive protein (CRP), and serum amyloid A are seen, and IgD levels greater than 100 IU/dL are sensitive but not specific for HIDS. In 1999, mevalonate kinase (MVK) gene mutations were found in patients with HIDS. Currently, tests for the MVK gene are the gold standard in diagnostic testing. HIDS is an autosomal recessive disorder, with defects in the gene encoding MVK, an enzyme central to cholesterol synthesis. Although colchicines and steroids are sometimes effective, anakinra has become the drug of choice because it has been more uniformly beneficial in observational reports.[1,10]

FAMILIAL MEDITERRANEAN FEVER

FMF is the most common of the ancestral or monogenic autoinflammatory disorders.[1–6] FMF preferentially affects Sephardic Jews, Armenians, Turks, North Africans, Arabs, Moroccans, and others whose familial origins can be traced to the Mediterranean basin. Although the vast majority of cases have Mediterranean roots, ancestry should not exclude this diagnosis or the need for genetic testing if the clinical picture is suggestive, because many non-Mediterraneans have been diagnosed with FMF. The disorder often begins in childhood or adolescence, and up to 20% may have their first attack after the age of 20 years. Younger cases usually have more striking features, and severity lessens with age. FMF is characterized by febrile episodes accompanied by cutaneous, serosal, or synovial/tenosynovial inflammation. Fevers are usually 38°C or higher and last 1 to 3 days, ending as abruptly as they begin. Bouts are unpredictable in their frequency and are usually without known triggers but may be provoked by infection, stress, exercise, or surgery. Cutaneous features are distinctive, if not pathonomonic, and manifest as unilateral, more so than bilateral, erysipelas-like erythema that is often painful and located on the extensor surface of the arms, legs, or dorsum of feet. Also distinctive is the occurrence of recurrent inflammatory, sterile, monarticular inflammatory joint effusions or tenosynovial swelling. Less commonly, myalgia, migratory arthritis, and destructive/erosive arthritis may occur. Serositis manifests as either pleuritis or peritonitis with abdominal pain and, less frequently, as pericarditis or scrotal swelling. Rare manifestations include aseptic meningitis, orchitis, and vasculitis. Laboratory findings include leukocytosis and marked elevations of the ESR and CRP during the attacks. Amyloidosis may complicate FMF with serum amyloid A deposition in the kidney or other organs. Amyloidosis is more common with M694V homozygosity, male patients, and the alpha/alpha serum amyloid A1 gene. Amyloidosis is unrelated to the severity of FMF and can be diagnosed by biopsy of the rectum, kidney, abdominal fat, or bone marrow.

FMF results from a recessive mutation of the MEFV or Mediterranean Fever gene 16p13. This recessive mutation is located on the short arm of the chromosome 16. The zygosity and type of mutation determines the severity of the disorder and age of onset in many. In FMF, there are more than 80, mostly missense, mutations with the 5 most common genotypes (M694V, M6941, M680I, V726A, and E148Q) accounting for nearly 80% of cases. The dominant mutation depends on the population: V726A is common among Ashkenazi and Iraqi Jews, Druzes, and Armenians; M680I is frequent in Armenians and Turks; M694I and A744S in Arabs; and R761H in Lebanese patients. MEFV is found in neutrophils and myeloid cells and encodes an 86-kDa protein, called pyrin (or marenostrin). Defective pyrin function leads to uncontrolled inflammation with elevated levels of IFN-γ and circulating proinflammatory cytokines, including TNF-α, IL-1, IL-6, and IL-8.

Many patients with FMF respond favorably to colchicine. Colchicine is effective in both aborting and preventing attacks and, when used chronically, decreases the risk of amyloidosis. Most patients respond well with only a minority refractory to colchicine—either because of dose-limiting gastrointestinal toxicity or more-aggressive disease. Steroids may be effective but are seldom needed. Refractory cases respond well to IL-1 inhibition (with anakinra, canakinumab, or rilonacept).[1,10]

The diagnosis of FMF should be a largely clinical one, based on recurrent 1- to 4-day bouts of fever with synovial, serosal, or skin inflammation and high acute-phase proteins. Confirmation by MEFV testing may be necessary in atypical cases and those evidently not of Mediterranean ancestry.

CRYOPYRIN-ASSOCIATED PERIODIC SYNDROMES (CRYOPYRINOPATHIES)

The CAPS are a distinct subset of autosomal dominant disorders etiologically connected by mutations of the NACHT domain of NLRP3, previously known as cryopyrin.[1–4,12] NLRP3 (which stands for NOD-like receptor family pyrin domain 3) includes the cold-induced autoinflammatory syndrome 1 (CIAS1) gene and, as such, much of the literature suggests that these disorders are related to defects in CIAS1. CIAS1 encodes for cryopyrin, a protein similar to pyrin that is also expressed primarily in neutrophils and monocytes. CAPS include familial cold autoinflammatory syndrome (FCAS), Muckle-Wells syndrome (MWS), and neonatal onset multisystem inflammatory disease (NOMID) also known as chronic infantile neurologic cutaneous and articular syndrome (CINCA). The severity of disease is milder in

FCAS and MWS but tends to be the most severe in NOMID, with often devastating neurologic complications. Common features of CAPS, regardless of the specific clinical entity, include fever, urticarial-like rash, conjunctivitis, bone and joint symptoms, and elevated inflammatory markers, such as CRP. There is little/no risk of amyloidosis with chronicity. CAPS patients have uniformly responded well to IL-1 inhibition (anakinra, rilonacept, and canakinumab).[11]

FCAS begins in infancy and is unique by being provoked by cold exposure, with brief episodes (lasting <24 h) of urticarial-like rash, fever, conjunctivitis, and joint/limb pain. Although some patients have significant disability related to these attacks, long-term prognosis is favorable for most.

MWS has an older onset (adolescents and young adults), with fevers lasting up to 7 days. Frequent attacks and chronicity may be accompanied by sensorineural hearing loss or deafness and a long-term risk of amyloidosis.[12]

NOMID is the most severe form of CAPS and differs from FCAS and MWS by being chronic, rather than episodic, in its manifestations. It is characterized by a neonatal or infantile onset of chronic urticarial rash, low-grade fever, otolaryngologic findings, sensorineural hearing loss, tinnitus, and, later, chronic aseptic meningitis, which may result in cerebral atrophy, seizures, hearing and vision loss, and mental retardation. NOMID patients may develop a distinctive overgrowth of the epiphyses in the long bones, with resultant deformity, leg length discrepancy, joint contractures, or premature degenerative arthritis. Late closure of the fontanel leads to frontal bossing. Amyloidosis is a known risk and mortality may be as high as 20%. Before administration of IL-1 antagonistic therapy, the prognosis for patients with NOMID was poor.

STILL DISEASE

Still disease is another name for systemic-onset juvenile idiopathic arthritis (SoJIA) and the adult continuum of that disease, adult-onset still disease (AOSD). AOSD and SoJIA are considered under the autoinflammatory syndromes, because they are often confused with these disorders, share many of the same clinical features, and seem uniquely responsive to IL-1 (or IL-6) inhibition. Still disease is a systemic inflammatory disorder of unknown cause or genetics that typically affects children under 16 years of age (SoJIA) or young adults from ages 18 to 35 years (AOSD). The classic triad includes quotidian (daily) spiking fevers (≥39°C), juvenile idiopathic arthritis or rheumatoid rash, and polyarthritis.[13,14] The cutaneous features associated with AOSD include pruritis, urticaria (<40%),

and salmon-pink evanescent (changes day to day) rash usually on the trunk, neck, and extremities and almost never on the face, palms, or soles. Other characteristic manifestations include a prodromal sore throat (in adults, not children), arthralgias, myalgias, rapid weight loss, serositis (pleuritis or pericarditis), generalized lymphadenopathy, hepatomegaly (often with elevated hepatic enzymes), and splenomegaly. Laboratory tests support the inflammatory nature of the disorder with neutrophilic leukocytosis, very high ESR and CRP, anemia of chronic disease, hypoalbuminemia, and absence of serum rheumatoid factor and antinuclear antibodies. The importance of hyperferritinemia has been overstated by most investigators because only 50% have elevated ferritin levels (compared with >90% ESR or CRP elevations) and extreme elevations, greater than 2000 mg/dL, are seen in 10% to 20% of patients with active systemic disease. These features are not intermittent (as they are in TRAPS or FMF) but instead are daily and quotidian, with a regular periodicity to the fever, rash, myalgias, and arthralgias.

The clinical course is marked by sporadic exacerbations of systemic inflammation (fever, rash, serositis, and inflammatory labs) and/or chronic inflammatory arthritis. There are no diagnostic clinical manifestations, serologic tests, or histopathologic findings; thus, the diagnosis can be based on criteria by either Cush[13] or Yamaguchi and colleagues[14] after exclusion of common infectious or neoplastic conditions.[13,14] Persistence of symptoms (fever rash, polyarthritis, hepatosplenomegaly, and so forth) beyond 6 weeks is necessary for considering a diagnosis of AOSD.

There is no known cause of AOSD or SoJIA, although several groups have noted polymorphisms in either the IL-18 or IL-1 genes. A minority of patients may respond to antiinflammatory doses of nonsteroidal antiinflammatory drugs but most require high-dose oral corticosteroids (ie, prednisone, 40–60 mg/d) with or without methotrexate or azathioprine to achieve partial control of systemic inflammatory activity. Refractory patients or those with recurrent systemic disease have shown a remarkable response to anakinra and other IL-1 inhibitors (canakinumab and rilonacept). TNF inhibitor therapy seems effective in patients with chronic inflammatory polyarthritis but is less successful in managing systemic manifestations.[15,16]

OTHER AUTOINFLAMMATORY DISORDERS

The PFAPA syndrome, also known as Marshall syndrome, affects children more than adults (from 5–35 y) and is predictable in the periodicity of febrile attacks that last an average of 4 to 5 days and recur approximately every 4 weeks.[17] In the interim, patients are healthy and asymptomatic. During febrile attacks, patients manifest aphthous stomatitis, pharyngitis, tender cervical lymphadenitis, abdominal pain, nausea, vomiting, and fatigue. There is no hearing loss or amyloidosis with the PFAPA syndrome. Treatment may include a single dose of corticosteroid (chronic cimetadine use is effective in less than 25%) or surgical removal of tonsils. Some patients have responded to anakinra. There is no known cause.

PAPA syndrome is an autosomal dominant disorder that affects children and adolescents with recurrent pyogenic, sterile arthritis with pustular skin lesions (eg, pyoderma gangrenosum and acne fulminans, cystic acne, and pathergy) but

no febrile episodes.[6,18,19] In some patients, the arthritis may be severe, destructive, or deforming. PAPA is the result of a missense mutation in the adapter protein proline-serine-threonine phosphatase-interacting protein (PSTPIP1) gene. The skin lesions of PAPA have responded to TNF inhibitors as well as IL-1 inhibitors.

The triad of PASH is included as an autoinflammatory syndrome that affects adults and adolescents and is similar to PAPA but differs by having hidradenitis suppurativa without pyogenic arthritis or fevers.[18] Early results suggest these patients may respond to IL-1 inhibitors. Gene mutations for PAPA and other autoinflammatory disorders (eg, PSTPIP1, MEFV, NLRP3, and TNFRSF1A) have been absent. The cause is currently unknown.

Table 1
Autoinflammatory syndromes: acronyms, meanings, and overview

Acronym	Meaning	Clinical Overview
AOSD	Adult-onset Still disease	Quotidian fevers >39°C, polyarthritis, rash, serositis, lymphadenopathy, organomegaly
CAPS	Cryopyrin-associated periodic syndromes	Includes FCAS, MWS, NOMID/CINCA
CINCA	Chronic infantile neurologic cutaneous and articular syndrome (same as NOMID)	Severe form of CAPS with infantile onset, chronic urticaria, neurologic involvement
DIRA	Deficiency of the IL-1Ra	Pustular lesions, periostitis, osteomyelitis, mucosal lesions
DITRA	Deficiency of the IL-36R antagonist	Chronic pustular psoriasis
FCAS	Familial cold autoinflammatory syndrome	Infants with cold induced fever, urticaria, conjunctivitis, joint/bone pain
FMF	Familial mediterranean fever	Periodic fevers, red painful rash, serositis
HIDS	Hyperimmunoglobulinemia D syndrome	Recurrent fever, cervical lymphadenopathy, abdominal pain, hepatosplenomegaly, arthralgia or arthritis, aphthous ulcers
MWS	Muckle-Wells syndrome	Adolescents/adults with fever, urticaria, sensorineural hearing loss, tinnitus
NOMID	Neonatal-onset multisystem inflammatory disease	Severe form of CAPS with infantile onset, chronic urticaria, neurologic involvement
PAPA	Pyogenic arthritis, pyoderma gangrenosum, and acne	Recurrent pustular skin lesiosn (pyoderma gangrenosum) with recurrent pyogenic, sterile arthritis
PASH	Pyoderma gangrenosum, acne, suppurative hidradenitis	Same as PAPA without the pyogenic arthritis
PFAPA	Periodic fever, aphthous stomatitis, pharyngitis, and adenopathy	Children with monthly fevers (last 4 d), aphthous stomatitis, pharyngitis, cervical lymphadenopathy, abdominal pain
SoJIA	Systemic-onset juvenile idiopathic arthritis	Children (3–16 y) with quotidian fevers >39°C, polyarthritis, rash, serositis, lymphadenopathy, organomegaly
TRAPS	TNF receptor–associated periodic syndrome	Toddlers with recurrent fever (>1 wk), arthralgia, myalgia, migratory rash, abdominal pain, pleuritis, conjunctivitis, periorbital edema

Table 2
Distinctive features among the autoinflammatory disorders

Disease	Genetics, Mutation	Onset Age	Fever/Flare Duration	Mucocutaneous	Musculoskeletal	Other Significant Findings	Effective Therapy[a]
TRAPS[b] (Hibernian fever)	Autosomal dominant, TNFR1	Infants, rarely adults	Usually 1–3 wk	Erthemous rash or dermal plaques on extremities	Myalgia Arthralgia (erosive synovitis is rare)	Serositis, abdominal pain, conjunctivitis periorbital edema	Etanercept Anakinra
FMF[b]	Autosomal recessive, MEFV gene	<20 y in 80% of patients	≥39°C 1–3 d	Erysipelas-like	Recurrent monarthritis, tenosynovitis, arthralgias, myalgia	Abdominal pain, serositis, scrotal swelling	Colchicine Anakinra Rilonacept
HIDS	Autosomal recessive, MVK gene	<2 y	3–7 d	Palmar/plantar rash, aphthous ulcers	Arthralgia Arthritis	Cervical adenitis, abdominal pain,	Anakinra
FCAS	Autosomal dominant, NLRP3	<1 y	<24 h	Urticaria	Arthralgias	Cold-induced conjunctivitis	Avoid cold Anakinra Rilonacept Canakinumab
Muckle-Wells[b]	Autosomal dominant, NLRP3	Variable; infants, teens, young adults	Low-grade fever 1–3 d	Erythematous rash, urticaria (sometimes cold-induced)	Myalgias, arthralgias, arthritis	Conjunctivitis, uveitis, sensorineural hearing loss, fatigue	Anakinra Rilonacept Canakinumab
NOMID[b]	Sporadic, NLRP3	<1 y	Mild fevers, constant	Chronic urticarial-like skin rash	Arthralgia, arthritis, bony overgrowth of epiphysis, bony hypertrophy/ deformity, frontal bossing	Chronic uveitis Conjunctivitis, chronic aseptic meningitis, sensorineural hearing loss, headaches, papilledema, optic atrophy, visual loss, mental retardation	Anakinra Rilonacept Canakinumab

Disease	Genetics	Age	Fever	Mucocutaneous	Arthritis	Prodromal/Other	Treatment
AOSD and SoJIA	Acquired; no known genetic link	3–35 y	≥39°C, daily quotidian fevers	Evanescent pink rash, 30%–40% pruritic or urticarial	Polyarthritis Polyarthralgia Myalgia Carpal anklyosis	Prodromal sore throat, serositis, lymphadenopathy, hepatospleno-megaly	Steroids Methotrexate Anakinra (IL-1 inhibitors)
PFAPA	Unknown	5–35 y	q 4 wk; Lasting 4–5 d	Aphthous ulcerations	None	Pharyngitis cervical adenitis, abdominal pain	Tonsillectomy Single steroid dose Cimetadine Anakinra
PAPA	Autosomal dominant, PSTPIP1 gene	Children adolescents adults	None	Acne Pyoderma gangrenosum Pathergy	Inflammatory arthritis mostly large joints (some erosive or deforming)		TNF inhibitors IL-1 inhibitors
Cyclic neutropenia	Autosomal dominant, neutrophil elastase gene (ELA-2 or ELANE)	Child to adult	10–14 d of low-grade fevers; recurs q 4–6 wk	Oral ulcers gingivitis periodontitis recurrent cellulitis or furunculosis	None	Malaise, pharyngitis, lymphadenopathy, LN, ST	G-CSF, steroids

[a] *Adapted from* Hoffman H, Patel D. Genomic-based therapy: targeting interleukin-1 for autoinflammatory diseases. Arthritis Rheum 2004;50:345–9.
[b] Associated risk for amyloidosis.

Schnitzler syndrome is a rare disorder of unknown cause and is thought to be an acquired autoinflammatory disorder because it typically affects older individuals (40–60 years). Of the more than 100 cases reported, few have been seen in the United States. Typical manifestations include nonpruritic urticaria and a monoclonal gammopathy (usually IgM kappa), with at least 2 of the following: periodic fever, arthralgia or arthritis, bone pain, hepatosplenomegaly, lymphadenopathy, elevated ESR, leukocytosis, and anemia. Other features include weight loss and pancreatitis. Dramatic responses have been seen with anakinra treatment. There is a rare long-term risk of developing a lymphoproliferative disorder (mainly Waldenström macroglobulinemia).[20]

DIRA is a rare, inherited disease that results from a deficiency of IL-1Ra and was initially described in patients from Newfoundland, Holland, Lebanon, and Brazil.[21] Lack of the IL-1Ra leads to unopposed IL-1 activity and chronic pustular skin disease. It begins in infancy and manifests as neutrophilic/pustular skin disease, pathergy, periostitis, multifocal osteomyelitis, oral mucosal lesions, nail dystrophy, and joint/bone pain. Laboratory results show elevated acute phase proteins. Radiographic changes include osteitis of the ribs and long bones and heterotopic ossification with periarticular soft tissue swelling. Treatment with anakinra leads to dramatic improvement and may abort significant morbidity and mortality if recognized early.

DITRA is a newly recognized entity wherein a mutation in the IL-35Ra gene results in either familial or sporadic cases of generalized pustular psoriasis that responds to IL-1 inhibition.[21] It is possible that this may be related to acrodermatitis continua

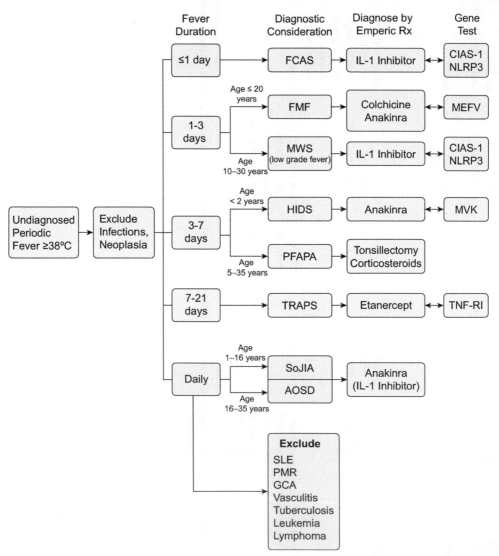

Fig. 1. The approach to undiagnosed periodic fever.

of Halloppeau that manifests as chronic, pustular eruptions involving the fingertips and nails.

Cyclic neutropenia is a disorder with recurrent fevers that last 5 to 14 days, recurs every 21 to 35 days, and coincides with episodic neutropenia (neutrophils $\leq 500/mm^3$). Common features include fatigue, pharyngitis, oral ulcers, stomatitis, cellulitis, and lymphadenopathy.[22] Such patients are at risk for infection and sepsis and this autosomal dominant disorder results from a mutation in the neutrophil elastase gene (ELA-2 or ELANE). Cyclic neutropenia differs from congenital neutropenia, which has more profound neutropenia and greater risk of infection. Effective treatments include granulocyte colony-stimulating factor (G-CSF), steroids and, in some cases, cyclosporine.

DIAGNOSTIC APPROACH TO PERIODIC FEBRILE DISORDERS

Advances in understanding of the pathogenesis and genetics of these disorders have led to testing, which may ultimately diagnose one of these rare disorders. To pursue genetic testing, however, clinicians need to have sufficient clinical grounds for ordering such tests. Hence, a complete clinical evaluation is necessary to characterize features that are most diagnostic. Although autoinflammatory disorders may have markedly elevated acute-phase reactants, anemia of chronic disease, neutrophilic leukocytosis, non-specific perivascular inflammation on skin biopsy, negative serologic tests for autoantibodies, or a clinical response to steroids, colchicines, or IL-1 inhibition, these findings are nonspecific. If a periodic fever or autoinflammatory condition is suspected, it is important to exclude possible infectious, neoplastic, or autoimmune disease based on the manifestations and pattern of organ involvement. Common adult causes of fever of unknown origin include polymyalgia rheumatic, giant cell arteritis and other systemic necrotizing vasculitides, lupus, tuberculosis and occult infections, lymphoma, leukemia, and inflammatory bowel disease. Once these are excluded, an autoinflammatory disorder can be considered.

The clinical features that are most predictive in making a diagnosis are (1) age of onset; (2) presence, magnitude, and duration of fever; (3) duration of attacks; (4) rash or urticaria; (5) distinguishing features (**Tables 1** and **2**) (eg, serositis, arthritis, organomegaly, ocular, or neurologic involvement); (5) ethnicity; and (6) family history of similar illness. **Fig. 1** details an algorithmic approach to patients with undiagnosed periodic fevers, initially focusing on the duration of febrile attacks and the age of the individual at onset. Once a differential diagnosis is

considered, confirmation may ensue by either an empiric trial of known effective therapy or the identification of a genetic mutation with commercially available tests. The downside of genetic testing is that not all patients with an apparent autoinflammatory disorder prove to have an identifiable known genetic anomaly. Moreover, widespread batteries of tests or screening for multiple gene mutations have not been shown to be either cost effective or diagnostically prudent.

SUMMARY

The autoinflammatory disorders can pose a significant challenge to pediatricians, internists, primary care physicians, dermatologists, rheumatologists, and infectious disease specialists. Affected individuals often have either dramatic clinical presentations of fever of unknown origin or puzzling episodic febrile/cutaneous disease without evidence of infection of malignancy. The diagnosis of an autoinflammatory disorder can be made based on clinical features and supported by either genetic testing or response to IL-1 inhibition or other specific therapy.

REFERENCES

1. Zeft AS, Spalding SJ. Autoinflammatory syndromes: fever is not always a sign of infection. Cleve Clin J Med 2012;79:569.
2. Fietta P. Autoinflammatory diseases: the hereditary periodic fever syndromes. Acta Biomed 2004;75:92–9.
3. Ozkurede VU, Franchi L. Immunology in clinic review series; focus on autoinflammatory diseases: role of inflammasomes in autoinflammatory syndromes. Clin Exp Immunol 2012;167(3):382–90.
4. Menu P, Vince JE. The NLRP3 inflammasome in health and disease: the good, the bad and the ugly. Clin Exp Immunol 2011;166:1–15.
5. Long SS. Distinguishing among prolonged, recurrent, and periodic fever syndromes: approach of a pediatric infectious diseases subspecialist. Pediatr Clin North Am 2005;52(3):811–35.
6. Lainka E, Bielak M, Lohse P, et al. Familial mediterranean fever in Germany: epidemiological, clinical, and genetic characteristics of a pediatric population. Eur J Pediatr 2012;171(12):1775–85.
7. Smith EJ, Allantaz F, Bennett L, et al. Clinical, molecular, and genetic characteristics of PAPA syndrome: a review. Curr Genomics 2010;11(7):519–27.
8. Toro JR, Aksentijevich I, Hull K, et al. Tumor necrosis factor receptor-associated periodic syndrome: a novel syndrome with cutaneous manifestations. Arch Dermatol 2000;136(12):1487–94.
9. Bulua AC, Mogul DB, Aksentijevich I, et al. Efficacy of etanercept in the tumor necrosis factor receptor-

associated periodic syndrome: a prospective, open-label, dose-escalation study. Arthritis Rheum 2012; 64(3):908–13.

10. van der Hilst JC, Bodar EJ, Barron KS, et al, International HIDS Study Group. Long-term follow-up, clinical features, and quality of life in a series of 103 patients with hyperimmunoglobulinemia D syndrome. Medicine (Baltimore) 2008;87(6):301–10.

11. Hoffman H, Patel D. Genomic-based therapy: targeting interleukin-1 for autoinflammatory diseases. Arthritis Rheum 2004;50:345–9.

12. Kuemmerle-Deschner JB, Koitschev A, Ummenhofer K, et al. Hearing loss in Muckle-Wells syndrome. Arthritis Rheum 2013;65(3):824–31.

13. Cush JJ. Adult onset Still's disease. Bull Rheum Dis 2000;49(6):1–4.

14. Yamaguchi M, Ohta A, Tsunematsu T, et al. Preliminary criteria for classification of adult Still's disease. J Rheumatol 1992;19(3):424–30.

15. Petryna O, Cush JJ, Efthimiou P. IL-1 Trap rilonacept in refractory adult onset Still's disease. Ann Rheum Dis 2012;71(12):2056–7.

16. Efthimiou P, Petryna O, Mehta B, et al. Successful use of canakinumab in adult-onset Still's disease refractory to short acting IL-1 inhibtors. EULAR 2012;THU0401.

17. Kyvsgaard N, Mikkelsen T, Korsholm J, et al. Periodic fever associated with aphthous stomatitis, pharyngitis and cervical adenitis. Dan Med J 2012; 59(7):A4452.

18. Lindor NM, Arsenault TM, Solomon H, et al. A new autosomal dominant disorder of pyogenic sterile arthritis, pyoderma gangrenosum, and acne: PAPA syndrome. Mayo Clin Proc 1997;72(7):611–5.

19. Braun-Falco M, Kovnerystyy O, Lohse P, et al. Pyoderma gangrenosum, acne, and suppurative hidradenitis (PASH)—a new autoinflammatory syndrome distinct from PAPA syndrome. J Am Acad Dermatol 2012;66(3):409–15.

20. Besada E, Nossent H. Dramatic response to IL1-RA treatment in longstanding multidrug resistant Schnitzler's syndrome: a case report and literature review. Clin Rheumatol 2010;29(5):567–71.

21. Cowen EW, Goldbach-Mansky R. DIRA, DITRA, and new insights into pathways of skin inflammation: What's in a name? Arch Dermatol 2012;148(3):381–4.

22. Dale DC, Welte K. Cyclic and chronic neutropenia. Cancer Treat Res 2011;157:97–108.

Autoinflammatory Diseases in Pediatrics

Jonathan S. Hausmann, MD*, Fatma Dedeoglu, MD

KEYWORDS

- Autoinflammatory diseases • Periodic fever • Pediatrics • Familial Mediterranean fever • PFAPA
- HIDS • TRAPS • CAPS

KEY POINTS

- Viral infections are the most common cause of recurrent fevers in children.
- Autoinflammatory diseases (AIDs) should be considered in a child with recurrent or persistent fever, when infectious and malignant causes have been excluded.
- AIDs are characterized by recurrent episodes of systemic and organ-specific inflammation, and are caused by defects in the innate immune system.
- Periodic fevers with aphthous stomatitis, pharyngitis, and cervical adenitis (PFAPA) is the most common AID in children and occurs at regular intervals.
- Familial Mediterranean fever (FMF) is the most common monogenic AID and presents with recurrent attacks of fever, abdominal pain, arthritis, and rash that last for 1 to 3 days.

INTRODUCTION

Repeated febrile illnesses are common in young children, especially in those attending daycare and school. Most often, these febrile episodes are caused by repeated viral infections. However, if there is continued recurrence of fever and other associated symptoms, it is important to maintain a broad differential that includes primary immunodeficiencies, anatomic and metabolic abnormalities, malignancies, and autoinflammatory diseases (AIDs). The diagnosis of an AID may be challenging, because there are numerous diseases, overlapping signs and symptoms, and lack of specific laboratory testing.

AIDs are characterized by recurrent episodes of systemic and organ-specific inflammation. Unlike patients with autoimmune disorders such as systemic lupus erythematosus, patients with AIDs do not have autoantibodies or antigen-specific T cells. Instead, AIDs result from inborn errors of the innate immune system.[1] They involve disorders of neutrophils, macrophages, and molecules of innate immunity that evolved to protect against external pathogens. These innate immune cells are activated by endogenous or exogenous stimuli, so-called pathogen-associated molecular patterns (PAMPs) and damage-associated molecular patterns (DAMPs), which lead to inflammation.

In contrast with most autoimmune diseases, AIDs usually present during childhood. Many are characterized by recurrent or persistent fever, and they are an important part of the differential diagnosis of the febrile child. It is essential for physicians who care for children to recognize these disorders, and to refer these children to specialists who can initiate treatment, improve quality of life, and avoid long-term complications.

Researchers over the last 10 years has identified many of the genes that cause AIDs. Most of these diseases are monogenic and inherited in an

---

No disclosures.

Program in Rheumatology, Division of Immunology, Boston Children's Hospital, 300 Longwood Avenue, Boston, MA 02115, USA

* Corresponding author.

E-mail address: jonathan.hausmann@childrens.harvard.edu

Dermatol Clin 31 (2013) 481–494

http://dx.doi.org/10.1016/j.det.2013.04.003

autosomal dominant or recessive pattern. However, our understanding of these diseases continues to evolve. Most children with periodic fevers (greater than 80% in some studies) do not have mutations in known periodic fever syndrome genes.[2] This article presents the differential diagnosis of recurrent fever in children. It discusses periodic fevers with aphthous stomatitis, pharyngitis, and cervical adenitis (PFAPA), the most common AID in children. It then focuses on the clinical presentation of monogenic AIDs that present with fevers in children, including familial Mediterranean fever (FMF), Hyper-IgD syndrome (HIDS), tumor necrosis factor (TNF) receptor–associated periodic syndrome (TRAPS), cryopyrin-associated periodic syndromes (CAPS), deficiency of interleukin-36 receptor antagonist (DITRA), Majeed syndrome, chronic atypical neutrophilic dermatosis with lipodystrophy and increased temperature syndrome (CANDLE), and deficiency of the interleukin-1 receptor antagonist (DIRA). Two granulomatous disorders, pyogenic sterile arthritis, pyoderma gangrenosum, and acne (PAPA) syndrome and Blau syndrome, are also discussed.

RECURRENT FEVERS

Fever is one of the most common reasons for a child to visit his or her pediatrician.[3] Some children present with recurrent or periodic fevers, defined as 3 or more episodes of fever in a 6-month period without a known illness to explain the fevers, and with at least 7 days between febrile episodes.[4] The approach to children with recurrent fevers should be different than that for children presenting with fever of unknown origin, because their etiologies differ.

To better create a differential diagnosis, the pattern of the fevers should be characterized precisely, especially whether there is a regularity to the intervals of fever. Episodes of fever occurring at regular intervals suggest a diagnosis of PFAPA or cyclic neutropenia. Other characteristics that should be noted include the age of fever onset, height of the fever, and pattern during the day. It is important to monitor for associated symptoms during an episode, including rashes, and involvement of the mucosa, joints, eyes, lung, or abdomen.

Viral infections are the most common causes of fevers occurring at irregular intervals in children.[4] Although most viral infections cause obvious symptoms, such as those of upper or lower respiratory tract infections, many viruses can also cause fevers without any other defining signs or symptoms.

Most children with occult bacterial infections present with prolonged rather than recurrent fevers. However, children with repeated bacterial infections should be evaluated for immunodeficiencies, cystic fibrosis, or anatomic abnormalities. Parasitic infections with *Plasmodium* may occur in children who have traveled to endemic areas.

Inflammatory bowel disease is a common cause of recurrent fevers, and the fevers may precede other signs of inflammatory bowel disease, such as abdominal pain, bloody stools, poor growth, and anemia, by weeks or months.

In Behçet disease, febrile children also present with recurrent oral and genital ulcers, uveitis, or skin rashes such as erythema nodosum. Systemic juvenile idiopathic arthritis presents with at least 2 weeks of daily fevers, along with a rash, lymphadenopathy, hepatosplenomegaly, or serositis. These two syndromes share many of the features of AIDs but no clear genetic causes have been identified.

After the diagnoses mentioned earlier have been excluded, AIDs should be considered, especially if there is a family history of recurrent fevers or if the child is of certain ethnic groups. One of the characteristics of AIDs is that the fever pattern and associated features are similar with each episodes. In most of these diseases, children are well between episodes, although some of AIDs follow a more chronic course and cause significant morbidity and mortality unless treated. Fever is not a part of all of the AIDs, although this article focuses on the ones in which fever is present, and briefly touch on several without fevers.

Clinical scoring systems have been created to determine the likelihood that a child will have an AID with a known genetic cause, and may help guide genetic testing (http://www.printo.it/periodicfever), although this needs to be validated in a diverse patient population.

PERIODIC FEVERS WITH APHTHOUS STOMATITIS, PHARYNGITIS, AND CERVICAL ADENITIS

The syndrome of PFAPA is the most common cause of periodic fevers in childhood. First described in 1987,[5] it is characterized by recurrent febrile episodes lasting 3 to 6 days, occurring every 3 to 6 weeks, in addition to the presence of the features that make up the name of this syndrome. Regular intervals (with almost clockwork regularity) between episodes are the cardinal feature of PFAPA, whereas the presence of associated symptoms is more varied. The disease is common in most ethnic groups.[6]

Cause

The cause of PFAPA is unknown. Genetic studies have failed to find a common genetic abnormality in patients with this syndrome. However, 17% to 45% of children with PFAPA have a family history of recurrent fevers, and 12% have a family history of PFAPA,[7,8] suggesting a genetic susceptibility. Some of these patients have heterozygous mutations in various genes known to be involved in other monogenic AIDs such as NRLP3, Mediterranean fever (MEFV), TNFRSF1a, or mevalonate kinase (MVK).[9]

The resolution of PFAPA with tonsillectomy suggests that the tonsils may provide a reservoir for a pathogen that causes an augmented innate immune response.[10,11] These patients show increase in molecules of the innate immune system including complement and interleukin (IL)-1β.

Clinical Presentation

PFAPA usually presents in children less than 5 years of age,[6] although cases have been reported to occur during adolescence[10] and adulthood.[12] Several studies have noted a slight male predominance of 1.2:1 to 2.3:1.[6,8,10,13] Characteristics of patients with PFAPA are shown in **Table 1**.

The interval between febrile episodes varies from 21 to 42 days between patients.[6,10] However, for a particular patient, fevers recur at regular intervals. Many families state that they can predict the onset of fever with remarkable accuracy. Over a period of years, the cycles may shorten or lengthen, and may even stop for several months before restarting again with their usual regularity.

Most patients have a prodrome before the episode of fever begins. This prodrome may include fatigue, headache, abdominal pain, or irritability.[6] Pharyngitis and cervical adenitis are the most common features. When aphthous stomatitis is present, it is usually limited to 1 to 4 superficial aphthae (<1 cm or less), or less frequently by a crop of small aphthae.

Additional symptoms may include chills, headache, nausea, diarrhea, abdominal pain, lethargy, poor appetite, myalgias, and arthralgias.[10,13] Patients are completely well between episodes and have normal growth and development.

Long-term outcome for patients with PFAPA is excellent. Most patients have resolution of episodes after 4 to 6 years.[8,13,14] Those patients who are still symptomatic after several years typically have a shortening of febrile days and a decrease in the frequency of the episodes.[10,14] Follow-up studies have shown good long-term outcomes in children diagnosed with PFAPA without increased risk for malignancy, autoimmune disorders, or chronic infectious diseases.[13,14]

Diagnosis

There are no laboratory or genetic tests to confirm the diagnosis of PFAPA. As such, it is a diagnosis of exclusion made clinically. However, monogenic AIDs can often overlap with PFAPA. A recent study showed that patients with monogenic AIDs such as HIDS or TRAPS, also met criteria for PFAPA.[2,15]

During attacks, children have leukocytosis with increased monocytes and neutrophils, and an increase in inflammatory markers including erythrocyte sedimentation rate (ESR), C-reactive protein (CRP), and serum amyloid A protein (SAA).[9] ESR may be normal at the onset of fever, but it increases within a few days.[6] Between attacks, all inflammatory markers normalize. Neutropenia during episodes should prompt evaluation for cyclic neutropenia. Diagnostic criteria are shown in **Box 1**.

Table 1
Characteristics of patients with PFAPA in various clinical studies

	Licameli 2012[10] (n = 102)	Feder and Salazar 2009[6] (n = 105)	Thomas 1999[13] (n = 94)
Pharyngitis	79%	61%	72%
Cervical adenitis	84%	46%	88%
Aphthous stomatitis	44%	21%	70%
Steroids abort fever	96%	97%	76%
Age at disease onset	NA	3.3 y	2.8 y
Duration of episode	NA	4.1 d	4.8 d
Days between episodes	NA	29.8 d	28.8 d
Tonsillectomy aborts PFAPA	97%	100%	64%

Abbreviation: NA, not applicable.
Data from Refs.[6,10,13]

Box 1
Modified diagnostic criteria for PFAPA

- Regularly recurring fevers with an early age of onset (<5 years)
- Constitutional symptoms in the absence of upper respiratory infection with at least 1 of the following clinical signs:
  - Aphthous stomatitis
  - Cervical lymphadenitis
  - Pharyngitis
- Exclusion of cyclic neutropenia
- Completely asymptomatic intervals between episodes
- Normal growth and development

Data from Thomas KT, Feder HM, Lawton AR, et al. Periodic fever syndrome in children. J Pediatr 1999;135(1):15–21.

Treatment

A single prednisone dose of 1 to 2 mg/kg at the onset of an attack may be sufficient to halt an attack. If the fever does not resolve, a second dose 12 hours later may be attempted. A recent study also found efficacy with a lower dose of prednisone of 0.5 mg/kg.[16] Other symptoms may take longer to resolve.[6,13] Although steroids have been effective in aborting episodes, they may paradoxically increase their frequency.[6,13]

Antipyretics are only partially effective in controlling the fevers.[10] Cimetidine has also been used for treatment, and seems to be effective in resolving fevers in 27% of patients.[6] Small case reports have shown good clinical responses with an IL-1 receptor antagonist (anakinra).[11]

Tonsillectomy has been shown to be successful in eliminating future episodes in several studies.[6,10,13] A recent report on 102 patients who underwent tonsillectomy showed excellent response in 97% of children, without any surgical complications.[10] However, tonsillectomy is still an invasive, expensive procedure, and may be considered unnecessary for an illness that is self-limiting and transient. On the other hand, the impact of monthly fevers on the daily lives of patients and families cannot be disregarded. As such, tonsillectomy can be an acceptable alternative for some patients.

FAMILIAL MEDITERRANEAN FEVER

FMF is the most common monogenic AID in the world. It presents as recurrent attacks of fever, serositis, arthritis, and rash, with completely asymptomatic episodes between attacks. The first case of FMF was described in 1908,[17] and the first series of patients was published in 1945.[18] It was initially thought to be a disease limited to certain populations living in the Mediterranean, including Sephardic Jews, Turks, Armenians, and Arabs. However, the discovery of the gene responsible for FMF in 1997[19,20] has allowed the identification of patients with FMF in other ethnic groups including Europeans, Americans, Australians, Indians, Chinese, and Japanese.[21,22]

Carrier frequencies as high as 1:3 to 1:5 have been described in certain populations.[23] The high frequency of carriers of this mutation suggests that heterozygous individuals may have an evolutionary advantage, perhaps by conferring a more potent immune response against certain pathogens.[24,25]

Cause

FMF is an autosomal recessive disease caused by mutations in the MEFV gene located in chromosome 16. MEFV codes for the protein pyrin (marenostrin), which is expressed predominantly in neutrophils, although it is also found in eosinophils, monocytes, dendritic cells, and fibroblasts of the synovium, peritoneum, and skin. The distribution of expression of pyrin within the body accounts for the sites of inflammation that are affected during attacks.[22] Mutated pyrin leads to increased activation of caspase 1 and uncontrolled release of IL-1β from phagocytes.[1]

Although it is an autosomal recessive disorder, genetic sequencing of patients with FMF has revealed substantial numbers of patients with only one mutated MEFV allele but full phenotype of the disease,[26] suggesting that FMF could also result from MEFV haploinsufficiency.

Clinical Presentation

FMF is characterized by recurrent, self-limited, febrile episodes accompanied by sterile arthritis, peritonitis, pleuritis, and skin involvement. The episodes occur suddenly, typically last 12 to 72 hours, or resolve spontaneously. They can be triggered by a variety of factors including infections, stress, exercise, or menses.[27] The frequency of attacks varies, occurring several times per month to once yearly. Each attack is associated with leukocytosis and increased inflammatory markers including increased ESR, CRP, and fibrinogen.

The disease usually starts during childhood. Thirty percent of patients present at less than 2 years of age,[28] and 80% of cases present before 20 years of age.[29] Most young patients are homozygous for the M694V mutation. Younger children may present with recurrent fevers as the only manifestation of FMF, making the diagnosis a challenge and delaying the initiation of treatment.[28] The frequency of the initial presenting symptom for FMF is shown in **Box 2**.

Abdominal attacks occur in 95% of patients.[30] Pain is usually severe, confining children to bed, and may be mistaken for appendicitis.[31] Radiologic examination may reveal air-fluid levels, leading to the suspicion of acute abdomen and the need for surgery.[32] In children, diarrhea is common, although constipation can also be seen.[30,32] Recurrent abdominal attacks may cause peritoneal adhesions.

Pleuritis, manifested as chest pain, is found in 23% to 62% of patients.[33] Pericarditis is only seen in a minority of patients.[34]

Arthritis is present in 37% to 77% of patients and may even be the presenting symptom.[30,33,35] The arthritis is of sudden onset, usually monoarticular, most often affecting the knees, ankles, and hips.[33,35] Joints may be red, swollen, warm, and tender, and may be mistaken for septic arthritis.[30] Although arthritis usually develops spontaneously, exertion and insignificant trauma can also precipitate an attack.[35] Short attacks of arthritis are most common and usually resolve within 1 week without sequelae. In a minority of patients, a chronic arthritis occurs, usually of the knee or hip. Sacroiliac involvement, presenting as inflammatory back pain, has also been described in several case series, and is thought to affect 0.4% to 7% of patients with FMF.[33,36–39] Sacroiliitis seems to be more common in FMF patients with positive human leukocyte antigen (HLA)-B27.

Skin manifestation of FMF is limited to an erysipelas-like rash that occurs in 7% to 34% of children with FMF.[33] The rash mainly presents in the lower extremities, especially around the ankles or dorsum of the feet, and usually fades within 1 to 3 days.[31]

Exercise-induced myalgias are also common.[33] Up to 20% of patients develop lower extremity pain after physical exertion, mostly in the evening, which can last from a few hours to 2 or 3 days, and resolves with rest.[40]

Protracted febrile myalgia syndrome is seen in a small percentage of patients with FMF and is characterized by high fever and severe, debilitating myalgias of the extremities.[41] It is occasionally accompanied by abdominal pain, diarrhea, arthritis, or a purpuric rash. Although there is extreme pain and tenderness on examination, laboratory work reveals normal creatine phosphokinase and nonspecific electromyogram changes.[42] Untreated, it typically lasts for 4 to 6 weeks, but resolves with steroids.

Other less-frequent features of FMF include orchitis and scrotal swelling, which most commonly occurs during childhood.[43] Splenomegaly may also occur.[31,33] Patients with FMF seem to be at increased risk of vasculitis including Henoch-Schonlein purpura, polyarteritis nodosa, and Behçet disease.[31,34]

Secondary amyloidosis is the most severe complication of FMF. It commonly affects the kidney, causing proteinuria or nephrotic syndrome. However, long-term use of colchicine in children prevents this potentially fatal complication.[44] Screening urinalyses are important to detect impaired renal function.

The clinical manifestation of FMF attacks may vary between individuals, and even among individuals through their lifetimes, which is likely related to the interplay between genes and the environment. For example, the most common mutation, M694V, is associated with earlier onset and more severe disease, including more frequent attacks, more joint disease, higher doses of colchicine required for control, and higher rates of amyloidosis is seen among patients not adequately treated.[45]

The environment also plays a role in the expression of the disease. A recent study compared disease severity of Turkish children with FMF living in Turkey, with Turkish children living in Germany.[46] Although there was no difference between the increase of acute phase reactants during attacks, the severity of the attacks was significantly higher in children living in Turkey, suggesting that microbes or other aspects of the environment may affect the final disease expression.

Diagnosis

Several clinical diagnostic criteria for FMF have been created; the Tel Hashomer criteria are the most widely used, and are shown in **Box 3**. There are efforts to create diagnostic criteria specifically for children, although these have yet to be validated in diverse populations.[47]

Box 2
Presenting symptoms of FMF

Symptom	Percentage
Abdominal pain	55
Arthritis	26
Chest pain	5
Fever	3

Data from Sohar E, Gafni J, Pras M, et al. Familial Mediterranean fever. A survey of 470 cases and review of the literature. Am J Med 1967;43(2):227–53.

Box 3
Simplified Tel Hashomer criteria for the diagnosis of FMF

Major criteria:

Typical attacks

- Peritonitis (generalized)
- Pleuritis (unilateral) or pericarditis
- Monoarthritis (hip, knee, ankle)
- Fever alone

Minor criteria

Incomplete attacks involving 1 or more of the following sites:

- Chest
- Joint

Exertional leg pain

Favorable response to colchicine

Diagnosis requires 1 or more major criteria or 2 or more minor criteria. Typical attacks are defined as recurrent (≥3 of the same type), febrile (≥38°C), and short (lasting between 12 and 72 hours). Incomplete attacks differ from typical attacks in lack of fever, being of shorter or longer length, lack of abdominal attacks, localized abdominal attacks, or arthritis in joints other than those specified.
Data from Livneh A, Langevitz P, Zemer D, et al. Criteria for the diagnosis of familial Mediterranean fever. Arthritis Rheum 1997;40(10):1879–85.

The use of genetic testing for the MEFV gene in countries with a low prevalence of FMF may be helpful. However, even complete sequencing of the MEFV gene sometimes fails to identify any abnormalities in a small subset of patients who exhibit symptoms consistent with FMF and respond appropriately to colchicine, suggesting that other genes may be involved.

Treatment

The simultaneous discovery of the efficacy of colchicine for FMF by Dr Ozkan in Turkey and Dr Goldfinger[48] in the United States changed the landscape of the disease. Before colchicine, up to 75% of patients developed amyloidosis during adulthood. However, this has become a rare outcome. Early introduction of colchicine during childhood is helpful to prevent painful, febrile attacks, avoid unnecessary interventions (laparotomy, antibiotics), and prevent amyloidosis.[49] Colchicine inhibits leukocyte chemotaxis and alters the expression of adhesion molecules. The exact mechanism of its efficacy in treating FMF is unknown.

Colchicine has been found to be safe and effective in children with FMF. Complete remission occurs in up to two-thirds of patients treated with colchicine; whereas a partial response, characterized as a significant decrease in frequency and severity of episodes, occurs in a third of patients.[50] Multiple studies have shown that amyloidosis can be prevented in children with regular use of colchicine, even if it does not completely prevent attacks.[33,51]

True colchicine resistance is rare (~5% of patients).[49,50] In patients who do not respond to colchicine, compliance should be evaluated, and alternative diagnoses should be sought. Newer biologics with anti–IL-1 activity (anakinra and canakinumab) have shown excellent responses in patients who do not tolerate, or are resistant to, colchicine.[52]

Treatment of acute attacks include nonsteroidal antiinflammatory drugs (NSAIDs) and opiates if pain is severe.[49] Increasing colchicine doses during attacks does not seem to have any beneficial effects.[29]

HYPER-IGD SYNDROME

HIDS is a rare, autosomal recessive AID characterized by recurrent episodes of systemic inflammation that includes fevers, abdominal pain, diarrhea, rash, arthralgias, aphthous ulcers, and lymphadenopathy. It is caused by mutations in the MVK gene, an enzyme involved in the synthesis of cholesterol and isoprenoids. Mutations of this gene cause a range of phenotypes, depending on the level of functioning enzyme. Reduced activity of the enzyme causes HIDS, whereas a complete deficiency results in mevalonic aciduria, a syndrome of severe febrile episodes and neurologic complications including ataxia, mental retardation, and early death. The exact mechanism of how mutations in MVK lead to periodic fevers is still unknown, but shortage of a product of the MVK pathway seems to activate of the inflammasome and secrete IL-1β.[53]

Half of the documented cases of HIDS are found in people of Dutch origin,[54] although cases have now been identified globally, with most patients being of European ancestry.[55] In the largest study of patients with HIDS, the average age of onset was 6 months, 78% of patients had their first attack within the first year, and all of them presented during childhood.[55] For most patients, childhood vaccinations precipitated their first attack. Emotional and physical stress can also precipitate attacks. The frequency of attacks decreased after age 20 years, although they still occurred at least every other month.

Attacks typically last 3 to 7 days and are characterized by lymphadenopathy, abdominal pain, vomiting or diarrhea, and arthralgia. Two-thirds of patients have a rash, usually maculopapular. Aphthous ulcers, sometimes with genital ulcers, occurred in about 50% of patients, mistaking this diagnosis with Behçet disease. Many features of HIDS are also seen in patients with PFAPA. However, HIDS can be differentiated by an earlier age of onset, longer periods of fever, longer intervals between episodes, and more frequent vomiting and abdominal pain. **Box 4** shows criteria to help make the diagnosis of HIDS.

Leukocytosis and elevation in inflammatory markers, including ESR and CRP, are seen during attacks. Urinary levels of mevalonic acid are increased during attacks, and are helpful in making the diagnosis.[56] IgD and IgA concentrations are increased in most patients, although 22% of patients with HIDS have normal IgD levels. IgD serum concentrations do not vary during acute episodes and are not correlated with severity of symptoms or frequency of attacks,[57] suggesting that the increased levels of IgD may be an epiphenomenon of the disease and, despite the name, not central to the pathogenesis of HIDS. Furthermore, 50% of patients with other periodic fever syndromes also have increased IgD levels.[58] Increases in IgD can also be seen in other conditions such as lymphoma and tuberculosis. Thus, genetic testing is probably the best way of diagnosing this disease.

Treatment is not standardized, and can include trials of NSAIDs, prednisone, anakinra, or etanercept.[50,59–61]

TNF RECEPTOR-ASSOCIATED PERIODIC SYNDROME

TRAPS is the most common autosomal dominant, inherited periodic fever syndrome.[62] It is characterized by prolonged, episodic fevers with systemic inflammation. Previously referred to as familial Hibernian fever because of its first description in an Irish family,[63] TRAPS has been found in other populations throughout the world.[64,65]

TRAPS is caused by mutations in the TNF receptor (TNFR1a), which is found mainly on monocytes and macrophages and responds to the inflammatory cytokine TNF. The pathogenic mechanism by which the mutation results in the phenotype of TRAPS is still not well understood.[66] Some mutations seem to result in impaired shedding of the soluble receptor.[62] Other mutations result in misfolding of the protein and retention of the receptor intracellularly.[64] The mutant receptor seems to accumulate within the cell and sensitizes the cell to produce inflammatory cytokines with little stimulation.[67] Most TRAPS mutations involve cysteine residues, which cause typical disease. However, two non-cysteine mutations, R92Q and P46L are associated with variable phenotypes and incomplete penetrance.[68]

Patients with TRAPS usually present at a median age of 3 years, although cases have been identified as early as 2 weeks and as late as 53 years.[65] Patients experience recurrent, prolonged episodes of fever, lasting an average of 3 weeks, but sometimes as long as 6 weeks.[26,65,69] Attacks may occur every 5 to 6 weeks and usually consist of myalgias, fever, and rash. The rash is usually a centrifugal, migratory, erythematous patch that overlies the area of myalgia. The rash is tender, warm, and blanchable. There is no increase of muscle enzymes.

Peritonitis causing abdominal pain is common, and may be mistaken for an acute abdomen. Patients may also have arthralgias, conjunctivitis, periorbital edema, uveitis, and iritis.[65]

Laboratory examinations show elevations in acute phase reactants including ESR, CRP, haptoglobin, fibrinogen, and ferritin.[65] There may be leukocytosis, thrombocytosis, and anemia from the chronic inflammatory disease.[66] Patients may

---

Box 4
Clinical criteria for the consideration of a diagnosis of HIDS

When to consider HIDS

Recurrent episodes of fever lasting 3 to 7 days for more than 6 months

And 1 or more of the following:

Sibling with genetically confirmed HIDS

Increased serum IgD (>100 IU/L)

First attack after childhood vaccination

Three or more symptoms during attacks:

• Cervical lymphadenopathy

• Abdominal pain

• Vomiting or diarrhea

• Arthralgia or arthritis of large peripheral joints

• Aphthous ulcers

• Skin lesions

Data from van der Hilst JC, Bodar EJ, Barron KS, et al. Long-term follow-up, clinical features, and quality of life in a series of 103 patients with hyperimmunoglobulinemia D syndrome. Medicine 2008;87(6):301–10.

also have polyclonal hypergammaglobulinemia. Acute phase reactants may remain increased between attacks, although at lower levels than during attacks.

Because of the persistent inflammatory state, children with TRAPS are at risk of developing amyloidosis, most commonly involving the kidneys.[65]

Treatment of TRAPS seems to be more challenging than for other AIDs, possibly due the heterogeneity of genetic mutations and clinical phenotypes.[66] NSAIDs and corticosteroids can be effective to treat acute attacks, especially if associated with certain mutations.[50,66] Etanercept has been shown to be beneficial in most patients, although a complete response is not always achieved.[50,70] Other anti-TNF agents seem to cause exacerbation of the disease.[66] Anakinra was shown to produce a complete response in most patients in one observational study.[50]

CRYOPYRIN-ASSOCIATED PERIODIC SYNDROMES

The CAPS are a set of rare, autosomal dominant AIDs that encompass a spectrum of severity from mild to severe disease. They are caused by mutations in nucleotide-binding domain, leucine-rich repeat family, pyrin domain containing 3 (NLRP3), which codes for cryopyrin. NLRP3 is a key component of the inflammasome and is expressed in neutrophils, monocytes, and chondrocytes.[71] Most patients with CAPS have gain-of-function mutations that activate the inflammasome and cause release of IL-1β, in response to reduced or absent stimuli.[26] The discovery of NLRP3 in 2001[72] linked 3 diseases (familial cold autoinflammatory syndrome [FCAS], Muckle-Wells syndrome [MWS], and neonatal-onset multisystem inflammatory disease [NOMID]), previously thought to be unrelated. Most cases of NOMID are associated with de novo mutations, whereas the mutated gene is usually inherited in FCAS and MWS.

CAPS is distinguished from other AIDs by the presence of an urticarial rash and cold exposure as a trigger for attacks. Unlike most of the AIDs, a third of patients do not have fever accompanying the episodes.[73]

FCAS is characterized by recurrent episodes of fever, urticaria, and arthralgia brought about by cold exposure. The rash is seen in the trunk and limbs, and individual lesions migrate and last less than 24 hours.[74] The rash is minimal during the morning and increases in severity in the evening.[75] Amyloidosis is a rare complication of this disease.

In MWS, in addition to fever, urticarial rash, and arthralgias, the episodes often lead to progressive neurosensory hearing loss secondary to cochlear inflammation,[26] which was present in 50% of patients in one study.[73] The urticaria is present most days, and tends not to be pruritic, or only mildly pruritic. Other commonly occurring symptoms include conjunctivitis, uveitis, headache, abdominal pain, and diffuse aching of the extremities. Amyloidosis can be seen as a late complication in 25% of patients with MWS.

The most severe form of the disease, called NOMID or chronic infantile neurologic cutaneous and articular syndrome (CINCA), includes all of the symptoms of MWS but presents during the newborn period. Episodes are nearly continuous and also associated with dysmorphic features, chronic aseptic meningitis, blindness, mental retardation, and bone deformation.[76] Patients with NOMID have significant arthropathy affecting large joints, resulting in functional disability with endochondral ossification and calcified masses in the joints.[74]

Laboratory abnormalities include increases in CRP and SAA, which usually remain increased even without attacks.[74] Urine should be checked for protein, to screen for amyloidosis. Biopsy of the urticarial lesion shows a sparse interstitial neutrophilic infiltrate in the reticular dermis,[75] and can help in the diagnosis of this syndrome.

Anakinra has been shown to be effective in resolution of fever, rash, conjunctivitis, and joint symptoms, as well as normalization of inflammatory markers.[77] It may even be effective in reversing amyloid deposits.[73] Canakinumab[78] and rilonacept[79] also seem to be effective in controlling the disease, again highlighting the importance of IL-1β in the pathogenesis of this AID.

A similar phenotype to that seen in FCAS, with arthralgias and myalgias in response to cold exposure, has been found as a result of mutations of a different gene, NLRP12, which also seems to enhance secretion of IL-1β.[80]

DEFICIENCY OF INTERLEUKIN-36 RECEPTOR ANTAGONIST

An autosomal recessive disease first described in 2011 in several Tunisian families, DITRA is characterized by generalized pustular psoriasis.[81] It is caused by mutations in IL36RN, the gene that encodes for interleukin-36 receptor antagonist. In the wild-type state, IL-36 receptor antagonist works to block several proinflammatory signaling pathways. Most patients present between birth and 11 years of age. Patients have repeated flares of sudden-onset, high-grade fever of more than 40°C, malaise, and weakness, in addition to a diffuse, erythematous rash associated with pustules, leukocytosis, and increased CRP.

MAJEED SYNDROME

Majeed syndrome, first described in 1989, is a rare, autosomal recessive condition that consists of 3 prominent features: chronic recurrent multifocal osteomyelitis (CRMO), congenital dyserythropoietic anemia, and an inflammatory dermatosis.[82] It has been identified in Kuwaiti,[82] Jordanian,[83] and Turkish[84] families. The gene responsible for this syndrome is LPIN2, although its function is still unclear.[83]

Majeed syndrome presents in children less than 2 years of age. It is characterized by recurrent fevers, occurring every 2 to 4 weeks and lasting 3 to 4 days. CRMO has an early age of onset; as many as 1 to 3 relapses per month; and short, infrequent remissions.[82] It eventually leads to delayed growth, joint contractures, or both.[83] Anemia severity can range from mild to severe requiring blood transfusions. The inflammatory dermatosis commonly presents as Sweet syndrome. Anakinra and canakinumab have been effective in 2 patients.[84]

CHRONIC ATYPICAL NEUTROPHILIC DERMATOSIS WITH LIPODYSTROPHY AND INCREASED TEMPERATURE SYNDROME

CANDLE syndrome is characterized by recurrent fevers, purpuric skin lesions, violaceous swollen eyelids, arthralgias, progressive lipodystrophy, anemia, delayed physical development, and increase of acute phase reactants.[85] It is caused by mutations in PSMB8, which leads to immunoproteasome dysfunction. The immunoproteasome is critical for protein degradation and generation of antigenic peptides for major histocompatibility complex class I presentation. Mutations within this structure cause inability to maintain cell homeostasis and results in increased interferon signaling.

Previously identified diseases, including Nakajo-Nishimura syndrome, Japanese autoinflammatory syndrome with lipodystrophy, and joint contractures, muscular atrophy, microcytic anemia, and panniculitis-associated lipodystrophy (JMP) syndrome, have been shown to result from mutations within this same gene.

The onset of this disease usually occurs shortly after birth, and is uniformly present by 6 months of age.[85] Fevers occur daily or almost daily and have poor response to NSAIDs.[86] In addition, children develop erythematous and violaceous, annular cutaneous plaques that last days to weeks and leave residual purpura. During infancy, children develop persistent periorbital erythema and edema, finger or toe swelling, and hepatomegaly.

During the first year of life, patients lose peripheral fat and develop failure to thrive, lymphadenopathy, and anemia. Use of high-dose steroids improves symptoms, but the disease rebounded with their tapering. Methotrexate, calcineurin inhibitors, TNF inhibitors, anti–IL-1 and anti–IL-6 therapy have limited success in managing this disease.[85]

DEFICIENCY OF THE INTERLEUKIN-1 RECEPTOR ANTAGONIST

First described in 2009 by Aksentjevich and colleagues,[87] deficiency of the interleukin-1 receptor antagonist (DIRA) is an inherited, recessive disease caused by mutations in IL1RN, the gene that codes for the interleukin-1 receptor antagonist. The endogenous IL-1 receptor antagonist normally inhibits the proinflammatory cytokines IL-1α and IL-1β. A mutation in IL1RN leads to overstimulation by proinflammatory cytokines. Although the mutation has been found in patients from Canada, the Netherlands, Lebanon,[87] Brazil,[88] and Turkey,[89] it seems to be particularly common in some areas of Puerto Rico as a result of a founder mutation, with an incidence as high as 1 in 6300 births.[87] DIRA usually presents within the first 2 weeks of birth with fetal distress, a pustular rash, arthritis, oral lesions, and pain with movement. Soon after birth, children develop cutaneous pustulosis, multifocal aseptic osteomyelitis, and periostitis. Fever is typically not present, but inflammatory markers, including ESR and CRP, are markedly increased. Neutrophilia is present in the blood and neutrophilic infiltrates can be found in skin and bones. DIRA is often confused with infections in the newborn period.[88] Untreated disease can lead to death from multiple organ failure[87]; however, treatment with anakinra has shown rapid and complete remission of the disease.[87,88,90]

PYOGENIC STERILE ARTHRITIS, PYODERMA GANGRENOSUM, AND ACNE

PAPA is a rare, autosomal dominant, inherited AID distinguished by painful flares of recurrent sterile arthritis with a prominent neutrophilic infiltrate.[91] The disease is caused by missense mutations in the proline-serine-threonine phosphatase-interacting protein 1 gene (PSTPIP1). PSTPIP1 is an adaptor protein that seems to interact with pyrin and the inflammasome. Mutations are thought to cause spontaneous activation of the inflammasome and release of IL-1β.[91]

The skin involvement is variable, and may present as ulcerations, pyoderma gangrenosum, cystic acne, or pathergy.[91,92] Arthritis usually presents during early childhood, and may begin after minor trauma or sporadically.[92] It is characterized by recurrent episodes that lead to accumulation of pyogenic, neutrophil-rich material within affected joints, which results in synovial and cartilage destruction. It typically affects 1 to 3 joints at a time. By puberty, joint symptoms tend to subside, and cutaneous symptoms become more prominent.

Laboratory findings reflect systemic inflammation. Treatment has been successful with anakinra[93,94] and infliximab.[95]

BLAU SYNDROME/EARLY-ONSET SARCOIDOSIS

The familial Blau syndrome is an autosomal dominant AID manifested as a triad of granulomatous dermatitis, arthritis, and uveitis. In 2001, mutations in NOD2 were found in Blau syndrome[96] and subsequently discovered in patients with early-onset sarcoidosis, now known to be the sporadic form of the same disease.[97] NOD2 acts as an intracellular sensor of bacterial cell wall components and activates nuclear factor kappa B (NF-κB) and enhanced autophagy. Gain-of-function mutations, as seen in Blau syndrome, lead to increased NF-κB activity and possibly to the release of inflammatory cytokines.

The average age of onset of the disease is between 2 and 3 years. Arthritis is polyarticular, often affecting the hands and feet, and produces a boggy synovitis and tenosynovitis as a result of granulomatous inflammation.[98,99]

The dermatitis is described as a tan, maculopapular rash with ichthyosiform desquamation and the presence of dermal granulomas.[100] Bilateral uveitis occurs in most patients between 7 and 12 years of age.[98] It presents as anterior uveitis with eye pain, photophobia, and blurred vision. Over time, eye inflammation can cause severe visual impairment and blindness. About one-third of patients also have other prominent features including fever, sialadenitis, lymphadenopathy, erythema nodosum, and vasculitis.

Diagnosis is made by finding noncaseating granulomas in skin, synovium, or conjunctiva.[100] Genetic testing for the NOD2 mutation has increasingly helped to make the diagnosis. There are no studies on the optimal treatment of the disease, but methotrexate, thalidomide, corticosteroids, TNF inhibitors, and IL-1 inhibitors have been tried with various levels of success.[99]

SUMMARY

Fever is one of the most common reasons for a child to present to a pediatrician. Repeated febrile episodes are most commonly caused by viral infections. However, in a child with recurrent fevers and other features of inflammation, AIDs should be considered. Although these diseases are rare, they have helped clinicians to understand the role of the innate immune system and inflammatory pathways that are ubiquitous in health and disease. Over the last decade, advances in genetics and molecular biology have focused attention on AIDs, and the pathways responsible for these rare syndromes have also been implicated to play a role in a variety of more common conditions such as gout, diabetes mellitus, and atherosclerosis. By continuing to study and improve the new treatment of children with AIDs, treatments may be discovered for many of the diseases that affect people in the modern world.

REFERENCES

1. Masters SL, Simon A, Aksentijevich I, et al. Horror autoinflammaticus: the molecular pathophysiology of autoinflammatory disease*. Annu Rev Immunol 2009;27(1):621–68.
2. Gattorno M, Sormani MP, D'Osualdo A, et al. A diagnostic score for molecular analysis of hereditary autoinflammatory syndromes with periodic fever in children. Arthritis Rheum 2008;58(6): 1823–32.
3. Finkelstein JA, Christiansen CL, Platt R. Fever in pediatric primary care: occurrence, management, and outcomes. Pediatrics 2000;105(1 Pt 3):260–6.
4. John CC, Gilsdorf JR. Recurrent fever in children. Pediatr Infect Dis J 2002;21(11):1071–7.
5. Marshall GS, Edwards KM, Butler J, et al. Syndrome of periodic fever, pharyngitis, and aphthous stomatitis. J Pediatr 1987;110(1):43–6.
6. Feder HM, Salazar JC. A clinical review of 105 patients with PFAPA (a periodic fever syndrome). Acta Paediatr 2010;99(2):178–84.
7. Cochard M, Clet J, Le L, et al. PFAPA syndrome is not a sporadic disease. Rheumatology (Oxford) 2010;49(10):1984–7.
8. Førsvoll J, Kristoffersen EK, Oymar K. Incidence, clinical characteristics and outcome in Norwegian children with PFAPA syndrome; a population-based study. Acta Paediatr 2013;102(2):187–92.
9. Kolly L, Busso N, Scheven-Gete von A, et al. Periodic fever, aphthous stomatitis, pharyngitis, cervical adenitis syndrome is linked to dysregulated monocyte IL-1β production. J Allergy Clin Immunol 2012. http://dx.doi.org/10.1016/j.jaci.2012.07.043.
10. Licameli G, Lawton M, Kenna M, et al. Long-term surgical outcomes of adenotonsillectomy for PFAPA syndrome. Arch Otolaryngol Head Neck Surg 2012;138(10):902–6.

11. Stojanov S, Lapidus S, Chitkara P, et al. Periodic fever, aphthous stomatitis, pharyngitis, and adenitis (PFAPA) is a disorder of innate immunity and Th1 activation responsive to IL-1 blockade. Proc Natl Acad Sci U S A 2011;108(17):7148–53.

12. Padeh S, Stoffman N, Berkun Y. Periodic fever accompanied by aphthous stomatitis, pharyngitis and cervical adenitis syndrome (PFAPA syndrome) in adults. Isr Med Assoc J 2008;10(5): 358–60.

13. Thomas KT, Feder HM, Lawton AR, et al. Periodic fever syndrome in children. J Pediatr 1999;135(1): 15–21.

14. Wurster VM, Carlucci JG, Feder HM, et al. Long-term follow-up of children with periodic fever, aphthous stomatitis, pharyngitis, and cervical adenitis syndrome. J Pediatr 2011;159(6):958–64.

15. Gattorno M, Caorsi R, Meini A, et al. Differentiating PFAPA syndrome from monogenic periodic fevers. Pediatrics 2009;124(4):e721–8.

16. Yazgan H, Gültekin E, Yazıcılar O, et al. Comparison of conventional and low dose steroid in the treatment of PFAPA syndrome: preliminary study. Int J Pediatr Otorhinolaryngol 2012; 76(11):1588–90.

17. Janeway TC, Mosenthal HO. An unusual paroxysmal syndrome, probably allied to recurrent vomiting, with a study of the nitrogen metabolism. Arch Intern Med 1908;2(3):214.

18. Siegal S. Benign paroxysmal peritonitis. Ann Intern Med 1945;23(1):1–21.

19. Consortium TIF. Ancient missense mutations in a new member of the RoRet gene family are likely to cause familial Mediterranean fever. The International FMF Consortium. Cell 1997; 90(4):797–807.

20. French F. A candidate gene for familial Mediterranean fever. Nat Genet 1997;17(1):25.

21. Ben-Chetrit E, Touitou I. Familial Mediterranean fever in the world. Arthritis Rheum 2009;61(10): 1447–53.

22. Chae JJ, Aksentijevich I, Kastner DL. Advances in the understanding of familial Mediterranean fever and possibilities for targeted therapy. Br J Haematol 2009;146(5):467–78.

23. Touitou I. The spectrum of familial Mediterranean fever (FMF) mutations. Eur J Hum Genet 2001; 9(7):473–83.

24. Fumagalli M, Cagliani R, Pozzoli U, et al. A population genetics study of the familial Mediterranean fever gene: evidence of balancing selection under an overdominance regime. Genes Immun 2009;10(8):678–86.

25. Lachmann HJ. Clinical and subclinical inflammation in patients with familial Mediterranean fever and in heterozygous carriers of MEFV mutations. Rheumatology (Oxford) 2006;45(6):746–50.

26. Park H, Bourla AB, Kastner DL, et al. Lighting the fires within: the cell biology of autoinflammatory diseases. Nat Rev Immunol 2012;12(8):570–80.

27. Rigante D. The fresco of autoinflammatory diseases from the pediatric perspective. Autoimmun Rev 2012;11(5):348–56.

28. Padeh S, Livneh A, Pras E, et al. Familial Mediterranean fever in the first two years of life: a unique phenotype of disease in evolution. J Pediatr 2010; 156(6):985–9.

29. Sohar E, Gafni J, Pras M, et al. Familial Mediterranean fever. A survey of 470 cases and review of the literature. Am J Med 1967;43(2):227–53.

30. Onen F. Familial Mediterranean fever. Rheumatol Int 2005;26(6):489–96.

31. Ozen S. Familial Mediterranean fever: revisiting an ancient disease. Eur J Pediatr 2003;162(7–8):449–54.

32. Bhat A, Naguwa SM, Gershwin ME. Genetics and new treatment modalities for familial Mediterranean fever. Ann N Y Acad Sci 2007;1110(1):201–8.

33. Majeed HA, Rawashdeh M, Shanti El H, et al. Familial Mediterranean fever in children: the expanded clinical profile. QJM 1999;92(6):309–18.

34. Group TFS. Familial Mediterranean fever (FMF) in Turkey. Medicine 2005;84(1):1–11.

35. Heller H, Gafni J, Michaeli D, et al. The arthritis of familial Mediterranean fever (FMF). Arthritis Rheum 1966;9(1):1–17.

36. Lehman TJ, Hanson V, Kornreich H, et al. HLA-B27-negative sacroiliitis: a manifestation of familial Mediterranean fever in childhood. Pediatrics 1978; 61(3):423–6.

37. Balaban B, Yasar E, Ozgul A, et al. Sacroiliitis in familial Mediterranean fever and seronegative spondyloarthropathy: importance of differential diagnosis. Rheumatol Int 2005;25(8):641–4.

38. Langevitz P, Livneh A, Zemer D, et al. Seronegative spondyloarthropathy in familial Mediterranean fever. Semin Arthritis Rheum 1997;27(2):67–72.

39. Kaşifoğlu T, Calişir C, Cansu DU, et al. The frequency of sacroiliitis in familial Mediterranean fever and the role of HLA-B27 and MEFV mutations in the development of sacroiliitis. Clin Rheumatol 2009; 28(1):41–6.

40. Cassidy JT, Petty RE, Laxer R, et al. Textbook of pediatric rheumatology E-Book. Philadelphia: Saunders; 2010.

41. Senel K, Melikoglu MA, Baykal T, et al. Protracted febrile myalgia syndrome in familial Mediterranean fever. Mod Rheumatol 2010;20(4):410–2.

42. Majeed HA, Al-Qudah AK, Qubain H, et al. The clinical patterns of myalgia in children with familial Mediterranean fever. Semin Arthritis Rheum 2000; 30(2):138–43.

43. Leung DY, Sampson H, Geha R, et al. Pediatric allergy: principles and practice E-Book. Philadelphia: Saunders; 2010.

44. Zemer D, Livneh A, Danon YL, et al. Long-term colchicine treatment in children with familial Mediterranean fever. Arthritis Rheum 1991;34(8): 973–7.

45. Dewalle M, Domingo C, Rozenbaum M, et al. Phenotype-genotype correlation in Jewish patients suffering from familial Mediterranean fever (FMF). Eur J Hum Genet 1998;6(1):95.

46. Ozen S, Aktay N, Lainka E, et al. Disease severity in children and adolescents with familial Mediterranean fever: a comparative study to explore environmental effects on a monogenic disease. Ann Rheum Dis 2009;68(2):246–8.

47. Yalcinkaya F, Ozen S, Ozcakar ZB, et al. A new set of criteria for the diagnosis of familial Mediterranean fever in childhood. Rheumatology (Oxford) 2009;48(4):395–8.

48. Goldfinger SE. Colchicine for familial Mediterranean fever. N Engl J Med 1972;287(25):1302.

49. Kallinich T, Haffner D, Niehues T, et al. Colchicine use in children and adolescents with familial Mediterranean fever: literature review and consensus statement. Pediatrics 2007;119(2):e474–83.

50. Haar Ter N, Lachmann H, Ozen S, et al. Treatment of autoinflammatory diseases: results from the Eurofever Registry and a literature review. Ann Rheum Dis 2012;72(5):678–85.

51. Zemer D, Pras M, Sohar E, et al. Colchicine in the prevention and treatment of the amyloidosis of familial Mediterranean fever. N Engl J Med 1986; 314(16):1001–5.

52. Caorsi R, Federici S, Gattorno M. Biologic drugs in autoinflammatory syndromes. Autoimmun Rev 2012;12(1):81–6.

53. van der Burgh R, Haar ter NM, Boes ML, et al. Mevalonate kinase deficiency, a metabolic autoinflammatory disease. Clin Immunol 2012. http://dx.doi.org/ 10.1016/j.clim.2012.09.011.

54. Korppi M, van Gijn ME, Antila K. Hyperimmunoglobulinemia D and periodic fever syndrome in children. Review on therapy with biological drugs and case report. Acta Paediatr 2010;100(1):21–5.

55. van der Hilst JC, Bodar EJ, Barron KS, et al. Long-term follow-up, clinical features, and quality of life in a series of 103 patients with hyperimmunoglobulinemia D syndrome. Medicine 2008;87(6):301–10.

56. Ryan JG, Kastner DL. Fevers, genes, and innate immunity. Curr Top Microbiol Immunol 2008;321: 169–84.

57. Simon A, Bijzet J, Voorbij HA, et al. Effect of inflammatory attacks in the classical type hyper-IgD syndrome on immunoglobulin D, cholesterol and parameters of the acute phase response. J Intern Med 2004;256(3):247–53.

58. Ammouri W, Cuisset L, Rouaghe S, et al. Diagnostic value of serum immunoglobulinaemia D level in patients with a clinical suspicion of hyper IgD

syndrome. Rheumatology (Oxford) 2007;46(10): 1597–600.

59. Demirkaya E, Caglar MK, Waterham HR, et al. A patient with hyper-IgD syndrome responding to anti-TNF treatment. Clin Rheumatol 2007;26(10): 1757–9.

60. Topaloglu R, Ayaz NA, Waterham HR, et al. Hyperimmunoglobulinemia D and periodic fever syndrome; treatment with etanercept and follow-up. Clin Rheumatol 2008;27(10):1317–20.

61. Bodar EJ, van der Hilst JC, Drenth JP, et al. Effect of etanercept and anakinra on inflammatory attacks in the hyper-IgD syndrome: introducing a vaccination provocation model. Neth J Med 2005;63(7): 260–4.

62. McDermott MF, Aksentijevich I, Galon J, et al. Germline mutations in the extracellular domains of the 55 kDa TNF receptor, TNFR1, define a family of dominantly inherited autoinflammatory syndromes. Cell 1999;97(1):133–44.

63. Williamson LM, Hull D, Mehta R, et al. Familial Hibernian fever. QJM 1982;51(204):469–80.

64. Kimberley FC, Lobito AA, Siegel RM. Falling into TRAPS-receptor misfolding in the TNF receptor 1-associated periodic fever syndrome. Arthritis Res Ther 2007;9(4):217.

65. Galeazzi M, Gasbarrini G, Ghirardello A, et al. Autoinflammatory syndromes. Clin Exp Rheumatol 2006;24(1 Suppl 40):S79–80.

66. Cantarini L, Lucherini OM, Muscari I, et al. Tumour necrosis factor receptor-associated periodic syndrome (TRAPS): state of the art and future perspectives. Autoimmun Rev 2012;12(1):38–43.

67. Simon A, Park H, Maddipati R, et al. Concerted action of wild-type and mutant TNF receptors enhances inflammation in TNF receptor 1-associated periodic fever syndrome. Proc Natl Acad Sci U S A 2010;107(21):9801–6.

68. Ravet N, Rouaghe S, Dode C, et al. Clinical significance of P46L and R92Q substitutions in the tumour necrosis factor superfamily 1A gene. Ann Rheum Dis 2006;65(9):1158–62.

69. Stojanov S, Dejaco C, Lohse P, et al. Clinical and functional characterisation of a novel TNFRSF1A c.605T>A/V173D cleavage site mutation associated with tumour necrosis factor receptor-associated periodic fever syndrome (TRAPS), cardiovascular complications and excellent response to etanercept treatment. Ann Rheum Dis 2007;67(9):1292–8.

70. Bulua AC, Mogul DB, Aksentijevich I, et al. Efficacy of etanercept in the tumor necrosis factor receptor-associated periodic syndrome: a prospective, open-label, dose-escalation study. Arthritis Rheum 2012;64(3):908–13.

71. Feldmann J, Prieur AM, Quartier P, et al. Chronic infantile neurological cutaneous and articular syndrome is caused by mutations in CIAS1, a

gene highly expressed in polymorphonuclear cells and chondrocytes. Am J Hum Genet 2002;71(1):198–203.

72. Hoffman HM, Mueller JL, Broide DH, et al. Mutation of a new gene encoding a putative pyrin-like protein causes familial cold autoinflammatory syndrome and Muckle-Wells syndrome. Nat Genet 2001;29(3):301–5.

73. Leslie KS, Lachmann HJ, Bruning E, et al. Phenotype, genotype, and sustained response to anakinra in 22 patients with autoinflammatory disease associated with CIAS-1/NALP3 mutations. Arch Dermatol 2006;142(12):1591.

74. Yu JR, Leslie KS. Cryopyrin-associated periodic syndrome: an update on diagnosis and treatment response. Curr Allergy Asthma Rep 2010;11(1): 12–20.

75. Shinkai K, McCalmont TH, Leslie KS. Cryopyrin-associated periodic syndromes and autoinflammation. Clin Exp Dermatol 2008;33(1):1–9, 071010075526003–???

76. Cuisset L, Jeru I, Dumont B, et al. Mutations in the autoinflammatory cryopyrin-associated periodic syndrome gene: epidemiological study and lessons from eight years of genetic analysis in France. Ann Rheum Dis 2011;70(3):495–9.

77. Hawkins PN, Lachmann HJ, Aganna E, et al. Spectrum of clinical features in Muckle-Wells syndrome and response to anakinra. Arthritis Rheum 2004; 50(2):607–12.

78. Lachmann HJ, Koné-Paut I, Kuemmerle-Deschner JB, et al. Use of canakinumab in the cryopyrin-associated periodic syndrome. N Engl J Med 2009;360(23):2416–25.

79. Hoffman HM, Throne ML, Amar NJ, et al. Efficacy and safety of rilonacept (interleukin-1 trap) in patients with cryopyrin-associated periodic syndromes: results from two sequential placebo-controlled studies. Arthritis Rheum 2008;58(8): 2443–52.

80. Borghini S, Tassi S, Chiesa S, et al. Clinical presentation and pathogenesis of cold-induced autoinflammatory disease in a family with recurrence of an NLRP12 mutation. Arthritis Rheum 2011;63(3): 830–9.

81. Marrakchi S, Guigue P, Renshaw BR, et al. Interleukin-36-receptor antagonist deficiency and generalized pustular psoriasis. N Engl J Med 2011; 365(7):620–8.

82. Majeed HA, Kalaawi M, Mohanty D, et al. Congenital dyserythropoietic anemia and chronic recurrent multifocal osteomyelitis in three related children and the association with Sweet syndrome in two siblings. J Pediatr 1989;115(5 Pt 1): 730–4.

83. Ferguson PJ. Homozygous mutations in LPIN2 are responsible for the syndrome of chronic recurrent multifocal osteomyelitis and congenital dyserythropoietic anaemia (Majeed syndrome). J Med Genet 2005;42(7):551–7.

84. Herlin T, Fiirgaard B, Bjerre M, et al. Efficacy of anti-IL-1 treatment in Majeed syndrome. Ann Rheum Dis 2012;72(3):410–3.

85. Liu Y, Ramot Y, Torrelo A, et al. Mutations in proteasome subunit β type 8 cause chronic atypical neutrophilic dermatosis with lipodystrophy and elevated temperature with evidence of genetic and phenotypic heterogeneity. Arthritis Rheum 2012;64(3):895–907.

86. Torrelo A, Patel S, Colmenero I, et al. Chronic atypical neutrophilic dermatosis with lipodystrophy and elevated temperature (CANDLE) syndrome. J Am Acad Dermatol 2010;62(3):489–95.

87. Aksentijevich I, Masters SL, Ferguson PJ, et al. An autoinflammatory disease with deficiency of the interleukin-1–receptor antagonist. N Engl J Med 2009;360(23):2426–37.

88. Jesus AA, Osman M, Silva CA, et al. A novel mutation of IL1RN in the deficiency of interleukin-1 receptor antagonist syndrome: description of two unrelated cases from Brazil. Arthritis Rheum 2011;63(12):4007–17.

89. Altiok E, Aksoy F, Perk Y, et al. A novel mutation in the interleukin-1 receptor antagonist associated with intrauterine disease onset. Clin Immunol 2012;145(1):77–81.

90. Schnellbacher C, Ciocca G, Menendez R, et al. Deficiency of interleukin-1 receptor antagonist responsive to anakinra. Pediatr Dermatol 2012. http://dx.doi.org/10.1111/j.1525-1470.2012.01725.x.

91. Smith EJ, Allantaz F, Bennett L, et al. Clinical, molecular, and genetic characteristics of PAPA syndrome: a review. Curr Genomics 2010;11(7):519–27.

92. Demidowich AP, Freeman AF, Kuhns DB, et al. Brief report: genotype, phenotype, and clinical course in five patients with PAPA syndrome (pyogenic sterile arthritis, pyoderma gangrenosum, and acne). Arthritis Rheum 2012;64(6):2022–7.

93. Schellevis MA, Stoffels M, Hoppenreijs EP, et al. Variable expression and treatment of PAPA syndrome. Ann Rheum Dis 2011;70(6):1168–70.

94. Dierselhuis MP, Frenkel J, Wulffraat NM, et al. Anakinra for flares of pyogenic arthritis in PAPA syndrome. Rheumatology 2005;44(3):406–40.

95. Stichweh DS, Punaro M, Pascual V. Dramatic improvement of pyoderma gangrenosum with infliximab in a patient with PAPA syndrome. Pediatr Dermatol 2005;22(3):262–5.

96. Miceli-Richard C, Lesage S, Rybojad M, et al. CARD15 mutations in Blau syndrome. Nat Genet 2001;29(1):19–20.

97. Borzutzky A, Fried A, Chou J, et al. NOD2-associated diseases: bridging innate immunity and autoinflammation. Clin Immunol 2010;134(3):251–61.

98. Sfriso P, Caso F, Tognon S, et al. Blau syndrome, clinical and genetic aspects. Autoimmun Rev 2012;12(1):44–51.

99. Rose CD, Martin TM, Wouters CH. Blau syndrome revisited. Curr Opin Rheumatol 2011;23(5):411–8.

100. Rose CD, Arostegui JI, Martin TM, et al. NOD2-associated pediatric granulomatous arthritis, an expanding phenotype: study of an international registry and a national cohort in Spain. Arthritis Rheum 2009;60(6):1797–803.

Type 2 Diabetes Mellitus
A Metabolic Autoinflammatory Disease

Thomas Mandrup-Poulsen, MD, DMSc[a,b,*]

KEYWORDS

- Beta-cell • Cytokines • Interleukin-1 • Insulin resistance • Islets • Low-grade inflammation
- Macrophage • Pancreas

KEY POINTS

- Type 2 diabetes mellitus shares features with autoinflammatory disorders and is known for its recurrent inflammatory skin complications.
- Inhibitory treatments of aberrant inflammasome activation that dramatically cure the diverse rashes, erythemas, hives, pustoloses, and pyodermas of rare autoinflammatory disorders may have a place in the therapy for common disorders, such as type 2 diabetes mellitus, and thereby it is hoped also reduce its dermatologic complications.

THE SKIN AND THE PANCREATIC ISLETS AS AUTOINFLAMMATORY TARGETS: HOMAGE TO PAUL LANGERHANS

To the dermatologist the name of the German histopathologist Paul Langerhans (1847–1888) is as inseparably connected with the dendritic epidermal Langerhans cells as it is with the pancreatic islets of Langerhans to the diabetologist. Langerhans trained at the Friedrich Wilhelm Universität in Berlin with his main mentors Rudolf Virchow (1821–1902) and Julius Cohnheim (1839–1884). While applying the gold chloride staining developed by Julius Cohnheim to study cutaneous innervation in Virchow's laboratory at the Charité Institute of Pathology in Berlin, Langerhans discovered already as an undergraduate student in 1868 the dendritic cells in the epidermis, which he erroneously classified as neuronal cells because of their stellate appearance.[1] Only a year later in his doctorate thesis he described the pancreatic islets and suggested that they were small intrapancreatic lymph nodes.[2]

Tragically, at the age of 41 Paul Langerhans succumbed to the inflammatory consequences of disseminated tuberculosis that he contracted as a 27-year-old Chair of Pathology at the University of Freiburg. He died unknowingly of the functions of the cells that to date bear his name. It would no doubt have been gratifying to him to realize that the Langerhans cells of the skin belong to the innate immune system, and that the pancreatic islets of Langerhans constitute the endocrine pancreas. Most certainly he would have been amazed if he had lived to take part in the progress that in the last decade has united the two anatomically remote and apparently functionally disparate cell types he discovered: that both the Langerhans cell of the skin and the pancreatic β-cell of the islets of Langerhans strongly express the protein complex that is the subject of this special issue of *Dermatologic Clinics* and caused much of the symptomatology that haunted him the last 14 years of his life: the inflammasome.[3–5]

Conflicts of Interest: None.
[a] Department of Biomedical Sciences, Faculty of Health and Medical Sciences, University of Copenhagen, 3 Blegdamsvej, DK-2200 Copenhagen N, Denmark; [b] Department of Molecular Medicine and Surgery, Karolinska Institutet, Solna, SE-17176 Stockholm, Sweden
* Department of Biomedical Sciences, Faculty of Health and Medical Sciences, University of Copenhagen, 3 Blegdamsvej, DK-2200 Copenhagen N, Denmark.
E-mail address: tmpo@sund.ku.dk

Dermatol Clin 31 (2013) 495–506
http://dx.doi.org/10.1016/j.det.2013.04.006

THE PATHOGENESIS OF TYPE 2 DIABETES MELLITUS

Before reviewing the growing evidence that type 2 diabetes mellitus (T2D) has an autoinflammatory origin, the following list summarizes inflammation in its metabolic context.

- T2D is the metabolic consequence of failure of the insulin-producing pancreatic β-cell to compensate for increased insulin needs.
- Most commonly, insulin resistance caused by obesity is the reason for increased insulin needs; puberty, pregnancy, and certain drugs are additional causes.
- Sedentary lifestyle and inappropriate quality and quantity of foods mediate inflammatory and neurohumoral alterations in appetite regulation, thermogenesis, satiety, and food choices believed to instigate a vicious cycle that contribute to obesity.
- The accumulation of fats, particularly in visceral depots, alters adipocyte differentiation and size that leads to alterations in adipose tissue blood flow, hypoxia, and shear stress activating the transcription, translation, and processing of proinflammatory cytokines and adipokines.
- Adipocytokines elicit a systemic low-grade inflammatory response characterized by discretely elevated C-reactive protein (CRP) driven in particular by circulating interleukin (IL)-1 and IL-6.
- Intrahepatic fat deposition contributes to local inflammation that may progress into nonalcoholic steatohepatitis and potentiate the systemic inflammatory response.
- Circulating proinflammatory cytokines may amplify insulin resistance by interfering directly with the insulin signaling cascade in liver, skeletal muscle, fat, and pancreatic β-cells and stimulate proinflammatory gene transcription in these tissues and in the hypothalamus, further contributing to neurohumoral dysregulation of metabolism; however, clinical proof-of-principle is lacking.
- The increased insulin need caused by insulin resistance is initially compensated by expansion of the functional β-cell mass and secretory hyperactivity leading to hyperinsulinemia.
- Insulin is a potent macrophage chemoattractant and compensatory hypersecretion may be a primary cause for increased recruitment of islet macrophages.
- With insulin, islet amyloid polypeptide (IAPP) and extracellular danger-associated molecular patterns (DAMPs), such as ATP, are secreted. IAPP and ATP are believed to activate the intraislet macrophage and β-cell inflammasomes leading to local secretion of IL-1, known for long to signal β-cell apoptosis.
- Once β-cell functional mass starts to decline, insulin secretory decompensation follows, leading to impaired glucose and lipid homeostasis and eventually overt T2D.
- Elevated extracellular glucose and lipids (glucolipotoxicity) in turn enhance insulin resistance and β-cell dysfunction, believed in part to involve inflammatory pathways and inflammasome activation in insulin-responsive and insulin-secreting cells. This accelerating process leads to the progressive metabolic deterioration of T2D.
- Blockade of IL-1 signaling improves glycemia and β-cell function, but not insulin resistance, in particular in patients genetically deficient in endogenous production of the naturally occurring IL-1 receptor antagonist. Thus, T2D shares properties with the genetic deficiency of IL-1Ra syndrome.
- T2D and Alzheimer's disease share genetic susceptibility genes, cooccur more frequently than expected, and in both diseases inflammasome activation by IAPP and β-amyloid has been implicated in β-cell and neuronal failure, respectively.

Thus, accumulating genetic, preclinical, and clinical evidence supports a primary role of inflammasome activation in T2D, justifying the inclusion of T2D to the group of autoinflammatory diseases. This appreciation may provide novel therapeutic options for the treatment of T2D.[6–9]

T2D AND THE DEFINITIONS OF AUTOINFLAMMATION

Autoinflammatory diseases are clinical disorders marked by abnormally increased sterile inflammation, mediated predominantly by the cells and molecules of the innate immune system, with a significant genetic or epigenetic host predisposition.[10]

With the recognition that T2D is characterized by sterile low-grade systemic inflammation, discrete but significant inflammatory cell infiltrates in fat, liver, and islets of Langerhans and in most organs affected by the late diabetic complications (ie, the vascular wall, the glomerulus, and the retina), a polygenetic predisposition, and significant and dynamic epigenetic changes, such as gene methylation/demethylation induced by inactivity, metabolic, and inflammatory factors, it is clear that T2D fulfills the definition of and should long have been recognized as an autoinflammatory disease. Reluctance to broadly accept this concept is probably more related to the nature of the definition than to professional conservatism; the current definition is, with purpose, indiscriminately inclusive to accommodate the many heterogeneous disorders that it attempts to cover.[10]

If the definition is narrowed to diseases associated with an aberrant activity of the inflammasome, the criteria become more stringent by focusing on the subset designated inflammasomopathies. Accordingly, the autoinflammatory diseases caused by mutations in the NLRP3 inflammasome are designated intrinsic and those caused by genetic variation in other activators or by aberrant activation of the inflammasome are named extrinsic inflammasomopathies.[10] Evidence to support the notion that T2D fulfills the requirements for a metabolically activated extrinsic inflammasomopathy is presented next.

THE ROLE OF THE INFLAMMASOME IN THE PATHOGENESIS OF T2D AND ITS COMPLICATIONS

The evidence of IL-1 as a type 2 diabetokine, listed in **Box 1**, suggests that IL-1 is the link between dysnutrition and obesity, obesity and insulin resistance, dysmetabolism and progressive β-cell failure, and dysmetabolism and late diabetic vascular complications.

The Inflammasome in Dysnutrition and Obesity

The laws of mass constancy and thermodynamics define that obesity arises from an imbalance between caloric intake and expenditure, but the pathophysiologic basis of this imbalance is debated. Hypothalamic neuron leptin and insulin resistance and dysnutrition-induced hypothalamic neuronal dysfunction by endoplasmic reticulum (ER) stress and the canonical inflammatory nuclear factor kappa B (NFκB) pathway have been implicated to disrupt the energy balance and lead to obesity in animal models.[11–13] Defective autophagic removal of dysfunctional mitochondria associated with increased formation of reactive oxygen species (ROS) contributes to the activation of the hypothalamic NFκB signaling pathway leading to obesity.[14] Of note, defective autophagy and ROS are activators of the inflammasome,[15] and the NLRP1 inflammasome is abundantly expressed in the brain in neurons and oligodendrocytes.[3] Because the inflammasome is activated by free fatty acids[16] it is

---

Box 1
Evidence for the pathogenetic role of IL-1 in T2D and its macrovascular complications

IL-1: a type 2 diabetokine

- Insulin-resistance and obesity
  - IL-1 is an adipokine
  - Regulates appetite and body weight homostasis
- Low-grade inflammation
  - Elevated circulating IL-1 levels in T2D
  - Drives IL-6, CRP, and IL-1Ra
  - Elevated IL-1 and IL-1 Ra predict development of T2D
- Diabetic macroangiopathy
  - Foam cell formation
  - Fibrous cap generation
- Progressive β-cell failure and destruction
  - Mediates glucose-induced human β-cell apoptosis
  - Expressed by β cells and islet macrophages in those with T2D
  - IL-1 Ra expression by β cells is reduced in those with T2D
  - Imbalance between IL-1 and IL-1Ra in the T2D islet

---

tempting to speculate that dysnutrition may instigate a vicious cycle of energy imbalance leading to obesity by hypothalamic inflammasome activation (**Fig. 1**). Formal experimental proof and direct evidence from human research of this hypothesis is lacking.

IL-1 in Obesity and Insulin Resistance

The concept of T2D as an inflammatory disorder long rested on epidemiologic associations between the disease and inflammatory biomarkers and on associations between the antidiabetic effects of drugs with anti-inflammatory properties as bonus to their specific actions, such as angiotensin-converting enzyme inhibitors, insulin sensitizers, or cholesterol-lowering statins.[6,17,18] The discovery of the expression of adipose tissue tumor necrosis factor (TNF)-α and the protective effects of TNF-α neutralization on glucose uptake in obese *fa/fa* rats[19] provided a mechanistic link in the inflammatory pathogenesis of insulin resistance.

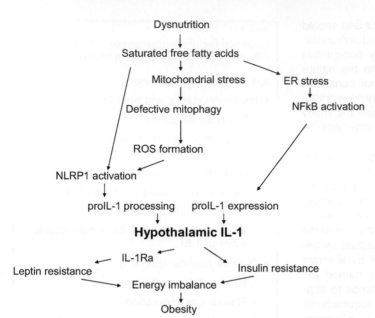

Dysnutrition
↓
Saturated free fatty acids
↓
Mitochondrial stress   ER stress
↓   ↓
Defective mitophagy   NFkB activation
↓
ROS formation
↓
NLRP1 activation
↓
proIL-1 processing   proIL-1 expression
↓   ↓
Hypothalamic IL-1

IL-1Ra
Leptin resistance   Insulin resistance
↓
Energy imbalance
↓
Obesity

Fig. 1. Model of IL-1 as link between dysnutrition, hypothalamic inflammation, and obesity. Inappropriate intake of saturated fats increase blood saturated free fatty acid levels, causing hypothalamic neuronal ER and mitochondrial stress, leading to NFkB activation and pro–IL-1 expression, and ROS generation and inflammasome activation, respectively. Hypothalamic IL-1 induces insulin resistance and by local induction of IL-1Ra leptin resistance that perturbs energy balance and satiety, instigating an obesogenic chain. NFkB, nuclear factor kappa B; ROS, reactive oxygen species.

The adipocyte as immunoendocrine cell

Evolutionarily, fat-storing cells have developed from the phagocytic monocyte lineage; macrophage precursors can develop into adipocytes and adipocytes can dedifferentiate into macrophages.[20] The adipocyte, traditionally viewed to have only a passive function as a fat depot, is now recognized to respond to the degree of fat storage by the synthesizing and releasing numerous humoral signals, including the growing list of adipocytokines. As the adipocyte differentiates and expands, adipocytokine gene expression is initiated by membrane stress or tissue hypoxia induced by compromised fat tissue microcirculation that is not compensated by angiogenesis.[21] Apart from secreting signals reflecting fat mass, such as leptin, a negative feedback regulator on appetite and caloric intake, the adipocyte secretes proinflammatory cytokines, such as IL-1, TNF, and IL-6, which interferes with insulin signaling in insulin-sensitive tissues (eg, by inducing the expression of suppressors of cytokine signaling, directly interfering with tyrosine kinase activity of the insulin receptor,[22] and by mediating the ubiquitination and proteasomal breakdown of the insulin receptor substrates IRS1/2).[23]

Furthermore, stressed adipocytes release factors that recruit monocytes, such as macrophage chemotactic protein 1; increase adipose tissue endothelial adhesion molecules; increase capillary permeability; and recruit inflammatory cells that build up as so-called crown-like structures around expanded adipocytes.

These cells phagocytose necrotic adipocytes and are further activated to produce inflammatory cytokines and chemokines, leading to adipositis constituted by cells of the innate and adaptive immune systems.[21]

The adipocyte inflammasome

The inflammasome is expressed by adipocytes and apart from processing pro–IL-1β is an important regulator of adipocyte differentiation, insulin sensitivity, and metabolism by mechanisms that are incompletely understood. NLRP3 or caspase 1 deletion reduces diet-induced obesity[24]; caspase 1 inhibitors, or genetic deletion, improve insulin sensitivity[25]; in obese mice NLRP3 deficiency reduces IL-18 and interferon-γ expression and effector T-cell numbers, and increases naive T-cell numbers in adipose tissue[26]; in obese humans with T2D, weight loss–induced improved insulin sensitivity is associated with reduced NLRP3 expression and adipositis[26]; free fatty acids activate the inflammasome in adipose tissue macrophages[16] probably by increasing intracellular ceramide,[26] but the precise molecular mechanisms are unclear; mitoNEET, an iron-containing mitochondrial outer membrane protein that enhances lipid uptake and storage and yet preserves insulin sensitivity in adiposity, was described to inhibit iron transport into the mitochondrial matrix, electron transport, β-oxidation, and thereby ROS production[27,28]; and reduced mitoNEET expression or deficient function may contribute to adipocyte inflammasome activation. Interestingly, mitoNEET expression is upregulated by catecholamines and downregulated by the antidiabetic drug glibenclamide, and binds the thiazolidinedione-class of insulin sensitizers.

Taken together this evidence suggests that the adipocyte inflammasome may have a primary role upstream to its metabolic activation and an amplifying action once circulating metabolite levels are elevated and cause secondary inflammasome activation (**Fig. 2**).

Counteracting effects of IL-18 and IL-33

Inflammasome processing by caspase-1 cleaves and activates pro–IL-18 and pro–IL-1β, but inactivates pro–IL-33, which is active in its full-length form, or even more so after cleavage by the neutrophil serine proteases cathepsin G and elastase. Circulating levels of IL-18 are reduced after weight loss[29] in accordance with the reduced adipose tissue NLRP3 expression.[26] Surprisingly, mice deficient for IL-18 or the IL-18 receptor and mice overexpressing the neutralizing IL-18 binding protein displayed hyperphagia, obesity, and insulin resistance associated with defective phosphorylation of STAT3 enhancing expression of genes associated with hepatic gluconeogenesis.[30] Intracerebral administration of IL-18 inhibited food intake and reversed hyperglycemia in IL-18 null mice through activation of STAT3 phosphorylation.[30]

IL-33 and its receptor are expressed in adipocytes[31,32] and expression is increased in severe obesity, in particular in adipose tissue endothelium.[33] IL-33 reduced genetic adiposity, fasting glucose, and glucose and insulin intolerance in ob/ob mice, associated with adipose tissue Th2

cell accumulation and M2 polarization of adipose tissue macrophages that are known to protect against obesity-related dysmetabolism. High fat diet fed mice lacking the IL-33 receptor exhibited higher body weight and fat mass and impaired insulin secretion and glucose homeostasis than their wild-type counterparts.[31] It may be anticipated that the beneficial metabolic effects of reducing IL-1 and IL-33 processing by therapeutic targeting of the inflammasome could in part be counteracted by reduced processing of IL-18; there is currently no experimental evidence to support this concern.

Clinical studies

Despite promising preclinical evidence in favor of an inflammatory pathogenesis of insulin resistance, clinical trials of specific biologics targeting TNF-α, IL-1, and IL-6 in subjects who are insulin-resistant nondiabetic, or who have T2D have generally been disappointing. There are several nonrandomized, open reports of improved insulin sensitivity in patients treated with TNF blockers for rheumatologic diseases,[34–36] whereas randomized open or placebo-controlled studies in healthy lean or obese or in subjects with T2D have largely been negative,[37–41] possibly by type II error caused by small sample sizes and low statistical power. Alternatively, in insulin-resistant humans TNF-α could be a biomarker of another inflammatory signal (eg, IL-1), causally related to insulin resistance and, at the same time, inducing TNF-α as an epiphenomenon. IL-1 does indeed induce adipocyte and hepatocyte insulin resistance in vitro by direct interference at multiple

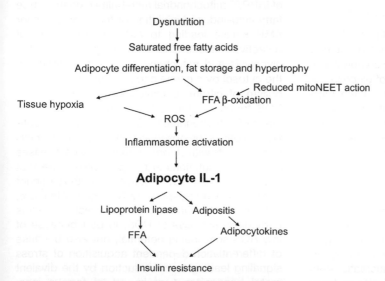

Fig. 2. Proposed role of inflammasome activation and IL-1 in the links between dysnutrition, adiposity, and insulin resistance. Inappropriate intake of saturated fats increases blood saturated free fatty acid levels that are stored in differentiating hypertrophic adipocytes. Adipocyte growth and inadequate compensatory angiogenesis lead to adipose tissue hypoxia. Reduced mitoNEET protein activity increases free fatty acid β oxidation leading to ROS formation, adipocyte inflammasome activation, pro–IL-1β processing, and IL-1β cellular export. IL-1 causes activation of adipocyte lipoprotein lipase liberating free fatty acids that contribute to insulin resistance by lipotoxicity. IL-1 attracts and activates monocyte-derived macrophages and T cells and perturbs Treg function, leading to accelerating adiposity and adipocytokine production causing low-grade systemic inflammation and aggravating insulin resistance. FFA, free fatty acid.

levels in the insulin-signaling cascade.[42–44] In T2D animal models IL-1 antagonism improves insulin resistance,[45] but in analogy to TNF-α antagonism, blocking IL-1 signaling in patients who are obese, insulin-resistant, nondiabetic, or who have T2D has failed to consistently improve insulin sensitivity.[46–50]

Expression and activation of the inflammasome seems to be an early and primary event in adipocyte differentiation, obesity, and insulin resistance, which introduces the difficulty that insulin-sensitizing therapies targeting the inflammasome or its products may have to be instituted very early in individuals at risk for the development of obesity and insulin resistance. It is possible that adipocyte hypertrophic stress and necrosis provokes the release of extracellular danger-associated molecular patterns that activate adipocyte inflammasome-dependent processing of IL-1β, which in turn stimulates lipoprotein lipase to liberate free fatty acids to induce insulin resistance by lipotoxicity.[9] Once insulin resistance is established, elevated circulating IL-1β may contribute to systemic inflammation; however, because systemic inflammatory markers, such as IL-6 or CRP, do not correlate with improved glycemia and β-cell function that follow IL-1 antagonism in T2D,[46,47] local rather than systemic inflammation may be more important for the inflammatory pathogenesis of T2D. This may explain the failure of blocking IL-1 (or other inflammatory cytokines) on overt insulin resistance in human studies, and also pertain to the role of inflammasome activation in the pancreatic islet, as reviewed in the next section.

IL-1, Dysmetabolism, and β-cell Failure

A unifying hypothesis implicating glucolipotoxicity as a common denominator of insulin resistance, β-cell dysfunction, and late diabetic complications suggested that chronic elevations of glucose and free fatty acids cause substrate-mediated mitochondrial ROS generation, activate the NFκB, p38, and JNK stress signaling pathways, eventually triggering the polyol-sorbitol, advanced glycation endproduct receptor and diacyl-glycerol/protein kinase C pathways in insulin-sensitive tissues, and causing cytokine and prostanoid production in pancreatic islets.[51]

In search for the inflammatory effector mechanisms mediating glucose-induced β-cell dysfunction and apoptosis, Donath and colleagues[52] discovered that high glucose induces Fas expression otherwise not detectable in pancreatic islets, raising the intriguing possibility of cis- or trans-ligation of this proapoptotic receptor by the Fas ligand, constitutively expressed on β-cells.

Because IL-1 was known to be a potent inducer of Fas in β cells,[53] these investigators next asked if IL-1Ra abrogated high glucose induced Fas expression and apoptosis in human islet cells and found that this was indeed the case. The following logical question was: what is the source of IL-1 in the T2 diabetic islet? High glucose induced release of mature IL-1β from human islets and IL-1β mRNA and protein expression in β cells, providing the first indirect demonstration of the presence of the inflammasome in the pancreatic islet. Subsequently, increased numbers of intraislet macrophages in animals and patients with T2D were described, providing an additional (and perhaps dominating) source of IL-1 in the endocrine pancreas.[54] These findings were confirmed and extended by the finding that high glucose activates the β cell NLRP3 inflammasome.[4] Later, other activators typical of the T2D state of the islet macrophage inflammasome (eg, IAPP and unsaturated free fatty acids) have been described,[55,56] as well as unfolded protein response-independent ER stress (**Fig. 3A**).[57–59]

Mechanisms of activation of the islet inflammasome

The precise molecular links between these stimuli and inflammasome activation are elusive and debated, as is the mechanism of inflammasome activation in general. TXNIP dissociated from TXN has been implicated as the ligand sensed by the leucine-rich repeat of the NLRP3 inflammasome. TXNIP dissociation from TXN is promoted by ROS,[4] which may be derived from several sources: cytosolic ROS induced by frustrated phagocytosis of IAPP,[55] mitochondrial metabolite oxidation, free fatty acid–induced inhibition of the energy sensor AMP kinase leading to reduced autophagy of defective mitochondria (mitophagy),[60] or aerobic glycolysis and mitochondrial export of citrate to the cytosol by a citrate carrier, allowing the metabolism of citrate to oxaloacetate with resulting ROS formation (**Fig. 3B**).[60,61] Against an importance of mitochondrial ROS in inflammasome activation speaks the observation that monocytic cells from patients with chronic granulomatous diseases caused by mutations in the p47-phox gene that have defective NADPH activity and thus cannot generate NADPH-dependent ROS generate more, not less, IL-1β. Of note, the pancreatic β cell is particularly sensitive to ROS, in part because of low ROS scavenging potential, but also because of differentiation-dependent acquisition of stress signaling leading to the induction by the divalent metal transporter 1 of import of ferrous ions, key catalysts of ROS formation.[62] In addition, purinergic P_2X_7 receptor activation by DAMPs as

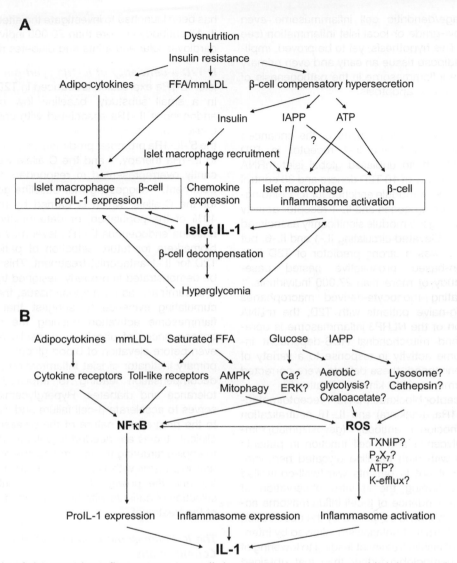

Fig. 3. Role of the intraislet inflammasome in β-cell decompensation. A suggested link between insulin resistance, β-cell failure, and diabetes. (A) Possible mechanisms of insulin resistance-mediated islet IL-1 expression and processing by islet inflammasome activation. β-Cell hypersecretion as a compensatory response to insulin resistance and increased insulin demands causes hyperinsulinemia-mediated macrophage chemoattraction and is associated with liberation of DAMPs, such as ATP, or islet amyloid polypeptide both cosecreted with insulin. These signals activate the inflammasome in islet macrophages/dendritic cells. Insulin resistance induced adipocytokines and elevated free fatty acids/minimally modified/oxidized low-density lipoprotein induce pro–IL-1β transcription in islet macrophages. Together these events lead to liberation of IL-1 that attracts monocyte-derived macrophages either directly or by induction of β-cell chemokine expression. This initiates a vicious cycle of low-grade islet inflammation and IL-1 secretion that contributes to progressive β-cell functional inhibition and apoptosis, causing β-cell decompensation and diabetes. (B) Suggested molecular pathways behind metabolic activation of pro–IL-1β gene expression and inflammasome activation. AMPK, adenosine monophosphate kinase; Ca, calcium; ERK, extracellular signal regulated kinase 1/2; K, potassium; MmLDL, minimally modified/oxidized low-density lipoprotein; P_2X_7, P2X purino receptor subtype 7; TXNIP, thioredoxin inhibitory protein.

potassium efflux or ATP release may synergize with the ROS-dependent pathway to activate the inflammasome.

Elevated free fatty acids and minimally oxidized low-density lipoprotein in insulin resistance may

deliver signal I to induce the expression of pro–IL-1 (see **Fig. 3**). Because ATP is cosecreted with insulin as is IAPP insulin hypersecretion to compensate for insulin resistance may deliver DAMPs as signal II to activate the β cell or resident islet macrophage/dendritic cell inflammasome even prior to low-grade or local islet inflammation (see **Fig. 3**).[63] This hypothesis, yet to be proved, implicates in adipose tissue an early and even primary role of the inflammasome in the pathogenesis of β-cell failure and apoptosis.

Clinical studies

There are now several reports of the enhanced expression of IL-1 and IL-1 receptor in T2D islets.[52,64–66] In an unbiased global islet mRNA expression study of 10 T2D donors and 38 control subjects, a gene module enriched for IL-1 binding-protein encoding genes and IL-1 receptor activity was the only gene module significantly associated with T2D.[66] Elevated circulating IL-1 and IL-6, but not TNF-α, was a strong predictor of T2D in a population-based prospective nested case-control study of more than 27,000 individuals.[67] In circulating monocyte-derived macrophages from drug-naive patients with T2D, the mRNA expression of the NLRP3 inflammasome is upregulated and mitochondrial ROS-dependent inflammasome activity in response to a variety of DAMPs enhanced; these defects were corrected by metformin by AMP kinase activation.[68]

IL-1 receptor blockade with IL-1 receptor antagonist (IL-1Ra, anakinra) and IL-1β neutralization with monoclonal antibody (gevokizumab) improved glycemia and β-cell function in patients with T2D with high baseline glycated hemoglobin,[46–48] but not in patients with well-controlled T2D,[50] confirming the in vitro observation of glucose-dependence of β-cell inflammasome activity.[4] This notion is supported by the observation that short-term IL-1 antagonism followed by intensification of insulin treatment leading to lowering of glycated hemoglobin further than that obtained with IL-1 blockade alone led to lasting reduction in CRP, IL-6, and β-cell function 39 weeks after the IL-1Ra therapy was withdrawn.[47] Notably, blinding was maintained during this follow-up phase of the study. Responders to IL-1Ra obtained the same reduction in glycemia at one-third of the insulin dose of the placebo-treated patients.[47]

Based on these collective data, it is tempting to speculate that breaking the vicious cycle of islet inflammation with IL-1 blockade may provide an intermittent remission induction therapy in T2D, allowing long-term stabilization of the metabolic state by conventional antidiabetic maintenance therapy until a hyperglycemic flare is encountered as a consequence of progressively reduced insulin sensitivity.

Large phase III studies confirming the findings in the phase I and IIa trials in patients with dysregulated T2D are needed. The so-called CANTOS trial has been launched to investigate the effect of anti–IL-1β antibody in more than 70,000 individuals on cardiovascular endpoints and diabetes risk.

Is T2D a deficiency of IL-1Ra syndrome?

Islet IL-1Ra expression is reduced in T2D islets.[69] In a small substudy, baseline low circulating endogenous IL-1Ra associated with carrying the C-allele of a single-nucleotide polymorphism in the 5′-IL-1Ra promoter predicted clinical response to IL-1Ra therapy,[46] and the C-allele was significantly overrepresented in responders to IL-1Ra treatment,[47] suggesting that baseline genotyping for the C-allele, which is carried by more than 40% of the population, or determination of the baseline endogenous IL-1Ra level may be useful biomarkers for future selection of patients with T2D for IL-1 antagonist treatment. This needs to be demonstrated in properly designed trials.

In summary, as for adipose tissue, there is accumulating evidence to suggest that islet inflammasome activation ensuing the metabolic consequences of obesity and insulin resistance even before elevation of blood glucose may be a primary instigator of islet inflammation and β-cell decompensation leading to impaired glucose tolerance and diabetes. Hyperglycemia in turn serves to accelerate β-cell failure and contributes to the progressive nature of the disease. Further clinical studies are needed to validate the use of therapies targeting the inflammasome or its products in patients with T2D with poor metabolic control and the power of biomarkers suitable for selection of patients with high likelihood of benefit of the treatment.

The Inflammasome in Late Diabetic Complications

Accelerated atherosclerosis in T2D is proposed to be mediated by inflammasome activation potentiated by the dysmetabolic state.[70] Cholesterol crystals and minimally oxidized LDL are potent activators of the NLRP3 inflammasome, and inflammasome activity is required for atherogenesis in some[71] but not all[72] animal models. IL-1Ra haploinsufficiency aggravates atherosclerosis in the ApoE null model.[73] A variable number of tandem repeats variation in the IL-1Ra gene, a two 86-bp-repeat in second intron termed A1 or the IL1RN*2 allele, increased risk of coronary artery disease in T2D but not in nondiabetics,[74] again emphasizing the importance of the IL-1/IL-1Ra balance for disease in patients with T2D with a metabolic drive on inflammasome activity. Whether IL-1 blockade is effective in reducing cardiovascular disease risk in T2D will be determined in the CANTOS trial.

The inflammasome seems to be implicated in diabetic microvascular complications. Caspase-1 inhibition or IL-1β blockade prevents diabetic degeneration of retinal capillaries,[75] and inflammasome activation involves a glucose-induced P1 and P2 purinergic receptor and cAMP signaling cascade.[76] Amyloid polypeptide is deposited in the diabetic glomerulosclerotic process,[77] and glomerular IL-1α secretion may contribute to inflammation in diabetic nephropathy.[78] Although NLRP3 inflammasome activation has been described in chronic nondiabetic kidney disease[79] this remains to be shown in diabetic glomerulosclerosis.

The inflammasome, T2D, and Alzheimer's disease

T2D and Alzheimer's disease are known comorbidities in aging populations.[80,81] Alzheimer's disease is caused by the formation of β-amyloid oligomers derived from a skew of the nonamyloidogenic α/γ-secretase cleavage of the transmembranous amyloid precursor protein toward the β/γ-secretase cleavage process leading to the liberation of β-amyloid peptide, which is now recognized to activate the inflammasome in microglia and astrocytes,[82] leading to IL-1 release and inflammatory and oxidative injury to neurons.[83] Insulin receptor signaling mediates amyloid polypeptide processing and β-amyloid accumulation.[84] Furthermore, the IL-1 RN*2 allele associated with the treatment response of T2D to IL-1 receptor blockade[47] is also associated with dementia severity of sporadic Alzheimer's disease.[85]

Taken together this evidence suggests that amyloid- and metabolite-stimulated inflammasome activation and imbalance between IL-1 agonism and antagonism is a common denominator of T2D and Alzheimer's disease and that therapies targeting the inflammasome or IL-1β may reduce this serious comorbidity in T2D.

SUMMARY

The past decade has offered amazing progress in the understanding of how low-grade inflammatory and oxidative stress pathways contribute to perturbed energy homeostasis and appetite regulation to aggravate sedentary lifestyle and overnutrition-mediated imbalance between caloric expenditure and intake of in particular energy-dense nutrients, such as saturated fats and alcohol. The conception of adipose tissue has developed from it being a passive fat depot to a highly complex immunoendocrine organ. Very recent discoveries suggest that inflammasome activation is an early and primary event, occurring even before and conditioning low-grade inflammation in adipose tissue and the endocrine pancreas. It should be noted that much of this evidence stems from in vitro and animal models, and that the relevance of these models is still unclear for human pathophysiology. Clinical proof-of-concept has been provided by trials either blocking IL-1 receptor signaling or neutralizing IL-1β, but interventional evidence supporting the causative role of inflammasome activation in the central and peripheral chain of events that lead to T2D is still lacking.

Many open basic and clinical questions need to be answered before rational therapies targeting these pathways can be developed and their potential fully exploited: What are the most important inflammasome subtypes in the relevant target tissues in obesity and T2D and how are they regulated? What are the precise mechanisms leading to inflammasome activation? What are the ligands sensed by the leucine-rich repeat? Are the stimuli discrete or overlapping between adipocytes, neurons, islet β cells and innate immune cells; if so why and what are pathologic consequences? How is IL-1 exported out of the producing cells, and how is this process regulated relative to inflammasome activity? What is the relative importance of the adipocyte, and the adipose tissue macrophages/dendritic cells, or of the islet endocrine and nonendocrine immune subtypes as sources of IL-1? How does the interplay between innate and adaptive immune cells in adipose tissue function and what are the consequences? Do IL-18 and IL-33 serve antagonizing functions to IL-1 and if so how can inflammasome processing of these cytokines be promoted at the expense of IL-1 processing? When should therapy targeting the production of IL-1 be initiated to be effective and safe; as early as in individuals at risk of adiposity, or in obese glucose-tolerant subjects; in patients with glucose intolerance or in patients with overt diabetes or high cardiovascular risk? Does such therapy depend on ambient glycemia or other dysmetabolic factors? What are the biomarkers useful for patient selection and surrogate end points for coming trials of anti–IL-1 therapies? These and many other gaps in knowledge should keep the scientific community interested in this important research area busy in years to come before the clinical potential of drugs targeting the inflammasome or its products in common metabolic disorders, such as T2D, is known.

REFERENCES

1. Langerhans P. Ueber die nerven der menschlichen haut. Virchows Arch Path Anat Physiol 1868;44: 325–37 [in German].

2. Langerhans P. Beitrage zur mikroscopischen anatomie der bauchspeichel druse. Inaugural-dissertation. Berlin: Gustav Lange; 1869.

3. Kummer JA, Broekhuizen R, Everett H, et al. Inflammasome components NALP 1 and 3 show distinct but separate expression profiles in human tissues suggesting a site-specific role in the inflammatory response. J Histochem Cytochem 2007;55:443–52.

4. Zhou R, Tardivel A, Thorens B, et al. Thioredoxin-interacting protein links oxidative stress to inflammasome activation. Nat Immunol 2010;11:136–40.

5. Mishra BB, Rathinam VA, Martens GW, et al. Nitric oxide controls the immunopathology of tuberculosis by inhibiting NLRP3 inflammasome-dependent processing of IL-1β. Nat Immunol 2013;14:52–60.

6. Kolb H, Mandrup-Poulsen T. An immune origin of type 2 diabetes? Diabetologia 2005;48:1038–50.

7. Kolb H, Mandrup-Poulsen T. The global diabetes epidemic as a consequence of lifestyle-induced low-grade inflammation. Diabetologia 2010;53:10–20.

8. Donath MY, Shoelson SE. Type 2 diabetes as an inflammatory disease. Nat Rev Immunol 2011;11:98–107.

9. Dinarello CA, Donath MY, Mandrup-Poulsen T. Role of IL-1β in type 2 diabetes. Curr Opin Endocrinol Diabetes Obes 2010;17:314–21.

10. Kastner DL, Aksentijevich I, Goldbach-Mansky R. Autoinflammatory disease reloaded: a clinical perspective. Cell 2010;140:784–90.

11. Meier CA, Bobbioni E, Gabay C, et al. IL-1 receptor antagonist serum levels are increased in human obesity: a possible link to the resistance to leptin? J Clin Endocrinol Metab 2002;87:1184–8.

12. Zhang X, Zhang G, Zhang H, et al. Hypothalamic IKKβ/NF-κB and ER stress link overnutrition to energy imbalance and obesity. Cell 2008;135:61–73.

13. Könner AC, Brüning JC. Selective insulin and leptin resistance in metabolic disorders. Cell Metab 2012;16:144–52.

14. Meng Q, Cai D. Defective hypothalamic autophagy directs the central pathogenesis of obesity via the IκB kinase β (IKKβ)/NF-κB pathway. J Biol Chem 2011;286:32324–32.

15. Salminen A, Kaarniranta K, Kauppinen A. Inflammaging: disturbed interplay between autophagy and inflammasomes. Aging 2012;4:166–75.

16. Wen H, Gris D, Lei Y, et al. Fatty acid-induced NLRP3-ASC inflammasome activation interferes with insulin signaling. Nat Immunol 2011;12:408–15.

17. Pickup J, Crook M. Is type II diabetes mellitus a disease of the innate immune system? Diabetologia 1998;41:1241–8.

18. Pickup JC. Inflammation and activated innate immunity in the pathogenesis of type 2 diabetes. Diabetes Care 2004;27:813–23.

19. Hotamisligil GS, Shargill NS, Spiegelman BM. Adipose expression of tumor necrosis factor-alpha: direct role in obesity-linked insulin resistance. Science 1993;259:87–91.

20. Charrière G, Cousin B, Arnaud E, et al. Preadipocyte conversion to macrophage. Evidence of plasticity. J Biol Chem 2003;278:9850–5.

21. Rutkowski JM, Davis KE, Scherer PE. Mechanisms of obesity and related pathologies: the macro- and microcirculation of adipose tissue. FEBS J 2009;276:5738–46.

22. Ueki K, Kondo T, Kahn CR. Suppressor of cytokine signaling 1 (SOCS-1) and SOCS-3 cause insulin resistance through inhibition of tyrosine phosphorylation of insulin receptor substrate proteins by discrete mechanisms. Mol Cell Biol 2004;24:5434–46.

23. Rui L, Yuan M, Frantz D, et al. SOCS-1 and SOCS-3 block insulin signaling by ubiquitin-mediated degradation of IRS1 and IRS2. J Biol Chem 2002;277:42394–8.

24. Stienstra R, van Diepend JA, Tack CJ, et al. Inflammasome is a central player in the induction of obesity and insulin resistance. Proc Natl Acad Sci U S A 2011;108:15324–9.

25. Stienstra R, Joosten LA, Koenen T, et al. The inflammasome-mediated caspase-1 activation controls adipocyte differentiation and insulin sensitivity. Cell Metab 2010;12:593–605.

26. Vandanmagsar B, Youm YH, Anthony Ravussin A, et al. The NLRP3 inflammasome instigates obesity-induced inflammation and insulin resistance. Nat Med 2011;17:179–88.

27. Kusminski CM, Holland WL, Sun K, et al. MitoNEET-driven alterations in adipocyte mitochondrial activity reveal a crucial adaptive process that preserves insulin sensitivity in obesity. Nat Med 2012;18:1539–49.

28. Sandra E, Wiley SE, Murphy AN, et al. MitoNEET is an iron-containing outer mitochondrial membrane protein that regulates oxidative capacity. Proc Natl Acad Sci U S A 2007;104:5318–23.

29. Esposito K, Pontillo A, Ciotola M, et al. Weight loss reduces interleukin-18 levels in obese women. J Clin Endocrinol Metab 2002;87:3864–6.

30. Netea MG, Joosten LA, Lewis E, et al. Deficiency of interleukin-18 in mice leads to hyperphagia, obesity and insulin resistance. Nat Med 2006;12:650–6.

31. Wood IS, Wang B, Trayhurn P. IL-33, a recently identified interleukin-1 gene family member, is expressed in human adipocytes. Biochem Biophys Res Commun 2009;384:105–9.

32. Miller AM, Asquith DL, Hueber AJ, et al. Interleukin-33 induces protective effects in adipose tissue inflammation during obesity in mice. Circ Res 2010;107:650–8.

33. Zeyda M, Wernly B, Demyanets S, et al. Severe obesity increases adipose tissue expression of interleukin-33 and its receptor ST2, both predominantly detectable in endothelial cells of human adipose tissue. Int J Obes 2012. http://dx.doi.org/10.1038/ijo.2012.118.

34. Gonzalez-Gay MA, De Matias JM, González-Juanatey C, et al. Anti-tumor necrosis factor-alpha blockade improves insulin resistance in patients with rheumatoid arthritis. Clin Exp Rheumatol 2006;24:83–6.

35. Kiortsis DN, Mavridis AK, Vasakos S, et al. Effects of infliximab treatment on insulin resistance in patients with rheumatoid arthritis and ankylosing spondylitis. Ann Rheum Dis 2005;64:765–6.

36. Stagakis I, Bertsias G, Karvounaris S, et al. Anti-tumor necrosis factor therapy improves insulin resistance, beta cell function and insulin signaling in active rheumatoid arthritis patients with high insulin resistance. Arthritis Res Ther 2012;14:R141.

37. Ofei F, Hurel S, Newkirk J, et al. Effects of an engineered human anti-TNFalpha antibody (CDP571) on insulin sensitivity and glycemic control in patients with NIDDM. Diabetes 1996;45:881–5.

38. Dominguez H, Storgaard H, Rask-Madsen C, et al. Metabolic and vascular effects of tumor necrosis factor-alpha blockade with etanercept in obese patients with type 2 diabetes. J Vasc Res 2005;42:517–25.

39. Paquot N, Castillo MJ, Lefèbvre PJ, et al. No increased insulin sensitivity after a single intravenous administration of a recombinant human tumor necrosis factor receptor: Fc fusion protein in obese insulin-resistant patients. J Clin Endocrinol Metab 2000;85:1316–9.

40. Bernstein LE, Berry J, Kim S, et al. Effects of etanercept in patients with the metabolic syndrome. Arch Intern Med 2006;166:902–8.

41. Wascher TC, Lindeman JH, Sourij H, et al. Chronic TNF-α neutralization does not improve insulin resistance or endothelial function in "healthy" men with metabolic syndrome. Mol Med 2011;17:189–93.

42. Lagathu C, Yvan-Charvet Y, Bastard JP, et al. Long-term treatment with interleukin-1β induces insulin resistance in murine and human adipocytes. Diabetologia 2006;49:2162–73.

43. Jager J, Grémeaux T, Cormont M, et al. Interleukin-1β-induced insulin resistance in adipocytes through down-regulation of insulin receptor substrate-1 expression. Endocrinology 2007;148:241–51.

44. Nov O, Kohl A, Lewis EC, et al. Interleukin-1beta may mediate insulin resistance in liver-derived cells in response to adipocyte inflammation. Endocrinology 2010;151:4247–56.

45. Ehses JA, Lacraz G, Giroix MH, et al. IL-1 antagonism reduces hyperglycemia and tissue inflammation in the type 2 diabetic GK rat. Proc Natl Acad Sci U S A 2009;106:13998–4003.

46. Larsen CM, Faulenbach M, Vaag A, et al. Interleukin-1 receptor antagonist in type 2 diabetes mellitus. N Engl J Med 2007;356:1517–26.

47. Larsen CM, Faulenbach M, Vaag A, et al. Sustained effect of interleukin-1-receptor antagonist treatment on beta-cell function in type 2 diabetes mellitus. Diabetes Care 2009;32:1663–8.

48. Cavelti-Weder C, Babiens-Brunner A, Keller C, et al. Effects of gevokizumab on glycemia and inflammatory markers in type 2 diabetes. Diabetes Care 2012;35:1654–62.

49. van Asseldonk EJ, Stienstra R, Koenen TB, et al. Treatment with anakinra improves disposition index but not insulin sensitivity in nondiabetic subjects with the metabolic syndrome: a randomized, double-blind, placebo-controlled study. J Clin Endocrinol Metab 2011;96:2119–26.

50. Ridker PM, Campbell P, Howard CP, et al. Effects of interleukin-1β inhibition with Canakinumab on hemoglobin A1c, lipids, C-reactive protein, interleukin-6, and fibrinogen. A phase IIb randomized, placebo-controlled trial. Circulation 2012;126:2739–48.

51. Evans JL, Goldfine ID, Maddux BA, et al. Are oxidative-stress activated signalling pathways mediators of insulin resistance and beta-cell dysfunction? Diabetes 2003;52:1–8.

52. Maedler K, Sergeev P, Ris F, et al. Glucose-induced beta cell production of IL-1beta contributes to glucotoxicity in human pancreatic islets. J Clin Invest 2002;110:851–60.

53. Yamada K, Takane-Gyotoku N, Yuan X, et al. Mouse islet cell lysis mediated by interleukin-1-induced Fas. Diabetologia 1996;39:1306–12.

54. Ehses JA, Perren A, Eppler E, et al. Increased number of islet-associated macrophages in type 2 diabetes. Diabetes 2007;56:2356–70.

55. Masters SL, Dunne A, Subramanian SL, et al. Activation of the NLRP3 inflammasome by islet amyloid polypeptide provides a mechanism for enhanced IL-1β in type 2 diabetes. Nat Immunol 2010;11:897–904.

56. Westwell-Roper C, Dai DL, Soukhatcheva G, et al. IL-1 blockade attenuates islet amyloid polypeptide-induced proinflammatory cytokine release and pancreatic islet graft dysfunction. J Immunol 2011;187:2755–65.

57. Menu P, Mayor A, Zhou R, et al. ER stress activates the NLRP3 inflammasome via an UPR-independent pathway. Cell Death Dis 2012;3:e261.

58. Lerner AG, Upton JP, Praveen PV, et al. IRE1α induces thioredoxin-interacting protein to activate the NLRP3 inflammasome and promote programmed cell death under irremediable ER stress. Cell Metab 2012;16:250–64.

59. Oslowski CM, Hara T, O'Sullivan-Murphy B, et al. Thioredoxin-interacting protein mediates ER stress-induced β cell death through initiation of the inflammasome. Cell Metab 2012;16:265–73.

60. Wen H, Ting JP, O'Neill LA. A role for the NLRP3 inflammasome in metabolic diseases—did Warburg miss inflammation? Nat Immunol 2012;13: 352–7.

61. Infantino V, Convertini P, Cucci L, et al. The mitochondrial citrate carrier: a new player in inflammation. Biochem J 2011;438:433–6.

62. Hansen JB, Tonnesen MF, Madsen AN, et al. Divalent metal transporter 1 regulates iron-mediated ROS and pancreatic beta-cell fate in response to cytokines. Cell Metab 2012;16:1–13.

63. Mandrup-Poulsen T. IAPP boosts islet macrophage IL-1 in type 2 diabetes. Nat Immunol 2010;11:881–3.

64. Böni-Schnetzler M, Thorne J, Parnaud G, et al. Increased interleukin (IL)-1β messenger ribonucleic acid expression in β-cells of individuals with type 2 diabetes and regulation of IL-1β in human islets by glucose and autostimulation. J Clin Endocrinol Metab 2008;93:4065–74.

65. Igoillo-Esteve M, Marselli L, Cunha DA, et al. Palmitate induces a pro-inflammatory response in human pancreatic islets that mimics CCL2 expression by beta cells in type 2 diabetes. Diabetologia 2010;53:1395–405.

66. Mahdi T, Hänzelmann S, Salehi A, et al. Secreted Frizzled-Related Protein 4 reduces insulin secretion and is overexpressed in type 2 diabetes. Cell Metab 2012;16:625–33.

67. Spranger J, Kroke A, Möhlig M, et al. Inflammatory cytokines and the risk to develop type 2 diabetes: results of the prospective population-based European Prospective Investigation into Cancer and Nutrition (EPIC)-Potsdam Study. Diabetes 2003;52:812–7.

68. Lee HM, Kim JJ, Kim HJ, et al. Upregulated NLRP3 inflammasome activation in patients with type 2 diabetes. Diabetes 2013;62:197–204.

69. Maedler K, Sergeev P, Jan A, et al. Leptin modulates β–cell expression of IL-1 receptor antagonist and release of IL-1β in human islets. Proc Natl Acad Sci U S A 2004;101:8138–43.

70. Masters SL, Latz E, O'Neill LA. The inflammasome in atherosclerosis and type 2 diabetes. Sci Transl Med 2011;3:81ps17.

71. Duewell P, Kono H, Rayner KJ, et al. NLRP3 inflammasomes are required for atherogenesis and activated by cholesterol crystals. Nature 2010;464: 1357–61.

72. Menu P, Pellegrin M, Aubert JF, et al. Atherosclerosis in ApoE-deficient mice progresses independently of the NLRP3 inflammasome. Cell Death Dis 2011;2:e137.

73. Isoda K, Sawada S, Ishigami N, et al. Lack of interleukin-1 receptor antagonist modulates plaque composition in apolipoprotein E–deficient mice. Arterioscler Thromb Vasc Biol 2004;24:1068–73.

74. Marculescu R, Endler G, Schillinger M, et al. Interleukin-1 receptor antagonist genotype is associated with coronary atherosclerosis in patients with type 2 diabetes. Diabetes 2002;51:3582–5.

75. Vincent JA, Mohr S. Inhibition of caspase-1/interleukin-1beta signaling prevents degeneration of retinal capillaries in diabetes and galactosemia. Diabetes 2007;56:224–30.

76. Trueblood KE, Mohr S, Dubyak GR. Purinergic regulation of high-glucose-induced caspase-1 activation in the rat retinal Müller cell line rMC-1. Am J Physiol Cell Physiol 2011;301:C1213–23.

77. Gong W, Liu ZH, Zeng CH, et al. Amylin deposition in the kidney of patients with diabetic nephropathy. Kidney Int 2007;72:213–8.

78. Vilaysane A, Chun J, Seamone ME, et al. The NLRP3 inflammasome promotes renal inflammation and contributes to CKD. J Am Soc Nephrol 2010; 21:1732–44.

79. Satirapoj B. Review on pathophysiology and treatment of diabetic kidney disease. J Med Assoc Thai 2010;93(Suppl 6):S228–41.

80. Peila R, Rodriguez BL, Launer LJ. Type 2 diabetes, APOE gene, and the risk for dementia and related pathologies. The Honolulu-Asia Aging Study. Diabetes 2002;51:1256–62.

81. Irie F, Fitzpatrick AL, Lopez OL, et al. Enhanced risk for Alzheimer disease in persons with type 2 diabetes and APOE ε4. The Cardiovascular Health Study Cognition Study. Arch Neurol 2008;65:89–93.

82. Halle A, Hornung V, Petzold GC, et al. The NALP3 inflammasome is involved in the innate immune response to amyloid-β. Nat Immunol 2008;9:857–65.

83. Heneka MT, O'Banion MK. Inflammatory processes in AD. J Neuroimmunol 2007;184:69–91.

84. Stöhr O, Schilbach K, Moll L, et al. Insulin receptor signaling mediates APP processing and β-amyloid accumulation without altering survival in a transgenic mouse model of Alzheimer's disease. Age 2011;35(1):83–101.

85. Bosco P, Guéant-Rodríguez RM, Anello G, et al. Association of IL-1 RN*2 allele and methionine synthase 2756 AA genotype with dementia severity of sporadic Alzheimer's disease. J Neurol Neurosurg Psychiatry 2004;75:1036–8.

Controlling Inflammation
Contemporary Treatments for Autoinflammatory Diseases and Syndromes

Gary Sterba, MD[a],*, Yonit Sterba, MD[b]

KEYWORDS

- Autoinflammation • Treatment • Anakinra

KEY POINTS

- The initial therapy for all of the autoinflammatory syndromes is the control of fever, pain, or the symptoms derived from the inflammatory reaction.
- The initial effort should focus on making the precise diagnosis. This strategy facilitates the choice of appropriate initial therapy, which has been defined for many of these syndromes and diseases.
- Accurate diagnosis is often difficult; rendering symptom management the mainstay of initial therapy while the definitive diagnosis remains elusive.
- Steroids are not considered useful in the autoinflammatory syndromes, yet they still play an important role in the early treatment of these diseases.
- Colchicine has been approved for the treatment of familial Mediterranean fever and its late complications.
- Antitumor necrosis factor therapy has been used and proved useful in several autoinflammatory diseases.
- The most recent acquisition for the treatment of autoinflammatory syndromes is anti-interleukin 1, anakinra, rilonacept, and canakinumab, with good results in many of the autoinflammatory syndromes.
- New molecules and pathways of disease will facilitate the development of effective therapies.

INTRODUCTION

The autoinflammatory disorders are an expanding group of diseases characterized by recurrent systemic inflammation in the absence of infection, autoantibodies, or antigen-specific T cells; they are thus probably related to a primary dysfunction of the innate immune system, with no adaptive immune deregulation. Dysfunction of the innate immune system includes abnormal responses to pathogens associated with the lipopolysaccharide and peptidoglycan of myeloid cells, such as neutrophils and monocytes in blood and tissues, in addition to the dysregulation of inflammatory cytokines and their receptors, like interleukin 1β (IL-1β), tumor necrosis factor α (TNF-α), and others[1]; thus, these substances and molecules have become the targets for present and future therapies.

The autoinflammatory diseases include hereditary disorders like: familial Mediterranean fever (FMF), mevalonate kinase (MK) deficiency, tumor necrosis factor receptor–associated periodic syndrome (TRAPS), cryopyrin-associated periodic syndrome (CAPS), familial cold autoinflammatory syndrome (FCAS), Muckle-Wells syndrome

Neither of the authors has any financial conflicts.
[a] Miami Medical Consult, 4950 South Le Jeune Road, Suite H, Coral Gables, FL 33146, USA; [b] Children's Hospital at Montefiore, 3415 Bainbridge Avenue, Bronx, NY 10467, USA
* Corresponding author.
E-mail address: gsterba@miamimedconsult.com

Dermatol Clin 31 (2013) 507–511
http://dx.doi.org/10.1016/j.det.2013.04.007

derm.theclinics.com

(MWS), chronic infantile neurologic, cutaneous, and articular (CINCA) syndrome, Blau syndrome, hyperimmunoglobulin D syndrome (HIDS), pyogenic sterile arthritis, pyoderma gangrenosum and acne (PAPA) syndrome, chronic recurrent multifocal osteomyelitis; some multifactorial disorders like Crohn and Behçet disease, juvenile idiopathic arthritis (JIA), adult Still disease, and macrophage activation syndrome (MAS) are considered autoinflammatory diseases; so are periodic fever, aphthous stomatitis, and adenopathy (PFAPA) syndrome and Majeed syndrome.

TREATMENT

The initial therapy for all the autoinflammatory syndromes is the control of fever, pain, or the symptoms derived from the inflammatory reaction. Antiinflammatory medications are the initial choice; nonsteroidal antiinflammatory drugs (NSAIDs) have been used with variable success for decades; so have systemic steroids.

The initial effort should focus on making the precise diagnosis. This goal facilitates the choice of appropriate initial therapy, which has been defined for many of these syndromes and diseases. Accurate diagnosis is often difficult, rendering symptom management the mainstay of initial therapy while the definitive diagnosis remains elusive.

Chronic management includes symptom management and prevention of complications of long-term disease and treatment, including amyloidosis and premature coronary artery disease (**Table 1**).

Nonspecific Medications

The initial drug management includes corticosteroids or nonsteroidal medications, as well as others with antiinflammatory effects, as follows.

Cimetidine

Cimetidine is a histamine 2 (H_2) receptor antagonist that inhibits stomach acid production. Used to treat and reduce the symptoms of gastritis and peptic ulcer disease, it has been shown debatably useful in the treatment of herpes simplex

1 and 2, herpes zoster virus, common warts, some inflammatory conditions associated with calcifications, and so forth. It has also been used to modify epidermal growth factor, vascular endothelial growth factor, and E-selectin, for the treatment of several cancers and their metastasis. Cimetidine was shown to be of some benefit in the pain of interstitial cystitis. Cimetidine has been used in PFAPA syndrome, with resolution of the fever and some of the other manifestations of the syndrome; at a dose of 20 mg/kg/d, cimetidine has a response greater than 50%; the mechanism of action is not known, but has been linked to inhibition of T-suppressor cells by blocking H_2-receptors, with minimal side effects.[2,3]

Statins

The involvement of MK in the cholesterol synthesis pathway encouraged the introduction of statins in the management of MK deficiency and HIDS; good results were obtained in a small group of patients.[4] MK plays an essential role in the cholesterol synthesis pathway; during cholesterol biosynthesis, 3-hydroxy-3-methylglutaryl-coenzyme A (HMG-CoA) reductase (the enzyme inhibited by statins) converts HMG-CoA to mevalonate. This conversion is blocked when a mutation in the MVK gene exists and mevalonate is not converted to mevalonate phosphate, causing an increase in mevalonic acid in serum, tissues, and urine. The absence of a negative feedback loop, naturally provided by the presence of the end products of synthesis, leads to increased HMG-CoA reductase activity, consequently increasing serum, tissue, and urine levels of mevalonic acid. The inhibition of MK also activates caspase 1 and decreases isoprenoids, which increase IL-1β. The blockade of these mediators may soon help to clarify the pathophysiology of these diseases.

NSAIDs

NSAIDs are nonselective inhibitors of cyclooxygenase, acting on both isoenzymes Cox1 and Cox2, causing a reversible inhibition, which is in contrast

---

Table 1
Overall summary of hereditary periodic fever syndromes

Feature	FMF	HIDS	TRAPS	MWS	FCU	CINCA
Treatment	Colchicine to prevent attacks and for long-term prevention of amyloidosis	Supportive NSAIDs, prednisone, simvastatin	NSAIDs and steroids, anti-TNF, anti-IL-1	NSAIDs and steroids, anti-IL1	Anti-IL-1	Anti-IL-1

Abbreviations: FCU, familial cold urticaria; HIDS, hyperimmunoglobulinemia D with periodic fever syndrome.

with that produced by aspirin, which is irreversible, with no formation of prostaglandins and thromboxane (mediators of inflammation). In crystal-induced arthritis, NSAIDs have been shown to inhibit urate crystal phagocytosis. The mechanism of action of NSAIDs is to block the formation of prostaglandin E_2, which regulates neurons within the hypothalamus responsible for the generation of temperature increase or fever.[5]

NSAIDS are used initially in the antiinflammatory syndromes to relieve constitutional symptoms or inflammatory signs like fever and arthritis, but in most instances, they are not the mainstay of therapy. Nonsteroidal and steroidal drugs have been used in Majeed syndrome for the control of symptoms, but the long-term management of the hematologic manifestations is accomplished by splenectomy and transfusions.[6]

Corticosteroids

Prednisone is a glucocorticoid converted in the liver to prednisolone, its active form. Isolated in 1950 and introduced for usage in 1955, it has been the mainstay of therapy for many autoimmune and inflammatory diseases in which steroids are helpful. Steroids are not considered useful in the autoinflammatory syndromes, yet they still play an important role in their early treatment.

Steroids are the main treatment option in acute attacks of HIDS. Patients with PFAPA syndrome are treated with prednisone for their fever. In some situations, PAPA syndrome responds well to oral glucocorticoids. Steroids are used in the febrile crisis of TRAPS, but their use in the chronic setting is best avoided. Low-dose steroids are recommended in JIA and in adult Still disease; prednisone 1 to 5 mg per day is used, although some patients may require 1 to 2 mg/kg/d, usually in divided doses.

In MAS, the usual starting dosage is pulse methylprednisolone at 30 mg/kg/d for 3 to 5 days or prednisone 1 to 2 mg/kg/d, usually in divided doses, 2 or 3 times a day.[7]

Colchicine

Historically, colchicine has been used for nearly all the rheumatic diseases. It was described for the treatment of rheumatism and swelling in the Egyptian Ebers Papyrus (ca 1500 BC). Extracted from the meadow saffron (*Colchicum autumnale*) in the early 1970s, colchicine was found useful in the acute management of FMF,[8] as well as in the prevention of its long-term complications like amyloidosis.[9] Colchicine was only approved by the US Food and Drug Administration (FDA) in August, 2009 for use in gout and FMF. The

mechanism of action of colchicine is believed to be inhibition of microtubule polymerization by tubulin binding, which blocks cell mitosis in neutrophils, and by antiinflammatory mechanisms involving altered expression of adhesion molecules and chemotactic factors, coming from the generation of reactive oxygen species occurring in crystal-induced arthritis.

Amyloidosis is a feared long-term complication of FMF; it results from accumulation of serum amyloid A (SAA) protein, deposited mainly in the kidney. A major manifestation of amyloidosis is renal injury, which may lead to proteinuria renal failure. Patients are normotensive, with no hematuria. Since the adoption of colchicine for FMF, the prevalence of amyloidosis among patients with FMF has decreased significantly. For adults, the dose of colchicine is 0.5 to 1 mg/d; for children, the starting dose should be 0.5 mg/d or less if younger than 5 years, 1 mg/d for children 5 to 10 years, and 1.5 mg/d for those older than 10 years; dosage can be increased in a stepwise fashion up to a maximum of 2 mg/d. A few patients do not respond to colchicine, usually because of poor treatment adherence; at the suggested dosage, it is a safe drug; side effects, including gastrointestinal, hematologic, and neuromuscular symptoms, are rare.

Bisphosphonates

These medications are being used and positive outcomes obtained with pamidronate and zolendronic acid in the treatment of SAPHO (synovitis, acne, palmoplantar pustulosis, hyperostosis, and osteitis) syndrome,[10,11] via their antiosteoclastic effect and supposed antiinflammatory action, may be related to the suppression of TNF-α.

Immunosuppressive Drugs

Methotrexate and cyclosporine have been tried in autoinflammatory disorders but proved ineffective in many, both as disease modifiers and steroid-sparing drugs. In TRAPS, they do not reduce the frequency or intensity of flares and have no effect in secondary amyloidosis.[12,13] In Blau syndrome, they have been used with limited success. Cyclosporine has been used in the treatment of MAS in association with steroids and is used for disease control, with good results[7]; anakinra in MAS has been shown to be effective.

TNF Inhibitors

In 1999, the cloning of the gene for the TNF receptor defined the cause of TRAPS.[11] Etanercept, a soluble antagonist of TNF, has proved useful in patients with TRAPS.[14] Worsening of disease has been seen in some patients treated with anti-TNF[15]; this phenomenon resembles the contradictory responses observed in some patients with JIA treated with anti-TNF medication who go on to develop MAS, when the MAS is induced or favored by the use of the anti-TNF medication, suggesting that it should be used with caution.[16] Infliximab, another TNF molecule and receptor antagonist, has been used in TRAPS and in Blau syndrome, with good responses, and in some cases, with reduced long-term complications; the response of amyloid deposition is controversial, and there is no definitive information on the effectiveness of anti-TNF in reducing long-term complications.

Anti-TNF medication has been described as useful in case reports for SAPHO syndrome.[17]

Anti-IL-1

Short-acting

Anakinra, a receptor antagonist for IL-1, showed no efficacy in sepsis and rheumatoid arthritis. IL-1 inhibition also occurs in systemic idiopathic arthritis and recurrent pericarditis of noninfectious origin. Anakinra has been used in systemic-onset JIA, with excellent results, and it has been used to prevent attacks and reduce systemic inflammatory markers in patients with colchicine-resistant FMF, HIDS, and even etanercept-resistant TRAPS. Similarly, remarkable responses were also reported in patients with Blau syndrome, PAPA syndrome, and deficiency of IL-1-receptor antagonist. Anakinra is effective during episodes of acute gout.[18]

Anakinra has been shown to prevent cold-induced symptoms when administered to patients with FCAS before a cold room challenge.[19]

Excessive production of IL-1 is seen in diseases like MWS, CINCA syndrome, and neonatal onset multisystem inflammatory disease (NOMID), and excellent therapeutic responses have been described.[20]

The dosage used of anakinra varies from 0.3 to 3 mg/kg/d, in divided doses.

Long-acting

Rilonacept is a recombinant fusion protein with a half-life of 8.6 days, it has a high affinity for IL-1β and also for IL-1α and IL-1 receptor accessory protein; it is used weekly at a dose of, for patients aged 12 years or older, 4.4 mg/kg, up to a maximum of 320 mg, delivered as 1 or 2 subcutaneous injections with a maximum single-injection volume of 2 mL. If the initial dose is of 2 injections, they should be given on the same day at 2 different sites; dosing should be continued with a once-weekly injection of 2.2 mg/kg, up to a maximum of 160 mg, administered as a single subcutaneous injection of up to 2 mL. Canakinumab is a humanized monoclonal antibody against IL-β; its half-life is 28 days and it may be dosed every 8 weeks; for body weights greater than 40 kg, the recommended dose is 150 mg as a single dose via subcutaneous injection; for body weights between 15 kg and 40 kg, the recommended dose is 2 mg/kg as single subcutaneous injections; for children 15 to 40 kg with inadequate response, the dose can be increased to 3 mg/kg as single subcutaneous injections.

Both rinolacept and canakinumab are useful in the treatment of NOMID, FCAS, MWS, HIDS, and, as recently reported,[21] JIA and in CAPS, both are FDA approved for this use.[22,23] Also, in crystal-induced arthritis, canakinumab was used with good results.[24] Recently, results of the treatment of Blau syndrome with canakinumab showed good responses.[25] Two randomized trials with canakinumab in JIA reported benefits.[26] Also, tozilizumab an anti-IL-6, used in JIA, was recently described as effective.[27]

Adverse Effects of Biological Therapies

Experiences with autoimmune disease have shown increases in the rates of mild to severe bacterial and viral infections, but the pathophysiology of these diseases is different and it is difficult to extrapolate. Nevertheless, at least a good history to exclude for tuberculosis, fungi, and viral diseases such as hepatitis C and B is mandatory; on the other hand, the use of immune-suppressive therapies might increase the risk of opportunistic infections in patients with autoimmune diseases.[28] The situation is different for the autoinflammatory syndromes. Increased rates of meningitis and urosepsis have been described in small CAPS trials with both rilonacept and canakinumab. Injection-site reactions are common with all antileukins.

SUMMARY

The continuous advance in the search for the cause and pathogenesis of the autoinflammatory syndromes, as well as reports of the efficacy of specific inflammation-mediator suppressors, has changed the way these syndromes are approached and treated; both the acute and long-term treatment of these diseases has improved significantly. Etiologic and pathophysiologic manipulation is and will be the future for controlling, even curing, this new and rare set of diseases.

REFERENCES

1. Masters SL, Simon A, Aksentijevich I, et al. Horror autoinflammaticus: the molecular pathophysiology of autoinflammatory disease. Annu Rev Immunol 2009;27:621–68.

2. Pillet P, Ansoborlo S, Carrere A, et al. (P)FAPA syndrome: value of cimetidine. Arch Pediatr 2000;7:54–7.

3. Schibler A, Birrer P, Vella S. PFAPA syndrome: periodic fever, adenitis, pharyngitis and aphthous stomatitis. Schweiz Med Wochenschr 1997;127:1280–4.

4. Simon A, Drewe E, van der Meer JW, et al. Simvastatin treatment for inflammatory attacks of the hyperimmunoglobulinemia D and periodic fever syndrome. Clin Pharmacol Ther 2004;75:476–83.

5. Aronoff DM, Neilson EG. Antipyretics: mechanisms of action and clinical use in fever suppression. Am J Med 2001;111(4):304–15.

6. Gatorno M, Federici S, Pelagatti MA, et al. Diagnosis and management of autoinflammatory diseases in childhood. J Clin Immunol 2008;28:73–83.

7. Stabile A, Bertoni B, Ansuini V, et al. The clinical spectrum and treatment options of macrophage activation syndrome in the pediatric age. Eur Rev Med Pharmacol Sci 2006;10(2):53–9.

8. Molad Y. Update on colchicine and its mechanism of action. Curr Rheumatol Rep 2002;4:252–6.

9. Zemer D, Revach M, Pras M, et al. A controlled trial of colchicine in preventing attacks of familial Mediterranean fever. N Engl J Med 1974;291:932–4.

10. Courtney PA, Hosking DJ, Fairbairn KJ, et al. Treatment of SAPHO with pamidronate. Rheumatology 2002;41:1196–8.

11. Kopterides P, Pikazis D, Koufos C. Successful treatment of SAPHO syndrome with zoledronic acid. Arthritis Rheum 2004;50:2970–3.

12. Hull KM, Drewe E, Aksentijevich I, et al. The TNF receptor-associated periodic syndrome (TRAPS): emerging concepts of an autoinflammatory disorder. Medicine 2002;81:349–68.

13. Mc Dermott MF, Aksentijevich I, Galon J, et al. Germ-line mutations in the extracellular domains of the 55kDa TNF receptor, define a family of dominantly inherited inflammatory syndromes. Cell 1999;97:133–44.

14. Bulua AC, Mogul DB, Aksentijevich I, et al. Efficacy of etanercept in the tumor necrosis factor receptor-associated periodic syndrome: a prospective, open-label, dose-escalation study. Arthritis Rheum 2012;64(3):908–13.

15. Nedjai B, Hitman GA, Quillinan N, et al. Pro inflammatory action of the anti-inflammatory drug infliximab in tumor necrosis factor receptor-associated periodic syndrome. Arthritis Rheum 2009;60:619–25.

16. Nádia EA, Carvalho JF, Bonfá E, et al. Macrophage activation syndrome associated with etanercept in a child with systemic onset juvenile idiopathic arthritis. Isr Med Assoc J 2009;9:635–6.

17. Burgemeister LT, Baeten DL, Tas SW. TNF blockade in the SAPHO syndrome. Neth J Med 2012;70(10):444–9.

18. Neogi T. Interleukin-1 antagonism in acute gout: is targeting a single cytokine the answer? Arthritis Rheum 2010;62(10):2845–9.

19. Hoffman HM, Rosengren S, Boyle DL, et al. Prevention of cold-associated acute inflammation in familial cold autoinflammatory syndrome by interleukin-1 receptor antagonist. Lancet 2004;364(9447):1779–85.

20. Goldbach-Mansky R, Daley NJ, Danna SW, et al. Neonatal-onset multisystem inflammatory disease responsive to interleukin-1beta inhibition. N Engl J Med 2006;355:581–92.

21. Ruperto N, Quartier P, Wulffraat N, et al. A phase II, multicenter, open-label study evaluating dosing and preliminary safety and efficacy of canakinumab in systemic juvenile idiopathic arthritis with active systemic features. Arthritis Rheum 2012;64(2):557–67.

22. Hoffman HM, Throne ML, Amar NJ, et al. Efficacy and safety of rinolacept (interleukin TRAP) in patients with cryopyrin-associated periodic syndromes. Results from two sequential placebo control studies. Arthritis Rheum 2008;58:2443–52.

23. Lachmann HJ, Kone Paut I, Kuemmerle-Deschner JB, et al. Use of canakinumab in the cryopyrin-associated periodic syndrome. N Engl J Med 2009;360:2416–25.

24. So A, De Meulemeester M, Pikhlak A. Canakinumab for the treatment of acute flares in difficult-to-treat gouty arthritis: results of a multicenter phase II, dose-ranging study. Arthritis Rheum 2010;62(10):3064–76.

25. Simonini G, Xu Z, Caputo R, et al. Clinical and transcriptional response to the long-acting interleukin-1 blocker canakinumab in Blau syndrome-related uveitis. Arthritis Rheum 2013;65(2):513–8.

26. Ruperto N, Brunner HI, Quartier P, et al, for the PRINTO and PRCSG. Canakinumab in systemic juvenile idiopathic arthritis: 2 randomized trials. N Engl J Med 2012;367:2396–406.

27. De Benedetti F, Brunner HI, Ruperto N, et al, for the Paediatric Rheumatology International Trials Organisation (PRINTO) and the Pediatric Rheumatology Collaborative Study Group (PRCSG). Randomized Trial of Tocilizumab in Systemic Juvenile Idiopathic Arthritis. N Engl J Med 2012;367:2385–95.

28. Botsios C. Safety of tumor necrosis factor and interleukin-1 blocking agent in rheumatic diseases. Autoimmun Rev 2005;4:162–70.

Index

Note: Page numbers of article titles are in **boldface** type.

Dermatol Clin 31 (2013) 513–520
http://dx.doi.org/10.1016/S0733-8635(13)00055-7
0733-8635/13/$ – see front matter © 2013 Elsevier Inc. All rights reserved.

Moving?

Make sure your subscription moves with you!

To notify us of your new address, find your **Clinics Account Number** (located on your mailing label above your name), and contact customer service at:

Email: journalscustomerservice-usa@elsevier.com

800-654-2452 (subscribers in the U.S. & Canada)
314-447-8871 (subscribers outside of the U.S. & Canada)

Fax number: 314-447-8029

Elsevier Health Sciences Division
Subscription Customer Service
3251 Riverport Lane
Maryland Heights, MO 63043

Printed and bound by CPI Group (UK) Ltd, Croydon, CR0 4YY

03/10/2024

01040346-0018